Mind, Body and

Rachel Charles grew up in the fells and coastland area of Cumbria. She studied drama and music at Bristol University and subsequently spent a few years in the theatre. She eventually settled in London and entered publishing, working mostly as a non-fiction editor. In search of a new way to express her creativity, she became a freelance writer and is now the author of five books.

Mind, Body and Immunity is the direct result of her own experience of cancer. Realising the enormous need among fellow-sufferers for emotional support, she decided to train as a counsellor at the Psychosynthesis and Education Trust and currently spends time working with the seriously ill as well as those with personal problems. In 1992 she appeared in the 'Free for All' film *Cancer Positive* shown on Channel 4 television.

Rachel's most absorbing hobbies are organic gardening and cello playing. She lives in a peaceful hamlet in Suffolk.

Mind, Body and Immunity

How to enhance your body's natural defences

RACHEL CHARLES

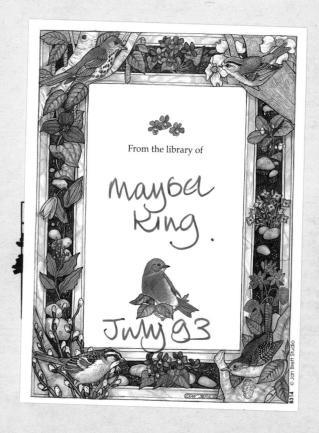

A Mandarin Paperback
MIND, BODY AND IMMUNITY

First published in Great Britain 1990
by Methuen London
This revised edition published 1993
by Cedar
an imprint of Reed Consumer Books Ltd
Michelin House, 81 Fulham Road, London SW3 6RB
and Auckland, Melbourne, Singapore and Toronto

Copyright © 1990, 1993 Rachel Charles
The author has asserted her moral rights.
The illustrations on pages 10 and 14 are taken
from *Understanding the Human Body*,
Tudor and Tudor (Churchill Livingstone, 1981).

A CIP catalogue record for this title
is available from the British Library
ISBN 0 7493 1544 X

Printed and bound in Great Britain
by Cox & Wyman Ltd, Reading, Berks

To Christoph,
who pointed the way

Contents

Acknowledgements	*page*	ix
Author's note		x
Foreword		xi
Introduction		1
1 The battle of the cells		8
2 How healthy is your personality?		43
3 Letting go of stress		87
4 Man-made threats		127
5 Moving for immunity		149
6 Feeding your defences		165
7 Recipes for peak immunity		214
Postlude		259
Addresses		261
Bibliography and further reading		265
Glossary		271
Index		275

Acknowledgements

I wish to give my thanks most especially to the Cancer Help Centre at Bristol and to the truly exceptional people there who set me on this journey of discovery. Dr Michael Wetzler has read every word of my manuscript and acted as my medical consultant, providing most helpful comments, as has Christopher Greatorex, psycho-therapist, who carefully went through the personality section. Gratitude is also due to my sister, Mary Pratt, MA (Oxon), MSc, biologist, who put me straight on some important facts about the body's defences and provided useful references. Additionally several willing friends and patients offered their personal responses, and David Francis kindly checked the manuscript. Ann Mansbridge at Methuen believed in my book from the very start, providing a much-needed boost to my confidence, and Sarah Hannigan con-tinued that support by giving it a new lease of life in this second edition. Last, but not least, special thanks must go to my friends and colleagues at the Psychosynthesis and Education Trust, without whose encouragement my own story would never have been told.

AUTHOR'S NOTE

The suggestions contained in this book are not intended to replace orthodox medical treatments, but are offered rather as complementary therapies. If you believe you may be unwell, always seek the advice of a qualified physician in the first instance.

For the sake of confidentiality, it has been necessary to change the names of some of the people who appear in the book and also to make slight amendments to their stories. Such alterations, however, do not fundamentally affect the psychological dynamics of their cases.

Foreword

We live in a crowded world. Pressures are increasing on each of us daily. Our lifestyles are busy. There is a compulsion to work harder and harder. We are encouraged to cram in ever more leisure activities. There is always more and more to read. And everywhere our environment is assaulted by polluting factors.

Despite, or perhaps because of, this expansion of activity, we find ourselves increasingly unwell. Coronary heart disease is becoming more common. Cancer maintains its level of threat. Diseases like multiple sclerosis, myalgic encephalomyelitis (ME) and Aids all infiltrate into our expectations of a healthy life. What are these incursions into our well-being? Are they different from previous times? Above all, what can we do about them?

Rachel Charles's book acknowledges these forces in a powerful, personal way. She tells her own story of cancer, and how, from it, she has learnt some important things about the life we lead in the twentieth century here in this 'civilised' world. Her own experiences, movingly described, run throughout the book, yet at the same time its focus is on helping readers to deal with their own outer and inner worlds in very practical ways. Perhaps it is the marriage of these two aspects that makes the book so successful. It leads readers through a series of questions to discover how 'immune' they are to the buffeting forces which they have to defend themselves against. Then the book draws from a wide variety of sources to give very helpful advice and positive suggestions as to how to develop immunity further, or redevelop it after it has suffered some major setback through disease.

Mind, Body and Immunity is, however, not only about practical steps, but is also about meaning. Perhaps because of some of the struggles we face in this century of material development our inner lives are frequently less nourishing than they might be. I feel that the core of this book delicately gives us pointers towards ways of re-nurturing ourselves, or indeed re-finding ourselves: a finding of our own meaningful and joyful paths in life. And what more important task could there be to fulfil?

This book has a prime place, therefore, in popular literature on health, and may just be what some readers need, to grope their way out of a darkness that they experience, perhaps through illness, into a new light.

MICHAEL J. WETZLER, MA (Cantab), MBBS, DCH, DRCOG

Introduction

A CRISIS

After leaving the hospital, I walked along the crowded London pavements towards the National Gallery in search of something to lift my flagging spirits. This was my fifth week of radiotherapy and my chest and neck were inscribed with strange purple hieroglyphs that indicated to the radiographers how their giant machine should be lined up before bombarding me with rays. Not being able to wash properly for more than a month, in case the gentian violet smudged, increased my discomfort. It was unnerving going through that thick door each day with its large red 'Danger' notice, lying bare-breasted on the couch with my arm strapped up to expose the lymph nodes, then watching the radiographers disappear into a well-protected room before switching on. This treatment was supposed to mop up any malignant cells that had escaped the surgeon's scalpel, but it was making me feel pretty wretched. Perhaps the soothing effects of Dutch landscapes would calm my jagged nerves.

I had found the lump just three months before, and spent the next ten days in agonies of apprehension, trying to summon up the courage to go to my doctor. I attempted to reassure myself – perhaps it was all right, perhaps it was just one of those insignificant little bumps that would go away again. But somehow I knew that it wasn't. Then came the mammography and ultrasound scan with needle biopsy, followed by an interminable week-long wait for the results. At that point I was more worried about radical surgery than about dying. I knew I could never face the trauma of losing my breast; mutilation of this order seemed appalling. It was only after finally deciding that I would refuse a mastectomy, come what may, that I felt strong enough to face the future. At last the registrar telephoned to inform me that the needle biopsy was clear, but that there was doubt about the mammogram. I must report to the hospital in two days' time for a lumpectomy.

I slept long and deep after the operation, and the following morning my consultant appeared with his white-coated entourage. He looked rather solemn. It must be difficult telling people that they have cancer – not that the word was ever mentioned. The verdict was primary carcinoma, with quite a good prognosis: no more surgery was needed, just radiotherapy for six weeks. I felt almost cheerful. Routine bone and liver scans were recommended to check that malignant cells were not spreading to other sites via the lymph or bloodstream.

Ten days later I was injected with radioactive material and placed in front of yet another vast machine that looked like some weird monster out of space. I had to chase the oncology department for the results. They seemed reluctant to reveal them to me. The liver scan was fine, but there were suspicions about a large 'hot spot' that had shown up across my left ribs. The doctor, a thin blonde woman with large spectacles, admitted that interpretation was difficult – either it was something insignificant that would clear up of its own accord, or else the cancer had metastasized. I felt alarmed. Whatever did that mean? Basically that the cancer had already spread out of control and any treatment would be merely palliative. Her voice was brittle. In other words, I would be incurable. She rattled on, but I was too devastated to take much more in, except that I would have to wait for three whole months before the scan could be repeated. Until then I was living with a possible death sentence hanging over me.

I ambled from gallery to gallery and soon found myself among some Christian religious paintings. Gentle scenes of the Annunciation, Nativity, Jesus's baptism, his Agony in the Garden and so on. Somehow, as I gazed at all this, I was filled with a sense of futility and the pointlessness of suffering. If there was such a being as a Christ, then I felt utterly abandoned by him. Why me? The inevitable question prodded away at the back of my mind. Why should I be faced with the reality of my own death when I had lived scarcely half of my life? But deep inside, there lingered a sense of why it should be me.

I had been pushing myself too hard for too long, working ridiculously long hours, always to tight deadlines and to a very high standard, with a lot of responsibility for both people and money. For years, there had been no time at all for myself and I had a vague feeling of having lost myself. I used to play the cello, but I was so exhausted by the time I arrived home after work that I rarely took it out of its case. Occasionally, I would consider ways of escaping the rat-race, but each time I could see no way out. I depended on my income to pay the mortgage, to mend the roof, meet the gas, electricity and phone bills, feed and clothe myself, run my car and so on and so on. How could I possibly give up my job, especially with my husband out of work? I might never find another as good. Then there was always the carrot dangled in front of me of future promotion and a higher salary. And so this life continued – if you could call it a life – and I imagined that, as I moved up the ladder, things would get better. But they didn't. They got worse.

By now, I was absorbing the Dutch landscapes. They were not at all peaceful, but foreboding and powerful. Storm clouds chased across the skies and strong winds weighed the trees down, while people and animals huddled in ditches for shelter. Forests, a favourite subject, seemed impenetrable and mysterious. I had an overwhelming longing for the countryside, to feel the rain and wind beat against me, to be close to nature and its elemental forces. I felt poisoned by my city environment, by the fume-laden air and the relentless noise. I felt dazzled by the constant glare of advertisements, oppressed by the crowds and threatened by the honking aggression of uncaring traffic.

Once again, the pains that had been troubling me on and off for the past three years tightened in an iron band across my chest. My breathing became restricted and the colours of the landscapes started to blur. Helplessness and panic overtook me. The pains became so intense that I felt I couldn't draw another breath. Somehow I forced myself to sit down, lowered my head and gradually the breathing returned. No, I wasn't suffering from heart disease; my doctor had done the necessary tests only a few weeks previously and could find nothing the matter with me. She prescribed the inevitable tranquillizers. Clearly, such intense pains were not imaginary. There was something desperately wrong with me and I had the feeling that all this was tied up with my cancer. The fact was that my body was beginning to complain furiously at the intolerable strain that I had imposed on it. How could I have treated myself with such lack of consideration? Yet I didn't know how to change myself or in what other way I could lead my life. I felt totally trapped.

Later, when I tried to explain to my husband that my chest pains had returned, indicating with difficulty my growing desperation, he looked perplexed. He didn't understand the state I was in. How could he? How could I describe it, when I didn't even understand it myself? I needed help – and quickly.

A couple of weeks later I walked through the doors of the Bristol Cancer Help Centre, and was warmly greeted. I had been counting the hours until my arrival. Somehow I sensed that here was a place where I might find some clues that would point me towards a more satisfactory way of living. And I was right.

AN OPPORTUNITY

Two and a half years later I was no longer in despair. In fact I had much to look forward to. My chest pains had vanished – hopefully for ever – and the world appeared less menacing. Most importantly, I felt glowingly well and energetic and usually (but not always!) moderately calm. Gradually I have come to understand how close the connection is between my thoughts and feelings and my physical body – how each affects and responds to the others. Chronic anxiety over a long period had caused immuno-suppressant hormones to course through my bloodstream, leaving me highly vulnerable to disease. Eventually my body succumbed, and the result was cancer.

The lifestyle I now follow is deliberately immunity-enhancing. Viruses pass me by, knowing they will have no easy place to flourish, and, I hope, my body is now hostile to secondary tumours. I have to admit that it hasn't been an easy programme to adopt, and for every two steps forward there has been at least one back. But the rewards are incalculable. Life, which previously was scarcely worth living, today seems rich and precious. I now know that change – though difficult – is possible, as long as the motivation is there. Yes, I was highly motivated. I was face to face with my own mortality. I was in a state of crisis, but somewhere in the midst of the anguish and confusion there was an opportunity to be found and nurtured. I would never even have noticed it if the wise and caring people at the Cancer Help Centre had not pointed me gently in the right direction. In saying goodbye to the old way of life that had led to my illness I was also saying hello to something new, and this was exhilarating.

The impact of my recent learnings has been tremendous. Previously, I had assumed that if there was something wrong with me

I would go to a doctor, who would prescribe pills that would cure me. But there are no pills to cure cancer. Nor are there any simple prescriptions to cure many other diseases from the common cold to Aids. What we so often fail to appreciate is that the body has a staggeringly complex system for healing and regulating itself. If you break a bone the doctor will set it, but the jagged ends will fuse without any further intervention until the bone is as good as new again. If a virus invades your body, your intricate immune system immediately goes on to the alert. It distinguishes that particular virus from literally billions of others, and special antibodies are formed to destroy it. Just as this delicately balanced system can be upset by poor diet, lack of exercise, long-term emotional problems and stress, so the opposite is also true: it can be positively encouraged to operate more effectively, so that the body is able to function efficiently and remain healthy.

If you are suffering from a serious disease, take heart in the knowledge that you can actively assist in your own healing. This book will show you many ways of doing that. If you are not ill, but feel that you might become so, then you will find in these pages the steps to take to fend off disease. Either way, this process involves looking deep within yourself. It means considering your personality, your emotions, your values and your lifestyle, as well as the more practical aspects of diet and exercise. It takes a great deal of courage to do this. There may be very good reasons why you need to be ill. Going to bed offers a safe retreat from life. You may also be earning a lot of sympathy and attention. If you become glowingly healthy, who will care for you then? The holistic road to health involves asking yourself difficult, personal questions. It is a road towards self-acceptance, self-knowledge and, yes, most especially self-love; it means that you will learn to respect and care for yourself in a very special way. If this sounds like a lot of hard work, then I can assure you from experience that the rewards far outweigh the pain and the effort.

A PROGRAMME FOR YOU

This book is not just for reading. Questions and self-scoring quizzes invite your involvement. They are devised to help you towards a greater understanding of yourself and your needs, so that you can work out a healthy-living programme that is absolutely right for you.

Before going any further, therefore, it is essential to consider how you are, now, at this very moment. So I am going to ask you to find a quiet place where you will not be disturbed. Sit comfortably in a straight-backed chair, close your eyes, relax as much as possible and ask yourself the three questions in the following exercise.

MY BODY, MY FEELINGS AND MY MIND

1 How is my body today?
Allow your mind to rest on this question and then experience your body fully. Start with your feet and work upwards. Are there any tensions? Any aches or pains, burnings or itchings or any other feelings of physical discomfort? Are you relaxed? Do you feel really fit? Don't make any judgments about all this. Simply note your observations. Then say to yourself: 'I am not just my body, I am more than that.'

2 How are my feelings today?
Do you feel angry, sad, anxious, happy? How closely in touch with your feelings are you? Allow yourself to experience your feelings fully. Don't repress them. Let them come to the surface and acknowledge them. When did you last express your feelings to someone fully and honestly? Yesterday, six months ago, or can you not remember when? Again, make no judgments; just observe how you are feeling today. Then say to yourself, 'I am not just my feelings, I am more than they are.'

3 How is my mind today?
Consider your own thoughts. What are they mostly involved with at present? Are you mentally alert or sluggish today? Notice the conversations and arguments that take place inside your head. What are they about? Who is speaking to whom? Again, make no judgments. Simply observe and note what is going on. Then say to yourself, 'I am not just my mind, I am more than that.'

You may be wondering what all this has to do with your immune system. In the first chapter you will be using your intellect to learn some of the basic principles about how this works; in chapters 2 and 3 you will spend time understanding how your feelings affect your body physiologically and how they can directly influence the workings of the immune system. After that you will be concentrating on your body, its environment and its nourishment. In order to appreciate this fully it is important to be able to distinguish between your feelings and your mind. Many people find this extraordinarily difficult. They are so out of touch with their emotions that if you ask them how they feel, they will tell you what they think. Unfortunately, our Western culture does not encourage us to honour our feelings. Repressing them can cause untold physical damage to your own body. Later in this book you will find ways of dealing with your feelings safely and effectively; you will also learn about the role that exercise plays in all of this.

Whenever you have a spare, quiet moment, practise the above meditative exercise and acknowledge to yourself how your body is, what you are feeling and what you are thinking. This is a very important first step towards taking control over your own healing.

A business colleague once said to me that whenever she walks into a hospital she feels like bursting into tears. I was surprised at this confession, because she is the sort of person who gives the impression of being fully in control of any situation. But I know exactly what she means. If you have to go to hospital you immediately feel at a disadvantage. You probably don't understand much of the medical jargon, the hierarchy is so complicated that it is difficult to make out who is who, you may have to face unpleasant treatments that make you feel anxious, and, above all, you feel as if you are handing over your body to some figure of authority who will take charge of it for you. In other words, you become a victim of the system.

As you work through this book, however, you will find that your active participation in working towards a positive state of health will become increasingly important to you. You will realise that you are the one who is in charge and you will feel empowered. So buy yourself a notebook and keep a record of your progress in building healthy immune defences. Use it for the exercises and quizzes and write down your thoughts, feelings and bodily condition, if possible on a daily basis. If you can persuade a friend or relative to follow the programme too, so much the better. You will be able to encourage each other and share experiences.

1 The battle of the cells

Before moving on to the main part of the programme it may be helpful for you to understand a little about how the immune system actually works. I have tried to explain this in as straightforward a manner as possible, but if you find the scientific information a bit heavy-going don't worry. Just skim over this chapter and move on to the more personal considerations in chapter 2. You can always refer back to the intricacies of the immune system later on if you wish.

So the first question to ask is, what is it? It is our body's natural defence system, that is triggered into action whenever it is threatened by foreign organisms, particles or other substances known as 'pathogens'. But how is the immune system able to recognise these pathogens? They contain, or bear on their surfaces, certain proteins and carbohydrates which act as alarm signals and cause the immune defences to react accordingly.

The term 'immune system' is used by some authorities to refer only to this specific type of response, which involves the production of antibodies against the alarm-signalling antigens presented by the invaders. Others, however, use the term more generally to refer to the whole battery of defences, including the external mechanisms such as the hairs in our noses that trap unwanted particles. For the purposes of this book, the broader definition will apply.

These two types of defences are quite distinct from our waste-disposal processes, which eliminate unnecessary or potentially harmful chemicals, such as toxic fumes that we may breathe in, or poisons in our food. This kind of 'cleaning up' is carried out by the liver and the kidneys.

We are not generally aware of it, but a myriad of minute organisms are present in, on and around us. Normally these cause no damage at all and live harmoniously with us, sharing our environment. Indeed, some are positively beneficial, such as the healthy bacteria that live in the intestine. Others, however, the pathogens, can invade and interfere with the body's mechanisms, and the result is often disease.

THE PATHOGENS

There are several categories of potential trouble-makers that the body has to deal with.

Bacteria are tiny organisms, invisible to the naked eye, which consist of just a single cell. They are neither animals nor plants. Very few actually cause disease. In fact, many are very useful, such as the ones that break down dead plant matter and help to produce rich compost.

Disease-causing bacteria, the pathogens, find a warm, moist environment in humans, ideal for reproduction and growth. They most commonly enter the body through the mouth or nose, then they may penetrate the epithelial surfaces (the linings) of the respiratory or digestive systems and colonise various organs. They can also enter through broken skin. If conditions suit them well, they can reproduce in vast numbers within hours, by simple division. Many double their population every five minutes, so one bacterium can create 4 million in only two hours! This explains how an illness such as cholera can kill within twenty-four hours.

Some types of bacteria produce chemicals which are harmful to the host. For instance, the toxin emanating from the tetanus bacterium paralyses the muscles. Other varieties of bacteria may actually invade cells and cause damage this way. If large numbers of cells are harmed, then disease will follow. Tuberculosis is the result of this kind of activity.

Viruses are even smaller and simpler than bacteria – so minute that many cannot be seen even under the most powerful light microscope. Because they are so simple they can reproduce only if they are inside the living cells of a host. As the thousands of new viral particles burst out of the host cell, they destroy it. Viruses are therefore always associated with disease and cause the familiar common cold and influenza as well as measles, mumps, smallpox, rubella and other serious infections. Because they live right inside the host cells it is more difficult for the immune system to attack them.

Fungi are very simple plants that thrive in damp areas. Many are useful; we are all familiar with yeast and blue cheese. Penicillin is

Barriers of defence on the body surfaces

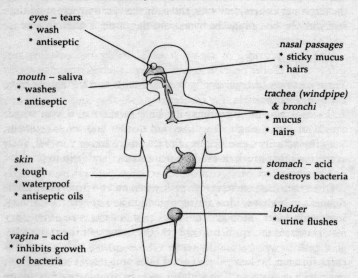

eyes – tears
* wash
* antiseptic

nasal passages
* sticky mucus
* hairs

mouth – saliva
* washes
* antiseptic

trachea (windpipe)
& bronchi
* mucus
* hairs

skin
* tough
* waterproof
* antiseptic oils

stomach – acid
* destroys bacteria

bladder
* urine flushes

vagina – acid
* inhibits growth
of bacteria

also produced by a mould. However, when fungi take up residence on or in a human they can cause infections such as athlete's foot and thrush.

Animal parasites are the largest of the pathogens, and depend on their host for food. Some are microscopic, single-celled organisms called protozoa and they can cause serious diseases in humans, such as malaria and sleeping sickness. Other parasites include tapeworms, roundworms and flukes, as well as insects such as fleas, lice and mites.

Other invaders

The body may react defensively to many other particles and substances which are foreign to it and may cause what are often referred to as allergic reactions. Pollen grains, cat hairs and certain foods are examples, and these are discussed in more detail at the end of this chapter and in chapter 6.

THE BODY'S EXTERNAL DEFENCES

Despite the innumerable organisms that share our environment, many of which attempt to invade our bodies, we are able to survive because our defence mechanisms are so effective. There are two ways in which our bodies deal with pathogens: either by preventing their entry in the first place, or by inactivating them if they do manage to find a way in.

The skin provides us with a flexible, waterproof covering that protects the tissues beneath in several ways, such as from damage by ultraviolet rays or from drying out. Although humans appear to be comparatively hairless, the sebaceous glands that open into the tiny hair follicle play an important role. They produce an oily substance which not only helps to keep the skin flexible and water-repellent, but it also forms a chemical barrier that discourages bacteria. Only when the skin is broken can bacteria find an easy entrance.

The respiratory passages provide a common pathway into the body for bacteria, but even here there are plenty of traps. Firstly, the flow of air is slowed down after entering the nose by the curving, narrowing tubes. Secondly, the hairs that line the nose catch many small, unwanted organisms, and, thirdly, most of the other pathogens become attached to the sticky mucus and are later expelled in this substance. At least 90 per cent of micro-organisms are effectively dealt with in this way. The few that manage to penetrate further are likely to be trapped by the cilia, the hair-like projections that line the windpipe and bronchi which lead into the lungs. The cilia are in constant movement, beating to and fro, and sweeping any foreign particles upwards into the mouth. Here the mucus is either expelled or swallowed, in which case any surviving bacteria will be quickly killed off by the acid in the stomach. The sneeze reflex is an efficient means of expelling invaders. Every sneeze or cough propels hundreds of millions of virus particles into the air.

Washing and flushing are also important natural processes that keep certain areas of the body clean and free from infection. Tears constantly wash the surfaces of the eyes, and other fluids – including saliva, bile and even urine – remove unwanted organisms by their flushing action. Like the oils in the skin, tears and saliva have antiseptic properties which are hostile to bacteria.

THE BODY'S INNER DEFENCES

Despite the protective qualities of the body's external surfaces, some micro-organisms do manage to slip through. If this happens, the body has many other resources to call on, and these fall into two main categories: general defence processes that attack any kind of foreign pathogens, and specific immune responses especially designed to fight and destroy particular invaders. If the general processes fail, then the specific responses come into operation. Let us look at the general processes first.

GENERAL DEFENCE PROCESSES

INFLAMMATION Suppose you accidentally cut your finger. Bacteria can now enter your body. So what happens? Almost certainly the area will become inflamed and painful. This may feel quite uncomfortable, but it is actually a sign that your immune system is mobilising one of its general forces. A cut causes injury to the tissues and cells beneath the skin, and, as a result, the cells release certain chemicals, in particular histamine and substances called kinins. These encourage the small blood vessels surrounding the wound to dilate, so that extra blood rushes to the area, causing the heat and redness that is so familiar. At the same time, the blood vessels become more permeable so that proteins from the blood plasma can actually pass through the walls into the tissue spaces. Plasma proteins not only help in defence; they assist with healing and repair work.

Attracted by the histamine and other chemicals released at the site of injury, white blood cells called 'scavengers' also squeeze their way through the walls of the blood vessels. Each one glides towards an invading bacterium which quickly becomes attached to its outer membrane. The jelly-like cytoplasm of the scavenger surrounds and swallows up the bacterium, which is then destroyed by digestive enzymes. This process of engulfing and killing bacteria is called phagocytosis.

You may wonder why your infected cut starts to ooze with pus. In the effort of overwhelming the bacteria, the scavengers themselves are very often killed also, and it is these dead white cells that contribute to the pus.

If the infection persists, even more lethal white cells called monocytes move into the attack. Each one of these can swallow up and annihilate up to 100 bacteria. The scavengers and monocytes do not always succeed, however, so the immune system has to call on other defence methods, one of which is the lymphatic system.

Scavenger cell destroys bacterium

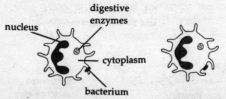

1. Bacterium is trapped by the tendril-like threads of cytoplasm.

2. Bacterium sticks to scavenger cell membrane.

3. Cytoplasm surrounds bacterium.

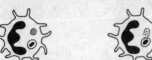

4. Bacterium becomes enclosed in cytoplasm.

5. Digestive enzymes attack bacterium.

6. Enzymes break up bacterium, some of which is metabolised. The dead waste is excreted.

THE LYMPHATIC SYSTEM   This is really the body's means of drainage, but it also plays an important part in the defence work against unwanted organisms. In addition to removing fluid from between cells, it picks up dead material and foreign bodies. It consists of a network of fine capillaries which are connected to the larger lymph vessels, which in turn drain into two main ducts. The walls of the capillaries are so thin that the tissue fluid is able to permeate through them, to form a pale yellow, almost colourless liquid called lymph. Unlike the circulation of the blood, which is kept in motion by the heart, the lymphatic system has no separate pump. However, because it is connected with the blood circulation, its movement is indirectly affected by the heart, as well as by muscular activity. Another type of white cell which is involved in immunity is carried by the lymph, and this is known as a lymphocyte.

Let us suppose that the bacteria that collected in your cut finger have not been entirely eliminated by the scavenger cells or monocytes, and that they are reproducing in the tissue fluid which fills the spaces between cells. As the fluid filters through the walls of the lymphatic capillaries it carries the bacteria along with it. But the bacteria have to face yet another trap: the lymph nodes. These are

Structure of a lymph node

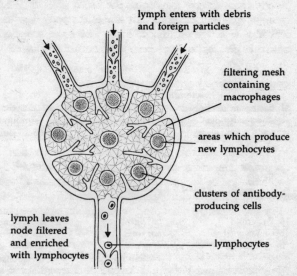

lymph enters with debris
and foreign particles

filtering mesh
containing
macrophages

areas which produce
new lymphocytes

clusters of antibody-
producing cells

lymph leaves
node filtered
and enriched
with lymphocytes

lymphocytes

situated in clusters along the larger lymphatic vessels, particularly in the armpit, neck and groin. Normally the size of a raisin, these glands become swollen when helping to deal with an infection. You may have been aware of the nodes under your jaw swelling up when you have been suffering from a sore throat. Inside each node is a fine meshwork of fibrous tissue which acts as a filtering bed to the lymph. As it passes through, any foreign bodies and bacteria become trapped. These are then devoured by large scavenger cells called macrophages. It is here in the lymph nodes that the white lymphocyte cells are produced. Some of them remain in the nodes, while others are carried by the lymph to the bloodstream. Therefore, after the lymph has passed through each node not only has it been filtered and cleaned of debris, but it has also been enriched with protective lymphocytes.

If particular types of micro-organisms enter the node, then specific immune responses may be set in motion: some of the white immune cells may produce antibodies, or chemicals, which will destroy the invaders. The lymph nodes, therefore, play a very important part in protecting the body from disease.

THE SPLEEN Occasionally, some bacteria outwit all the defence mechanisms described so far and travel via the lymph into the bloodstream. Others may enter the blood directly. The spleen, a spongy organ located on the left side of the body near the stomach, acts as a filter for the blood. Here, the large scavenger cells, or macrophages, capture and destroy any other unwanted organisms.

SPECIFIC IMMUNE RESPONSES

Sometimes the body is attacked by particularly aggressive pathogens that cause highly infectious diseases, and these are able to survive the general defence processes already discussed. However, the body has yet other defences to call upon that are even more ingenious. Particular immune responses are individually designed to deal with particular types of invaders. Even more amazing, these have a memory, so that we are unlikely to suffer from, say, chickenpox more than once. On the second or subsequent occasions the pathogen is recognised and dealt with so quickly that the disease has no time to take a hold on the body.

ANTIGENS AND ANTIBODIES   How is it possible for our immune systems to distinguish between thousands of different micro-organisms? As described in the introduction to this chapter, each of these has on its surface tiny molecules, known as antigens, and these are individual to each particular type of pathogen. These antigens stimulate the immune system to produce antibodies, which then combine with the antigens. However, they will only combine with the type of invader that evoked their production in the first place, so that chickenpox antibodies will only attack chickenpox antigens and not, for instance, measles antigens.

How then do the antibodies prevent the disease from spreading? Pathogens operate in different ways, so the antibodies vary their responses accordingly. Some antibodies assist the white scavenger cells in their work: having combined with the pathogen, the antibodies cause it to stick more easily on to the membrane of the scavenger cell, which can then readily engulf and destroy it. Other antibodies, when they combine with the surface antigens, cause a weakening in the wall of the bacterium, which then disintegrates. Yet others operate by attracting more than one corresponding antigen. For instance, if each antibody combines with two antigens, one invader on either side, then this causes clumping of the pathogens.

The scavengers can now more easily devour them. Some pathogens cause disease by producing toxins. In this case, antibodies will engulf the toxins and render them harmless.

B-CELLS There are two main types of protective white lymphocytes: the B-cells and the T-cells, so called because they mature in the bone marrow and thymus respectively. It is the B-cells that produce the antibodies. How exactly they do this has not yet been conclusively proved, but the evidence suggests that individual white B-lymphocytes are programmed to create one type of antibody only. Indeed, they carry receptor molecules on their membrane surfaces, which can identify and bind to specific antigens. When an invading pathogen enters the lymph and filters through the nodes, it will come into contact with thousands upon thousands of protective lymphocytes. Sooner or later it will meet its opposite number – the lymphocyte that will bind to its antigens – and produce the correct antibody to annihilate it. This works almost like lock and key; the lymphocyte receptor will fit into the invader's antigen. When this happens, the lymphocyte enlarges and then divides repeatedly into many other cells, known as plasma cells and B-memory cells. The memory cells are copies of the original lymphocyte, and these will rapidly provide immunity against that specific antigen in the future. The plasma cells are the ones that manufacture the correct antibodies and they secrete these into the bloodstream. Now they can effectively attack the disease-producing pathogen.

T-CELLS All white blood cells start their existence in the liver of the foetus. As the baby develops, they migrate to the bone marrow, the soft interior of the large bones of the limbs. Some of these, the T-cells, move on to the thymus, which is a pyramid-shaped gland beneath the breast bone, extending up to the base of the neck. These T-lymphocytes provide immunity in a different way from the B-cells, sometimes referred to as 'cell-mediated immunity'. The main difference is that T-cells don't make antibodies. You may recall that viruses operate by getting right inside the cells of the host, so that it is very difficult for antibodies to deal with them. Instead, the T-lymphocytes called T-killer cells recognise the infected cells and attack them directly with a cell poison.

Other T-cells are triggered into action by particular antigens and produce certain chemicals. These in turn stimulate the white scavenger cells, otherwise known as phagocytes, to do their job of gobbling up the invaders. Because of their cooperative role, these T-lymphocytes have earned the name of T-helper cells.

WHITE CELLS

LEUCOCYTES
The most common white cells, divided into three main types:

MAST CELLS
Tissue cells that release histamine in allergic and inflammatory reactions.

MONOCYTES
Large white cells in the blood and tissues. Develop into feeding cells, called *macrophages*. Their tendrils hook in the bacteria which are then engulfed. 'Cannibalistic' in that they also feed on dead microphages.

LYMPHOCYTES
Formed mostly in the bone marrow, but multiply in the lymphatic tissue. Of two types: B- and T-cells.

Neutrophils
(microphages). Small feeding cells that are fast moving. Dead ones, together with their foes, form the pus of wounds.

Basophils
Action not well understood, but thought to defend against inflammatory illnesses. Involved in allergy.

Eosinophils
Defend against parasites. Involved in allergy.

B-cells
Mature in the bone marrow. They produce antibodies that fight bacteria and viruses.

T-cells
Mature in the thymus gland. They deal with invaders that get inside the body's cells.

T-helper cells
Communicate with B-cells and feeding cells via chemical signals to rouse them to battle. They also modify the action of T-suppressor cells.

T-suppressor cells
Keep immune response in balance by curbing aggression of other white lymphocytes.

Natural killer cells
Kill invaders directly with a cell poison. Attack tumour cells.

Plasma cells
Large B-cells that are antibody 'factories'.

Memory cells
Live for many years and mount a quick response to any attack from a recognisable microorganism.

OTHER ELEMENTS OF THE IMMUNE SYSTEM

Complement system
Proteins with enzyme activity that dissolve infected cells. Can destroy bacteria by shooting holes in them. Help to increase the efficiency of antibodies and feeding cells.

Interferons
Proteins produced when the body's cells are under viral attack. Prevent multiplication of viruses and cancer cells.

There is another category of T-lymphocytes called T-suppressor cells, which have an opposite function to the helper cells. Rather than stimulating a B-cell into producing antibodies, for example, T-suppressor cells may inhibit this process. Perhaps you are wondering why two sets of lymphocytes should have apparently opposite functions. The reason is that once the plasma cells have finished their job of producing antibodies and have succeeded in dealing with the disease-producing organisms, they have to be 'switched off'. At this point, the T-suppressor cells intervene and the antibody level subsides to normal. The balance between T-helper and T-suppressor cells is crucial to the health of the individual, and their ratio indicates the effectiveness of the immune system. There should be almost twice as many helpers as suppressors, 1.8:1 to be exact. If the number of helpers falls, then serious immune disorders can result. Aids patients have a ratio of 1:1 or even less, indicating that the suppressor cells are actually destroying the body's own immunity.

THE ROLE OF THE LIVER

What happens to bacteria and viruses after they have been rendered harmless by the immune system? They will eventually end up in the liver, along with unwanted cellular matter including dead cancer cells, hormones (both natural and artificial), drugs and toxins. Of the five hundred or so functions of the liver, detoxification is a major one. In addition to toxins and debris, one of two entries to the liver, the hepatic portal vein, carries all the nutrients absorbed from the intestines. The liver has an ingenious screening system that enables it to defend the body against any micro-organisms and toxins that enter it from the gastro-intestinal tract. The portal vein sends off branches into the hundreds of lobules that make up the liver, and these branches subdivide into minute sinusoids. These have permeable walls lined with phagocytes, which destroy the unwanted matter as the blood filters through.

Additionally, enzymatic pathways convert drugs, noxious chemicals and hormones into harmless compounds. Waste substances that can be dissolved in water are eliminated via the kidneys in the form of urine. Otherwise they are dissolved in fat and returned to the digestive tract in the bile and eventually excreted. If faced with 'unrecognisable' toxic substances, such as pesticide residues, the liver will avoid metabolising them, but will instead store them in fat.

The liver is the largest gland in the body, weighing some 3 to 4 lbs (1.5kg) in an adult. It lies behind the lower right ribs, close to the diaphragm, and is shaped like a wedge. Life is impossible without it. Not only is it an efficient detoxification system, but it is also a vital processing plant and storehouse. There are many important metabolic activities that take place in the liver, including the formation, breakdown and storage of proteins, fats and carbohydrates from the variety of nutrients received through the portal vein. Certain substances, notably glucose, plasma proteins and cholesterol, are released into the bloodstream in order to maintain a constant level. Other compounds, such as vitamins, are made available when the body requires them. The waste product, urea, is transported from the liver to the kidneys to be excreted.

The vitamins that are stored by the liver are fat-soluble, namely A, D, E and K. These need bile for their absorption. This substance, which acts like a sort of detergent in that it is able to break down and assist with the digestion of fats, is produced in the liver, kept in the gall bladder and released into the duodenum when needed. Here it will deal with the fats swallowed in food.

A healthy liver is vital to immunity. If it is working efficiently it will be able to supply quickly the raw ingredients that the immune defences need to operate effectively. The processing of nutrients, essential for cell and tissue building, takes place here. Blood proteins (that in turn produce antibodies), as well as blood-clotting agents, are all manufactured in the liver. If it is overloaded with too many poisonous substances it will not be able to respond as quickly when the body is under attack by an infection. So take good care of this vital organ by feeding yourself with wholesome, nutritious food and avoiding environmental pollutants; then it will serve you well.

HOW DO WE BECOME ILL?

You will appreciate by now that a healthy immune system is truly impressive. With such a barrage of defences, how is it possible that any invader ever succeeds in establishing itself in the host and causing disease? This is mainly a question of time. When the body becomes infected by a particular micro-organism, there is a race between the multiplying microbes and the B-cells producing the antibody. A healthy human can usually beat off the attack, but the battle can be lost if the invasion force is extra-large, or if the immune system is in some way impaired, because of a depleted number of protective white cells. This can happen through stress, poor nutrition or environmental factors, all of which are discussed at length in this book. Hormonal imbalances, injury, surgery and drugs can also contribute to lowered immunity.

Then there are genetic considerations. Occasionally, a child can be born with a weak immune system as a result of damage to chromosome number 6. This is the one which contains the genes that control immunity, especially the T-lymphocytes. Such a child will be subject to recurring infections and possibly an early death. It is also interesting that people of Afro-Caribbean origin are able to resist diphtheria and influenza more effectively than Whites, but are more vulnerable to TB. A tendency to succumb to a particular disease, for example juvenile-onset diabetes, can also be inherited.

Viral epidemics do occur among healthy populations. Viruses have a cunning habit of confusing the human immune system by casting off the old, easily recognisable antigens through mutation and acquiring new ones, a process known as 'antigenic drift'. Influenza, for instance, gains a sure grip in this way. Yet in every epidemic, it is always noticeable that some people are only slightly affected by the pathogen or even not at all, while others succumb very easily. It is common knowledge that if you are feeling 'low' or 'run down' you are more susceptible to an infection. All the more reason to keep your immune system operating at peak efficiency by taking very good care of yourself.

SELF AND NON-SELF

You may have followed in the newspapers the development of transplant surgery. Despite the sophistication of techniques, the main problem that scientists have had to deal with all along is the patient's own immune system. Instead of assisting in the healing process, as is usual, the response is to regard the new organ as 'foreign' and reject it. To prevent this from happening, it is necessary to administer powerful immuno-suppressive drugs to the patient. How the body knows what is self and what is non-self is still something of a mystery, but the theory is that, during development, any lymphocytes able to produce antibodies against self are rapidly destroyed. In some cases this knowledge of self, or 'immune tolerance' as it is called, can go awry. The lymphocytes start to produce antibodies, not against invaders, but against the body's own cells. Severe damage can result, either to a single organ such as the thyroid gland or stomach, or else to cells or tissues present in, say, a whole network – like the small blood vessels. The illness that follows is described as an 'auto-immune disease'. One of the best-known of these is rheumatoid arthritis, in which the lining of the joints and tendons is destroyed. This and other auto-immune diseases will be discussed later in the chapter.

VACCINATION AND INFECTIOUS DISEASES

The word vaccination comes from the Latin *vacca*, which means cow. 'Whatever have cows to do with immunisation?' you may ask. At the end of the eighteenth century, an Englishman called Edward Jenner discovered a safe means of inoculating people against the dangerous and disfiguring disease of smallpox. He had noticed the smooth, unblemished skin of milkmaids and had recognised the truth in the old belief that people who had been infected with cowpox, a relatively mild disease, were less likely to catch the deadly disease of smallpox. To test this theory, he prepared an injection from an infected cow and inoculated a person with this cowpox material. He finally proved the theory to be correct when he later injected smallpox material into the same person, who, happily, proved to be immune.

Vaccination relies on the extraordinary process of immune memory in order to be effective. The antigen – the part of the invading organism that stimulates immune response – is modified in the laboratory so that it will not actually cause disease. Thus, a vaccine will contain either weakened or killed organisms, or the toxins they produce. This is then injected into the person and antibodies are formed in response. Memory cells subsequently circulate in the bloodstream and are available for a rapid reaction if the person is affected by that particular antigen in the future. The disease is therefore unable to take a hold on the body.

Only fifty years ago, many thousands of children in Western societies were dying from infectious diseases. In 1939 there were about 45,000 cases of diphtheria every year in Britain, resulting in around 2,500 deaths. It begins with a simple sore throat, but quickly blocks the respiratory passages, making it very difficult for the child to breathe. It also produces a poison that attacks the heart and nervous system. After the introduction of immunisation in 1940 the number of fatalities rapidly declined until there were only twenty-six cases between 1979 and 1986, with just one death. Smallpox has been eradicated altogether, and other common childhood diseases such as measles, mumps and rubella (German measles) are under control, as are tetanus and polio.

Measles is highly infectious, starting with a bad cold that develops into a fever, with red spots appearing behind the ears. These later spread to the rest of the body. It can cause encephalitis (inflammation of the brain), bronchitis and pneumonia and is still fatal in a few cases. Mumps is another viral disease that can result in encephalitis as well as viral meningitis (inflammation of the soft membranes of the brain), but it mainly affects the salivary glands. German measles, although a mild disease in itself, can seriously damage an unborn baby. It is safer, therefore, for adolescent girls to be vaccinated to protect the next generation. Both tetanus and polio can be fatal. In the case of tetanus, bacteria from the soil enter an open wound and then produce a toxin which attacks the nervous system. Painful muscle spasms follow, often in the jaw and neck – hence the name 'lockjaw'. Polio also attacks the nervous system and muscles become paralysed, especially in the legs. If breathing muscles are affected, the child may die.

In the mid-1970s there were stories in the media which suggested that the whooping-cough vaccine could cause brain damage. A study carried out since then is moderately reassuring: only one child in 330,000 is likely to suffer any such damage and even then it may not be severe. Because of the scare, only one-third of babies were being immunised and as a result a serious epidemic broke out, with at least 2,000 children going down with whooping cough every week. More than thirty children died and others were left with long-term effects, such as lung damage. It seems that, as with other vaccines, it is safer to have it than not to.

Sometimes you may need booster jabs of certain vaccines. The prepared antigens do not provide such long-lasting immunity as the original organisms, but successive inoculations raise the antibody population and give more effective protection.

It is not only the success of immunisation that prevents thousands of childhood deaths. Improved housing, clean water and better hygiene have all discouraged the spread of infections. In the Third World, where social conditions are poor, infant mortality rates from disease are still very high.

Recommended vaccination schedule (UK)

From 3 months:	Triple vaccine of diphtheria/tetanus/pertussis (whooping cough) by injection; poliomyelitis by mouth.
5 to 6 months:	Repeat of above.
9 to 11 months:	A further repeat.
12 to 24 months:	Measles.
At school entry:	Diphtheria, tetanus and polio boosters.
10 to 14 years:	Tuberculosis; rubella (girls only).
Before leaving school:	Tetanus and polio boosters.
Every 10 years:	Tetanus and polio boosters.

Before travelling abroad, it may be necessary to be immunised against diseases prevalent in the country you are visiting. In addition to those mentioned above, vaccines also exist against cholera, influenza, Rocky Mountain spotted fever and yellow fever.

So far, induced active immunisation has been described here, as well as natural immunity acquired through direct exposure to the infection. There is also passive immunisation in which the pathogen is first introduced into another organism, which then manufactures the necessary antibodies for the recipient. Babies acquire ready-made antibodies naturally: during the foetal stage they receive essential immunoglobulins straight from their mothers' blood. After birth they ingest further antibodies from the breast milk, which protects against infections of the stomach and intestines.

ANTIBIOTICS

It was not until early in this century that the first antibiotic drug was discovered. By 1911 Paul Ehrlich had developed salvarsan to treat syphilis. Later, another German, Gerhard Domagk, produced drugs effective against Streptococcal bacteria and against the killer disease tuberculosis. In London, at St Mary's Hospital, Sir Alexander Fleming discovered that a mould, *Penicillium notatum*, contained a vital healing property, active against the Staphylococcal bacteria, yet it was not until 1945 that a means of producing it in bulk had been perfected.

Many lives have been saved thanks to potent antibiotics such as penicillin, tetracycline and sulpha drugs, but like many powerful medicines they have their drawbacks, and doctors are now using them with greater caution. Basically, they are selective poisons designed to combat bacteria (not viruses) without harming the host. A few also fight other micro-organisms such as fungi and protozoa. Ironically, they can cause immune suppression, and some can induce anaemia. Additionally, the useful natural flora of the intestine may be upset by antibiotics, allowing harmful bacteria, such as *Candida albicans*, to flourish. Most worrying of all has been the finding that a number of pathogens are becoming resistant to them. Clearly, they should not generally be used for minor ailments, but principally be reserved for the fight against the life-threatening infections.

THE BRAIN AND IMMUNITY

Only in the last few years have scientists begun to appreciate how much the brain is involved in immune function. Previously, it was believed that immunity was a completely separate system that responded directly to harmful organisms. But it is now known that several of the chemicals called neurotransmitters, which pass messages from one nerve cell to the next (an essential part of the nervous system), can also regulate immunity.

A fascinating discovery has recently emerged: lymphocytes carry minute receptors that respond to a variety of neurotransmitters. It now seems probable that the messages received by these receptors from the brain can alter the way in which the lymphocytes behave. Additionally, peripheral nerves have been identified that run out to the key organs of the immune system, the thymus gland, the spleen, the lymph nodes and the bone marrow.

It has been known for some time that expectations can have a significant effect on the immune system. Two doctors from the University of Rochester in America, Robert Ader and Nicholas Cohen, proved that the immune system could be conditioned, or 'trained' to respond to a placebo (for example, a simple sugar pill). They administered an immune-suppressing drug together with the placebo and, naturally, when the blood was tested the immune response was low. After a while (unbeknown to the recipients), they removed the real drug altogether and gave only the placebo; yet, amazingly, the white cells did not revert to normal but still continued to show lowered immunity. Thus, as long as the recipients believed that they were receiving an immune-suppressing drug their white cells showed low responsiveness. This experiment pointed conclusively towards a link between the brain and immunity. The advantages of this kind of conditioning are considerable, especially for patients who are obliged to take immuno-suppressive drugs for a long time. If at least some of the medication could be harmless placebos, side effects would be greatly reduced. Indeed, the possibilities of the research are exciting. At present, mice with auto-immune disease are being conditioned, or 'taught', to reduce the attack of their own white cells against themselves.

The pieces of this enormous puzzle are gradually coming together. There is still a huge gap in our knowledge about exactly how the immune system relates to the nervous system, but it is now clear that the anatomical and physiological connections are numerous. At last, theories long held by psychotherapists about the way the mind can influence the health – immunity included – are beginning to be more precisely explained in scientific terms.

IMMUNE-DEFICIENCY DISEASES

These diseases are divided into two types: primary and secondary. The first class results from a genetic defect, and infants suffering from such a condition usually die at an early age from severe infections which their bodies have no means of resisting. An exception is Bruton's Syndrome, which is treatable with regular injections of antibodies. Owing to defective B-cells, sufferers are unable to produce their own antibodies, yet T-cell production is normal.

Secondary immune deficiency diseases can develop at any time in life as the result of environmental or emotional factors, stress, aging, poor nutrition, drugs (for example steroids), other diseases (such as hepatitis B), malignancies or unknown causes. Sometimes, immunity may become depressed due to a combination of factors. Some of the diseases that result are described below.

Aids

The catastrophic effects of Aids (acquired immune deficiency syndrome) have been well publicised. It is caused chiefly by strains of a virus called HIV (human immunodeficiency virus) which attacks the immune system directly by breeding inside the protective white cells and also in brain cells, all of which are destroyed. It attaches itself in particular to T-helper and natural killer cells, the very ones that are normally able to fight off harmful viruses. Guzzling macrophages also become infected, as do dendritic cells, which introduce invaders to the T-cells in the first place. The victim usually dies of diseases hitherto rarely seen. Typical are an unusual form of pneumonia and Kaposi's sarcoma. This cancer generally only appears among elderly men as a mild skin disease. The depleted white cells of Aids patients, however, allow this cancer to become aggressively invasive, causing widespread damage to many organs. Quite often, Aids patients are attacked by several infections at the same time, such as TB, herpes and candida. Perhaps most distressing of all is the brain damage that can result from the ravages of the HIV, which can manifest itself as increasingly severe dementia.

One of the reasons why it is so hard to produce an effective vaccine against the HIV is because it rapidly changes both its genetic material and its antigens as it reproduces. Equally, the human immune system finds it difficult to deal with, because as soon as a certain antibody has been produced it is already out of date. Indeed, some patients are found to be infected by several variants of the virus at the same time. Even more worrying to scientists has been the diagnosis of Aids in some patients who, inexplicably, do not seem to be infected with the HIV.

Despite the aggressive nature of this virus, people with high levels of immunity can resist succumbing to fatal infections for a very long time – perhaps indefinitely – although no one can yet be sure of this. On the other hand, those whose lifestyles result in compromised immunity may succumb very quickly. Drug addicts are especially vulnerable, particularly those who inject themselves intravenously, because the virus will go straight into the bloodstream. Since the HIV is passed on through body fluids, usually through sex, blood transfusions or contaminated needles, it is possible to be fairly sure of avoiding it. People who limit their sex lives to one partner in a long-term, stable relationship are at low risk. Before transfusion, all blood is now tested, and of course any needles used for injections must always be carefully sterilised.

During the first decade of the epidemic, some 13 million infections have been identified worldwide and the World Health Organization forecasts 40 million by the year 2000 – although it could rocket to 120 million – with the largest percentage in

Asia. This is due mainly to ignorance among prostitutes and their clients about the simple avoidance of infection through the safe use of condoms. In 1991 it was reported that up to 15 per cent of new army recruits from the northern provinces of Thailand were HIV-positive.

Chances of a medical cure being found look rather slim, owing to the nature of the virus, although the drug Zidovudine can slow down its effects. However, people who are HIV-positive can do a great deal to prevent themselves from submitting to the syndrome by altering their lifestyles and following the immunity-enhancing programme laid out in these pages.

Cancer

Imagine a jumbo jet crashing every day for a whole year and killing all its passengers. In the UK, the annual total of deaths from cancers directly caused by smoking alone is of this order. All of these cancers are quite literally self-induced and are totally avoidable. And yet people continue to smoke! It is generally not realised that habitual use of tobacco increases the risk not just to the lungs and respiratory system, but also to the cervix, pancreas, liver, stomach and other organs. Smokers additionally exposed to asbestos and radiation have a higher likelihood of contracting cancer and are more susceptible to carcinogens in polluted air. The same applies to women on the Pill. Excessive use of alcohol (especially spirits) when combined with smoking can result in cancer of the liver and digestive tract. As many as 30 per cent of all cancers could probably be avoided if everyone gave up smoking and drinking.

Causes of many other cancers are much less obvious. It seems that some people may be genetically predisposed to the disease. So, if it runs in your family, there is all the more reason to get your immune system into good shape. Radiation, whether from over-exposure to the sun or from nuclear plants or X-rays, can damage cells, which results in mutation and eventually cancer. Viruses can also cause cancer through infection of cells; the most common of these is the genital wart virus (*Herpes genitalis*) which can lead to cervical cancer. Unopposed oestrogens (without progesterone) in the Pill have now been conclusively linked with breast cancer, although protection against cervical cancer may be enhanced. It is certain that at least two agents have to be present to cause malignancy: an 'initiator' that results in abnormal cell division (mutation), and a 'promoter' that encourages the cancerous growth. In fact, there are probably several predisposing factors, one or more of which lower the immune response, so the body is even less able to deal with it.

A healthy immune system can generally detect abnormal cells and destroy them with cytotoxins (cell poisons). Macrophages, the large, devouring scavenger cells, are also called into action by certain T-cells. Additionally, natural killer cells may destroy cancer cells directly with the assistance of the immunoglobulin IgG, a certain kind of antibody. There is yet another weapon in the arsenal against abnormal cells, and that is interferon, which is a protein produced by white blood cells. This inhibits the reproduction of any offensive virus or cancer cell. As a matter of interest, some doctors believe that large doses of vitamin C can encourage the production of interferon. With such a barrage, how does any cancer become established? Indeed, most do not. But if the immune system is for some reason not as effective as it might be, and if the carcinogen (the cancer-causing agent) or virus is particularly vicious, then abnormal cells can quickly multiply until a tumour develops.

Our cells are so minute that it is virtually impossible to imagine them. To give you an idea of how small they are, think of a pinhead, then divide it into ten million fragments and you have the size of a single cell. It is truly fantastic that such vast numbers manage to live in balance with each other as well as they do. But just occasionally one errant cell mutates, manages to evade the immune system and starts to reproduce by division.

Of the two hundred or so cancers there are four main varieties: carcinomas (affecting the skin and linings of organs); sarcomas (cancer of the muscle and bone); lymphomas (of the lymphatic system) and leukaemias (affecting the blood). Very often the tumours themselves are not so deadly, but they can cause severe problems when they start to obstruct essential passageways. Other cancers can prevent vital organs from working properly, or some may cause a general weakening of the body.

As far as conventional medical treatment is concerned, some forms of cancer carry a better prognosis than others, in particular Hodgkin's disease, tumours of the testes, the rare cancer of the placenta (choriocarcinoma) and lymphoblastic leukaemia in children. Cancers of the cervix, skin, lip and larynx are also curable if caught in the early stages. Indeed, it is reckoned that some 30 per cent of all cancers are successfully treated by either drugs (chemotherapy), radiotherapy or surgery, or by a combination of these. It is therefore very unwise to refuse any orthodox treatment which has a good success rate in favour of an alternative approach, since the opportunity of a cure may be thrown to the winds. Thus, the ideas contained in this book are complementary to standard medical practice, to give the patient the best possible chance of recovery.

If the cancer is no longer medically treatable, improvement in the quality of life must be the prime concern during whatever time may be left. Such improvement may unexpectedly result in more years of life. The well-known psychotherapist Dr Lawrence LeShan tells an amusing story of a woman client who was terminally ill with cancer. He asked her what the one thing was that she most wanted to do. Her reply was to go round the world, but that it was too expensive. He pointed out that she might as well do it, since she was unlikely to need her savings now that she was so ill. So off she went. She arrived back home in excellent spirits and in complete remission, but furious with her therapist because he had encouraged her to spend all her money!

The main problem with many cancers is that metastases can occur i.e. secondary spread appears in other parts of the body some time (and this can be many years) after the primary cancer has apparently been cured. It is for this reason that common diseases such as breast cancer become fatal – and no one can tell for sure whose disease is likely to progress in this fashion. As far as my own experience of cancer is concerned, I believe that a lifestyle which is deliberately immunity-enhancing helps to provide me with an insurance policy against metastases. At the same time the quality of my existence has improved beyond recognition. I am now concentrating on living a rich and fulfilling life rather than worrying all the time about succumbing to a fatal recurrence.

Candidiasis
This is a fungal disease, generally known as thrush, that has become prevalent in the West in recent years, especially among women. Its invasive form also frequently affects Aids patients, clearly indicating its association with immune deficiency. Fortunately, it responds well to an immunity-enhancing régime. There are several factors that have contributed to its rapid spread: the Pill creates a chemical environment favourable to its growth; medically prescribed antibiotics kill the microbes that keep normal amounts of the yeastlike

organism *Candida albicans* in balance; ingestion of antibiotics in factory-farmed meat and eggs appears to have a similar effect; and although chlorine in drinking water kills off the unwanted bacteria, it can also damage intestinal flora.

Most commonly, the infection appears on the skin, under the nails, in the mouth or vagina. It can also invade the bronchial tubes or lungs. In chronic cases, the harmless, single-celled form changes into an invasive fungus which produces long thread-like tendrils that can penetrate through the mucous membranes of the gut and enter the bloodstream. The infection can then reach many other parts of the body. Noticeable symptoms can be varied and include extreme food and environmental allergies, migraine, recurring cystitis, indigestion, depression and lethargy.

Ideally, the yeastlike organism should live in appropriate symbiosis with the human being, and proper diet will help to ensure that chances of it progressing to disease are minimised (see chapter 6: 'The PI Diet and special conditions'), as will an immunity-enhancing lifestyle. The nutritional supplements (available without prescription) Capricin, which is derived from coconut oil, and sorbic acid, made from mountain ash berries, have been successfully used in treating even chronic forms of candida. Nystatin is also helpful.

Herpes

Most adults have several different types of herpes virus lying dormant in their body cells. When the immune system is depressed they become active, reproduce, and symptoms appear, generally in the form of the familiar cold sore on one lip (*Herpes simplex*). If immunity is severely compromised, as for instance with Aids patients, sores can occur all over the body. When they appear in the genital region, the disease is known as *Herpes genitalis*.

Chickenpox is caused by another virus of the same group, *Herpes zoster*. It can affect adults in the form of shingles, usually when they are feeling at a low ebb. The Epstein-Barr virus that produces glandular fever also belongs in the same family. This actually attacks the B-cells and often results in an extended illness with swollen glands, fever and lethargy.

There is a positive epidemic of *Herpes simplex* at the present time, no doubt the result of extra pressure on our immune systems as a result of our modern way of life. Many sufferers link the appearance of symptoms with especially stressful times at home or work. It is therefore worth spending time lowering stress levels and consciously including relaxation in your régime. There is plenty of advice about this later in the book.

As herpes is infectious it is best not to share towels, nor for that matter to touch sores, because the virus can be transferred to another part of the body on the fingers.

The most effective deterrent against herpes is to keep your immune system functioning at peak efficiency, then you will not be troubled by these unpleasant symptoms. Supplements of the vitamins A, C and E are also helpful, as is live yoghurt. Vitamin E oil can be applied directly to the skin.

AUTO-IMMUNE DISEASES

As we have seen, an auto-immune disease occurs when the body fails to distinguish between self and non-self and starts to produce antibodies against its own cells. The T-cells can malfunction as well as the B-cells; sometimes both go wrong. It is not known why this happens, why the system starts to see its own tissue as foreign. Apart from a failure in discrimination, it may be due to mutation. Another theory is that there are so many new environmental toxins causing an extra burden on our liver and kidneys that our immune and metabolic functions are not receiving the healthy back-up they need. There does seem to be a genetic connection; auto-immune diseases tend to run in families. However, it is not enough to be predisposed towards a certain disease. Something has to trigger it off. This may be a virus, or emotional and psychological factors, or maybe radiation or drugs.

Women are far more susceptible to auto-immune diseases than men, but no one understands why this should be so. Psychotherapists have noticed that these patients tend to have great difficulty in expressing anger and store it up inside themselves. Mounting tension of this sort over a long period of time can certainly result in physical disorders. Whatever the reason, expressing one's feelings directly, combined with a positive, cheerful outlook, will help to prevent auto-immune disorders. High immunity will also keep potentially dangerous viruses at bay.

There are two types of auto-immune diseases. The first affects one organ, such as the pancreas, as in the case of diabetes. The second affects parts of cells or tissues present in more than one organ. The following are the most common auto-immune diseases, but a large number of other diseases have auto-immune manifestations, such as Hashimoto's thyroiditis and pernicious anaemia.

Diabetes

Women are the main sufferers, with 50 per cent more female diabetics than male. One simple reason for this may be that women live longer, and the risk of developing diabetes increases with age. A poorly balanced diet and obesity are contributing factors for either sex, as is a sedentary lifestyle which probably accounts for at least a quarter of cases. There is also evidence that a virus can trigger off diabetes in children by causing damage to the pancreas.

This organ is a large gland close to the stomach, which has particular cells known as beta-cells. These produce the hormone insulin that regulates the sugar in the blood. It is the more serious *Diabetes mellitus*, the juvenile-onset type, that is considered to be auto-immune in nature, because the beta-cells are systematically destroyed by the patient's own antibodies. The result is excess glucose in the blood. The kidneys now have the job of getting rid of it, so they make more and more urine to flush it out, and the strain put on these organs can result in serious damage. There is also loss of minerals from the body and dehydration.

It is the insulin that acts as a catalyst for the use of the blood sugar by the muscles. If there is no insulin they have to burn up fat to function, and this can lead to fatty acid deposits in the arteries. The diabetic now has an increased risk of heart disease. This burning of fat can also lead to the condition called acidosis, resulting in coma or even death. Blindness, owing to problems with blood vessels, is another possible complication.

Happily, the disease can be effectively regulated by self-administered injections of insulin, combined with careful testing of blood-sugar levels. Diet is extremely important, and there is more about this under chapter 6: 'The PI Diet and special conditions'. As for regular exercise, this reduces the development of adult-onset diabetes, even in the overweight.

Multiple sclerosis

This is a complex disease which mainly affects the central nervous system. The nerve fibres in our bodies are insulated by a substance called myelin, and it is this which becomes damaged in the course of the disease, resulting in hardened patches or scarring. The name of the illness means 'many scars'. Nerve signals are unable to travel normally when demyelination occurs, and this leads to loss of coordination. Other symptoms can include poor balance, tingling, numbness or coldness in the extremities, fatigue and blurring of vision.

There is a definite auto-immune component in MS. When examined under the microscope, macrophages can be seen actually gobbling up the myelin. Normally, macrophages (white scavenger cells that remove unwanted debris and bacteria) are an important part of the immune system. Why they should turn against the body's own tissue in this way is a mystery. It seems that T-lymphocytes may also behave in a hostile way. Then there are astrocytes, the cells that form the scarring. These produce enzymes which, under normal circumstances, would assist in the healing process by cleaning away surplus dead matter. In a person suffering from MS, however, the enzymes seem to contribute to the damage to the myelin, wherever there is an area of inflammation.

It is thought that there is a genetic component in multiple sclerosis – i.e. some people are born with a susceptibility to the disease. Certainly, MS sufferers seem to have difficulty in metabolising fats. Stress appears to be a contributing factor. The progress of the disease varies considerably from patient to patient: it can be benign with no further deterioration after a one-off attack; or it can be the relapsing-remitting type, with intermittent attacks; otherwise there is the chronic progressive variety when the patient becomes gradually worse. The galloping form, in which the person dies within a few years, is rare.

Since there is no medical cure for MS, management of the disease in natural ways can make a lot of difference. It is possible, through careful diet, gentle exercise and a positive, stress-free outlook, to keep the most debilitating aspects of MS at bay for many, many years, especially if the natural therapies are implemented at an early stage. There are numerous anecdotal reports of MS sufferers continuing to live full and useful lives, and not becoming permanent cripples and succumbing to wheelchairs. There are one or two excellent books on the subject (see Bibliography) and the suggestions for immune efficiency in these pages will certainly help you.

Rheumatoid arthritis

No one knows the precise cause of RA, although various theories have been put forward. Recent research at King's College, London, indicates that a bacterium called Proteus, which causes urinary tract infections, could be a culprit. Many people who suffer from RA have the tissue type HLA-DR4, and there is a similarity between this tissue and the Proteus bacterium. It is therefore possible that the immune system mistakes the human tissue for the bacterium and reacts accordingly. Certainly, it has been shown that RA patients have much higher levels of antibodies to Proteus in their blood than healthy people. Two-thirds of sufferers are women, perhaps because they are anatomically more prone to urinary tract infections.

Whatever the precise cause, at some point the cells of the immune system turn against the lining of joints and tendons. The destruction spreads to the cartilage and bone itself, causing deformity, also to the fibrous connective tissues around the joint, resulting in wastage of the muscles.

The progress of this painful disease is hard to predict. Sometimes it will confine itself to one or two small joints for a long time, but then may suddenly spread to many other joints. It can even affect the heart and lungs, causing widespread inflammation.

Rheumatoid arthritis often strikes adults in their prime during their thirties and forties. Stress, especially if it is unexpected and severe, is often linked with its onset, so if RA runs in your family it is wise to follow a regular routine of relaxation and meditation (see suggestions at the end of chapter 3), and to keep anxiety levels as low as possible. High immunity to keep bacteria at bay is obviously vital.

The condition can be somewhat alleviated by anti-inflammatory drugs, but there is as yet no medical cure, so general maintenance of health is very important. Take plenty of sleep and rest, making sure you include sufficient gentle exercise to keep you mobile, and eat very nutritious food as described under 'The Peak Immunity Diet' in chapter 6.

Systemic lupus erythematosus

Lupus erythematosus is Latin for 'red wolf'. This seems an odd name for a disease, but it comes from one of the symptoms – a red rash across the nose and cheeks. 'Systemic' indicates that the disease penetrates to every part of the body, with the patient's own antibodies attacking all kinds of tissue, including the vital organs, joints, lymph nodes and digestive tract. This happens because the antibodies are formed against DNA, an essential genetic component of every cell. Even the central nervous system can be affected, causing fits and psychosis.

Nearly all lupus patients are females, but the reason for this is unknown. Psychological factors include stress or a major loss of some kind. Typical patients also seem to be excessively independent. If it is caught in the early stages symptoms can be controlled with anti-inflammatory drugs. Needless to say, an immunity-enhancing régime is vital.

Ulcerative colitis

This is a debilitating illness which often afflicts young adults, especially those under stress. The main symptoms are abdominal pain and tenderness accompanied by diarrhoea and bleeding. Naturally, the patient is liable to become depressed as a result of the incapacitating nature of the symptoms, which are difficult to control. Chronic inflammation and ulceration occur in the colon, which appears to be attacked by the sufferer's own antibodies. Remissions can occur from time to time, but this is generally a persistent disease.

Stress levels need to be kept as low as possible, and adequate rest is essential. A high-protein diet is often prescribed, so patients may like to refer to Chapter 6: 'Poor digestion'. Plenty of liquid will offset possible dehydration, preferably in the form of fresh vegetable juices, and an iron supplement may be advisable if anaemia results, with extra vitamin C to aid its absorption; folic acid can be helpful, too. Nutritionally this is a draining disease, so a rich intake of vitamins and minerals from natural sources is essential.

ALLERGIES

Allergies are similar to auto-immune diseases in that the immune system responds inappropriately: in the case of allergies there is an over-reaction to external stimuli (the allergens) and in auto-immune diseases there is an unsuitable response to internal stimuli. The word 'allergy' in fact means altered capacity to react.

While healthy bodies are perfectly capable of coping with normal allergens such as dust, mites, pollens, and spores from moulds, our detoxification systems have had no chance to evolve a tolerance to man-made substances such as those described in chapter 4. It was only when hyperactivity and behavioural disorders in children were finally traced to colouring in drinks that the scientific community started to take the problem of food intolerances seriously. These are discussed further in chapter 6.

Lining the membranes open to the environment, for example the nose and intestine, are mast cells. These are similar to B-cells, but they are unable to move around. They can produce specialised antibodies called immunoglobulins and they also have a memory system. When a person becomes sensitised to an allergen, immunoglobulins are formed and these bind to receptor sites on the mast cells. As soon as the allergen reappears, it forms a complex with the immunoglobulin and this activates enzymes; these in turn cause histamines and other chemical mediators to be released and the symptoms of irritation, swelling and running nose and eyes occur. This 'allergic reaction' typical of hay fever seems to be the body's way of attempting to rid itself of the invader. Drugs can alleviate these symptoms, but there is no medical cure as such. Avoidance of the offending allergen is really the best tactic.

Records taken during the ten years between 1971 and 1981 showed a marked increase in the incidence of allergies. Numbers per thousand of asthma cases almost doubled, and hay fever was nearly as bad. Yet hay fever was unknown up to the start of the nineteenth century. Cases of dermatitis, eczema and conjunctivitis also increased. City-dwellers suffer the most, while those who live in the mountains or by the sea are less likely to be afflicted. It is clear that allergies are the product of modern times. In less developed communities, where people have followed the same way of life in the same locality for many generations, they have become well adapted to their environment and allergies are rare.

Sadly, Western babies are now having a poor start in life as far as allergies are concerned. A mother's breast milk contains important immunoglobulins (antibodies) that strengthen the baby's immune system while it is still developing. Another important constituent is gammalinolenic acid (GLA), an essential fatty acid, discussed in chapter 6, which is known to protect against eczema. Previously, breast-fed babies were unlikely to suffer allergies, whereas those fed on cow's milk were prone to them. Now, however, babies who are breast-fed for long periods are showing an increased susceptibility to allergies because their mothers' milk is so contaminated with pesticides and other chemicals. It has been noticed that failure of immune discrimination early in life leads to recurring allergic problems later on.

Many millions of people suffer from the serious condition of asthma, in which the bronchioles (airways to the lungs) become blocked. This can be due to an excess of mucus, swollen mucous membranes, or tightening of the muscles. Not all asthma is the result of an allergic reaction, although this is more common in children. Stress is certainly a factor. Indeed, the psychological connection has been well documented. Perhaps the best-known case is that of a person allergic to roses who developed an asthmatic attack when shown artificial flowers, believing them to be real. Like hay fever, asthma can be triggered off by allergens such as dust mites or animal danders. Pesticides or household chemicals can often be the culprits. Here again, avoidance is the best tactic. Careful vacuuming, especially of bedrooms, will keep dust levels low.

Some sensitive people are violently allergic to insect bites and stings, in particular to bee stings. The condition called anaphylaxis can result, which consists of extreme asthma, a swollen throat and a dramatic drop in blood pressure. Emergency treatment, consisting of adrenalin by injection, is vital. Susceptible people are wise to carry a syringe with them if they are ever likely to be in contact with insects. Desensitisation treatment may also be worth considering.

Allergy sufferers are well advised to keep pollution levels as low as possible, so that the body's defences are not overstretched. Look at the questionnaire at the end of chapter 4 and see how many chemicals you can cut out of your environment altogether. You will be surprised how many are unnecessary. Stress levels need to be kept to a minimum also, with the assistance of a suitable psychotherapist in severe cases.

FOOD POISONING

The risk of eating contaminated food has always been present, but in recent years technology has outstripped legislation, with intensive farming and convenience foods becoming more and more common. Sometimes these can provide favourable conditions in which the deadly bacteria can thrive, and as a result food poisoning is reaching epidemic proportions, with listeria and salmonella in particular hitting the headlines. In 1983 an estimated 375,000 people suffered from food poisoning in the UK, but seven years later it reached the 1 million mark, with around 300 deaths annually. Since 1985 listeriosis has increased threefold, and the 1989 salmonella figures were up 17 per cent on those of 1988, despite the fact that egg-eating (the main source of contamination) had dropped 20 per cent.

Apart from viruses that cause gastro-enteritis or hepatitis, food poisoning is generally caused by a bacterium. The following are the most dangerous.

Botulism

This is particularly nasty, since it produces a vicious poison that enters the bloodstream and then prevents nervous impulses from reaching the muscles. This causes total collapse and a high probability of death. It may take only a hundred-millionth of a gram of the poison to kill someone. At this rate, botulinum toxin the size of a bean could eliminate the entire population of the UK. Yet the bacterium is widespread in the form of hard spores, being present in about 5 per cent of soil samples. Conditions have to be just right for the bacterium to flourish and produce its poison, and these are nutrients, warmth and moisture, but no oxygen. The centre of a sausage has proved an ideal spot, as have tinned vegetables and fish. Happily, high standards in the canning industry have ensured the rarity of botulism.

If you keep to the Peak Immunity Diet, as described in chapter 6, you will be very unlikely to suffer from this frightening illness, as meats and tinned foods are not recommended. However, if you do resort to buying the odd can, make sure that it is not dented, rusted or punctured, and heat any tinned vegetables very thoroughly.

Salmonella

These bacteria thrive particularly well in birds, without necessarily harming them, and therefore it is chickens and their eggs, turkeys and ducks that can cause trouble as far as human food is concerned. One of our defence mechanisms is the acid in our stomach, which is capable of destroying many bacteria – salmonella included. If the acid is weak, for example in invalids or babies, then the bacteria will survive. Alternatively, if the bacteria are consumed in large numbers, some will invade the intestines, where they form an enterotoxin resulting in illness. Occasionally they can enter the bloodstream and cause blood poisoning or septicaemia, accompanied by a very high temperature. In this case, the patient may collapse and die. Normally, however, the main symptom is diarrhoea – another defence mechanism, designed to rid the body of bacteria as quickly as possible. This is followed by a feeling of exhaustion. Some salmonella can remain in the gut without causing further disease, and such people can become carriers. This is why personal hygiene is so important, since bacteria can be transferred from unwashed hands to any food. As many as 1 million bacteria can be harboured around a single fingernail!

How does salmonella get into eggs? Bacteria can pass through shells, but the main route is directly from the egg-laying apparatus in breeding stocks. Some small chicks may die from it, but others will not and may be viewed as healthy. Egg-producers are unwilling to slaughter breeding stocks unless infection can be positively proved, so contamination continues. The problem is perpetuated by feeding the birds on recycled chickens, at least 50 per cent of which will probably be infected with salmonella. Biologists view this as a dangerous and unnatural practice, because chickens do not prey on their own species.

Since even free-range chickens cannot be guaranteed to be infection-free, safety measures need to be followed. Salmonella bacteria are killed by cooking for a reasonable length of time at a high temperature, so make sure that scrambled eggs are very well done. Boil eggs from room temperature for seven or eight minutes. Cook omelettes and fried eggs on both sides. Do not poach eggs. Soufflés and eggs used in baking should be fairly safe. Even so, vulnerable people such as babies, pregnant women, the sick and the elderly should avoid eggs altogether, at least until stricter legislation is brought in. Chickens should be very thoroughly thawed before cooking, otherwise temperatures inside the bird whilst in the oven may not be high enough to kill bacteria.

Listeriosis
Because the incubation period of the listeriosis bacterium in the gut is anything from five days to six weeks, tracing the source of the contamination is extremely difficult. By then, the incriminating evidence in the form of food scraps will almost certainly have been thrown away. Although it has been known for some time that animals

could harbour the bacteria, the way in which they were passed on to humans remained a mystery. Only in 1981, in Canada, was a definite cause finally established. In this case it was contaminated coleslaw. The cabbage involved had been cultivated with sheep manure and then stored in a cold shed. Unlike most bacteria, listeria flourishes at a low temperature. The addition of the mayonnaise to the cabbage provided moisture and nutrients that further encouraged the listeria to grow and to produce a toxin called listeriolysin. This damages the large white scavenging cells of the immune system, the macrophages. People with reduced immunity, such as those on steroids, or with an illness such as diabetes, are especially vulnerable to the toxin. Recent figures published in America suggest that the risk of adults dying from the disease is 25-30 per cent. Pregnant women who suffer from it are likely to lose their babies. The main symptoms are 'flu-like, accompanied by a high temperature.

In 1985 there was a serious outbreak in Los Angeles involving 142 cases. This time Mexican soft cheese made from unpasteurised milk was identified as the cause. The high temperature of pasteurisation would normally kill listeria, although contamination could still occur at a later stage. It is thought that soft cheeses with a crust, such as brie and camembert, are the most risky, and possibly those made from goats' and ewes' milk. Hard cheeses are less likely to provide a fertile environment for listeria.

Ready-made convenience foods that have been cooked and then chilled are recipes for disaster. Listeria can recover from damage by heat if refrigerated for a few days. In a recent survey carried out in Leeds, 7 out of 12 cook-chill chickens contained listeria, and of 100 cook-chill meals, nearly one-quarter had the bacteria. The answer is to cook your own food and eat it fresh. Salads are perfectly safe as long as they are well washed and any mayonnaise is kept separate.

Safety points
If you should be unfortunate enough to suffer from food poisoning, and diarrhoea is the main symptom, drink half a glass of filtered or bottled water mixed with fruit juice approximately every half hour. This will replace lost fluid. Avoid preparing food until you are better.

The following questionnaire will help you sort out a few more safety points related to the kitchen.

1 Do you keep eggs in the refrigerator?

2 Should you store cooked and raw food separately?

3 Should you have individual chopping boards for cooked and raw food?

4 Are your chopping boards deeply scored?

5 Do you know how cold your fridge and freezer should be?

6 How long should you allow for a chicken to thaw out?

7 Why should flies be kept out of the kitchen?

8 How often should you change your tea cloth and hand towel?

9 Do you use the tea cloth to wipe your hands?

10 Do you leave cooked food at room temperature for more than 1$\frac{1}{2}$ hours?

11 Is your kitchen very warm?

12 If you have to keep food hot for a while, do you know how hot it should be?

13 While preparing food, do you dip your fingers in to test it?

14 Why are powdered gravies and custards hazardous?

15 Does cooking in a microwave oven destroy bacteria?

16 Does freezing kill bacteria?

17 Should you allow your cats on to the table and work surface?

18 Do your pets use the same dishes and cutlery as you?

Answers

1 If you do, remove them at least half an hour before cooking, otherwise the temperature in the centre will not be hot enough to destroy salmonella. Preferably, keep in a cool place and eat within a week.

2 Yes, you should. Otherwise bacteria from the raw food may contaminate the cooked food.

3 It is better if you do, for the same reason as 2.

4 If they are, throw them out. Crevices can harbour bacteria.

5 A safe temperature for a fridge is 0 to 3°C (32 to 37°F) and for a freezer -18 to -23°C (0 to -9°F).

6 A chicken takes 24 hours in a cool room; a turkey 48 hours.

7 All insects can transfer bacteria between foods.

8 The ideal is every day, since bacteria can multiply on cloth.

9 If you do, bacteria can be transferred to crockery and cutlery.

10 After this time, bacteria will proliferate. With the exception of listeria, refrigeration halts their growth.

11 Keep your kitchen as cool as possible. This will help to keep food fresh.

12 Above 63°C (145°F). Most bacteria multiply fastest between 10°C (50°F) and 63°C (145°F). Keeping food warm for too long within this range is the commonest cause of food poisoning from restaurants and take-aways.

13 Not a good idea – a likely route to contamination.

14 Powdered ingredients often harbour bacteria. Keep temperatures high during cooking and discard left-overs.

15 Microwaves do not kill bacteria, although the heat generated by molecular agitation may do. Microwave ovens cannot be relied on to sterilise food.

16 No, it only arrests their growth, so they will start to multiply after thawing. It is hazardous to re-freeze items after slight thawing.

17 Bacteria from animals can infect humans.

18 It is better to keep pets' dishes and cutlery separate for the reason given in 17.

2 How healthy is your personality?

THE CANCER-PRONE PERSONALITY

I settled myself gratefully into the comfortable chintz-covered arm-chair. It was our first morning at the Bristol Cancer Help Centre and it had already proved exceedingly busy, with meditation first thing, followed by a talk outlining the holistic concept of the pro-gramme and then an introduction to the special diet. All sorts of new thoughts and ideas were buzzing around my brain. Any visit to a doctor induces feelings of shakiness inside me, and today was no exception. But Dr Michael was very different. He had come to work at the Centre because, as a GP, he had been obliged to see hundreds of patients at five-minute intervals with never enough time to talk to any of them. The result was frustration. As a trained psychotherapist also, he had cultivated a true understanding of the profound effect that the mind and emotions have on the body. Modern medics are taught only to treat the physical symptoms, without consideration of the whole person, despite the fact that around 70 per cent of all patients who turn up in their GP's surgery are suffering from psychosomatic complaints. Any doctor who leaves the system to find his own path must be truly special, and I had a strong sense of this man's uniqueness as I gazed into his warm brown eyes.

He started by asking me questions about my illness and treatment, and suggested a soothing, natural ointment for the irritating rash caused by the radiotherapy. Then he asked me about my family. I was feeling vulnerable and faltered when I mentioned that I used to have a brother. He looked suddenly alert. There was a persistent pricking sensation behind my eyelids. 'Go with the tears', he said gently.

'He wasn't just my brother; he was my closest friend.'

'And what happened?'

'His passion was rock-climbing. We were brought up in the Lake

District, so I knew all about the dangers of mountains. As a child he had always been reckless and accident-prone – not a safe mixture. With training, he became a superb athlete, but I always used to be filled with dread whenever he went out climbing. I remember one night some fellows were trapped on a ledge near the top of Coniston Old Man. It was dark and the weather was bad, so bad that the mountain rescue team refused to go out. But my brother insisted on helping them and abseiled down a rope in hazardous conditions. Eventually he and his friends managed to haul them to safety.'

My breathing came in gasps as I recalled the tortuous suspense of waiting for him to return home in one piece. 'That was the sort of thing he used to do. The next challenge was snow- and ice-climbing in the Alps. On his last expedition he was with two other climbers, one very reliable and experienced, the other much younger and new to Alpine conditions. As far as we know they were approaching a ridge near the top of Mont Blanc when there was a freak storm and all three disappeared without trace. The helicopters went out to search for them, but it was hopeless. We'll never know what happened to them. Perhaps one slipped and pulled the others down too, or they lost their way and fell into a crevasse, or were swept away by an avalanche.' My tears plopped on to my skirt, making little damp pools, as images filled my mind of his poor broken body trapped for ever under the ice. 'It was agonising waiting for news. I lost my voice completely. I couldn't speak at all for a week.'

'How long ago did this happen?'

'Oh, years ago.'

'It's still very fresh, though, isn't it?'

'Yes. I often have nightmares that I am up in the mountains searching for him. It is always dark and cold and I am attempting to scale terrifying precipices. But . . . I never find him.' I could hold back the sobs no longer and a handful of tissues was thoughtfully passed to me.

'What is most distressing you now?'

'I want to know how he died – that he didn't suffer.'

'Close your eyes. Imagine you are talking with him in the mountains. Can you see him there?'

'Yes.'

'What does he look like?'

'He's holding his ice axe and has a rope slung across his body. He has rumpled dark brown hair and hazel eyes with tiny flecks of green in them. He's a bit taller than I am. Athletic, with broad shoulders and slender hips.'

'Ask him how he died.'

I gulped down the sobs again. These recollections were unbearable. All I could hear was something about hypothermia. My brother was a doctor and knew about the effects of extreme cold. I remembered him telling me once that it was a reasonably pleasant way to die – like sinking into a long sleep.

But what on earth had all this to do with my illness? I was beginning to feel confused. Another question from Dr Michael: 'Were you angry with him for dying?' Angry? How could I ever be angry with the one person I loved most of all? But I recalled extreme feelings of rage towards the women at base camp, who had delayed so long before contacting the mountain rescue team. Then there were feelings of guilt. Perhaps if I had been a better sister to him in some way, he might never have been killed. I knew he wanted to die on a mountain. He often talked about it.

'Are you angry with him for *wanting* to die?' I hesitated. It was true that I was the one who was left behind to struggle on on my own. Maybe there was a little resentment there. 'It is quite natural to feel angry after the loss of a loved one, along with the grief. I feel it is important for you to complete the mourning process in order to achieve inner healing.' But time was up. He kissed me on the cheek. 'You may like to discuss this with your counsellor later in the week.'

'Yes.' I thanked him.

During the tea break I took the opportunity of looking at some of the books in the library. One in particular caught my eye – *You Can Fight For Your Life: Emotional Factors in the Treatment of Cancer* by Lawrence LeShan. As I read through its pages later in the evening, my session with the doctor began to make more sense. I also realised with a shock that the typical cancer personality that emerged bore an uncanny resemblance to my own.

According to LeShan's observations, the childhood or adolescence of his patients was invariably marked by feelings of isolation. My early years were carefree and happy, and I was an energetic, fun-loving kid. But at the age of ten I was sent to boarding school, where I spent six years of unremitting misery. Nothing I did ever seemed right and in the end I withdrew into a deep depression. In mid-adolescence my best friend was taken away from the school because, as I discovered some years later, the headmistress was an alcoholic and had been seducing members of the sixth form. The holidays were never long enough to establish lasting friendships at home, and at that stage I and my brother, being younger than myself, shared few interests. My sister was several years older, and our parents were eternally busy, so I spent the time largely on my own, comforted by my music and my dog.

The second phase of the typical cancer patient, says LeShan, involves an important relationship in early adulthood. Alternatively, or additionally, a deeply satisfying activity or job is found that adds meaning to life, and emotional energy is poured into this. My brother had caught up with me in maturity by the time we reached our early twenties and we suddenly discovered what an enormous amount we had in common. It was very exciting. Here at last was someone I could relate to, someone with whom I could share my most secret thoughts – my own brother. Somehow this seemed safe. Boyfriends might come and go, but my brother was always my brother. Nothing could change that. Whatever happened, we were always there for each other. Meanwhile I had finally managed to emerge from my shell by joining a theatre company and derived much enjoyment from working closely with a group of people. Creating something together in a team was fun and rewarding, and at last I was finding a way of expressing some of those bottled-up feelings. Perhaps I was instinctively making up for my arid adolescence.

The third phase involves the loss of the central relationship and/or the meaningful activity. Before my brother's accident, I had been obliged to give up the theatre. Although I was doing fairly well with many leading roles to my credit, it was constantly difficult for me to make ends meet and I needed to find a more secure way of earning my living. A careers analyst suggested a secretarial training and a job in publishing, but I found office work tedious and felt alienated and lonely. And then I lost my beautiful brother and a hollow despair set in.

After that, relationships seemed to be fraught with difficulties. LeShan says that people prone to cancer feel that 'to be loved they must be untrue to themselves'. In adolescence, I had become so used to behaving in a way that would earn at least some approval from teachers and parents that it seemed inconceivable that anyone could love me for my true self. The bouncy, fun-loving me had been unacceptable to the adults around me since the age of ten. She made a brief reappearance during my theatre days, but with the rigid routine of office work she once again retreated into obscurity. So my life seemed false and without meaning. Yet on the surface I appeared to cope well. I stuck at the dull job, hoping that, as I climbed the ladder, the work might become more interesting – and in some ways it did. Here again, this is typical of the cancer personality: dutiful, sweet-natured, patient and obliging on the surface and a secret desperation beneath. Linked to this is a total inability to express any anger in self-defence. So resentment builds up and starts to gnaw away inside. Such people never learnt in childhood how to cope with life's blows. They gave up and gave in – just like I did at boarding school: I could no longer race round on my bike or climb trees; I had to behave like a 'young lady', and so the energy became imploded.

Then later on, to lose the most precious thing of all is somehow only to be expected. This is what life is like. Reinforcing this negative attitude is an all-pervading sense of worthlessness, of never being good enough for anyone or anything. Music was my best subject at school, and at the age of sixteen I gained distinction in grade VIII piano, winning a prize for the highest mark in the north-west of England. My real ambition was to go to music college but, despite invitations to apply for scholarships, nothing would convince me that I was up to scratch. At the same time, says LeShan, in a futile attempt to make up for that inner feeling of worthlessness, other people's approval is keenly sought after. How desperately I tried to please other people! But living up to other people's expectations is a constant drain on the energy. So life has simply to be got through as best one can and the possibility of dying early is often accepted without surprise and even with relief. I always 'knew' that my brother would kill himself on a mountain, just as I always 'knew' that I would find myself with breast cancer. Neither of these events surprised me.

At lunch the next day, I started to test out these theories. Sitting next to me was a beautiful young woman with long, blonde hair. She had a rare sort of leukaemia and the prognosis was not good. During our conversation I was astounded to discover that she, too, had been close to her brother and he also had been killed in an accident. I particularly noticed how sweet, kind and well-behaved all the people around me were. All of us were quite extraordinarily 'nice'.

It has been accepted for some time by psychologists that bereavement can lower the immune response. In 1979 a paper was presented to the Psychosomatic Society in Dallas that described a study of men whose wives had died from breast cancer. Within the month following their bereavement, the responsiveness of the husbands' lymphocytes had declined significantly. When tested again a year later, this reaction remained equally low in several cases.

In LeShan's study, 76 per cent of his cancer patients shared this same emotional history, whereas only 10 per cent of the control group had a similar personality structure. Other studies, notably one carried out over a period of thirty years by Caroline B. Thomas, a psychologist at Johns Hopkins University in America, have confirmed LeShan's theories. Her findings concluded that people who later developed cancer had a history of lack of emotional closeness with their parents, seldom demonstrated strong emotions (especially in relation to their own needs), and generally appeared benign and low-gear. Through a test involving drawings, she also found that she could predict which parts of the body would develop the cancer.

Other emotional factors

Helplessness and hopelessness are qualities that are particularly noticeable before the onset of cancer. In 1971 Drs A.H. Schmale and H. Iker published a paper entitled 'Hopelessness as a predictor of cervical cancer'. They devised psychological tests to identify a 'helplessness-prone personality', and used these to study a group of women who were thought to be biologically predisposed to cervical cancer. With these measures alone they were able to predict which women would develop the cancer, and had a 73.6 per cent success rate.

Classically, people find themselves in a situation to which there appears to be no solution. Illness then presents itself as the only way out. For instance, a friend of mine had agreed with her boyfriend, who lived in her flat, that she should give up her job and go to university to study for a degree. He offered to give her financial support during this period. Unfortunately, their sexual relationship, which had never been especially satisfactory, deteriorated until it came to a complete halt. For Donald security and companionship were the most important elements, but for Jennifer physical expression of love was also a key factor. Yet she was totally unable to speak about her feelings and to ask for what she needed. Additionally, she longed for a child, but was already in her late thirties. As time passed, she became more hopeless. What could she do? Part of her realised that she ought to leave him, yet she was genuinely fond of him and couldn't bear to hurt his feelings. She was also mid-way through her course and wanted to finish it. Donald seemed quite content and would clearly be most unwilling to move out of the flat. Yet all the money that she had saved had gone into buying it. She had no spare cash at all of her own and was financially dependent on him. She felt trapped, stuck. Meanwhile she saw her last reproductive years dwindling and her womanhood being denied. She became depressed and unable to concentrate on her work. The following year she developed cancer.

PERSONALITY AND OTHER DISEASES

If there is a personality type that is more likely to succumb to cancer, are there then different personalities that tend to be associated with other illnesses?

The link between a 'Type A' personality and heart disease is now very well established. Such people are strongly competitive and have a desire for success and recognition. They are impatient and do things in a rush, cramming in far too many activities in too short a time. They maintain a high level of mental and physical alertness for long periods and find it hard to relax. They rarely appreciate things of beauty. This constantly over-aroused state appears to raise blood pressure and cholesterol levels, and increase the likelihood of forming blood clots, leading to a higher risk of coronary attack. Interestingly, researchers have shown that patients who modify their behaviour by relaxing and becoming calmer are less prone to a second attack than those who carry on as before.

Psychoneuroimmunology is a discipline still in its infancy, but useful studies have recently been carried out on people suffering from auto-immune diseases. What is it that turns the body against itself, causing it to attack its own tissue? How significant are psychological factors?

In 1981 Dr G.F. Solomon published a paper on this subject in the book *Psychoneuroimmunology*, with a special emphasis on people suffering from rheumatoid arthritis. A previous researcher had concluded that 'the arthritic process is . . . the expression of a personality conflict'. Other studies showed that, like cancer patients, arthritics tend to turn their anger inwards instead of expressing their feelings freely. A psychoanalyst found that, underneath, they are dependent types with feelings of inadequacy, yet they have an effective outward show of being able to cope. Either they overcompensate for these unworthy feelings by taking on too much responsibility, or else they do the opposite and rely totally on others for guidance. They are extremely sensitive to criticism, and avoid close personal contact. A critical factor in the onset or sudden worsening of the disease is the loss of a key figure upon whom they depend for support.

Solomon tested this profile by comparing sixteen female RA patients with their sisters who did not have RA. Thus, factors such as genetic inheritance and family background were as close as possible. The RA sufferers scored high on perfectionism, compliance and subservience, nervousness, introversion, depression and sensitivity to anger. By contrast, their healthy sisters described themselves as 'liking people, easy to get acquainted with, enjoying life in a generally unruffled manner'. A particular feature of the RA patients was their martyrlike or even masochistic relationship with their husbands, whereas their sisters were able to express anger directly and openly to family members when appropriate.

As you will remember from chapter 1, it is particularly noticeable that women suffer far more from auto-immune diseases than men, and the theory is that role conflicts could be a contributing factor. Many apparently dedicated housewives feel underneath that they are 'sacrificing' themselves for their families. They have taken on the role of wife and mother exclusively and have denied their other creative energies. As a result, hostility and resentment can build up over the years, and if turned inwards, as it so often is, can cause physiological changes to take place, finally resulting in degenerative disease. Culturally, women are not allowed to be aggressive and express anger and, instead, they tend to dissolve into tears and retreat to the safer position of victim. Assertiveness can be extraordinarily difficult for many women. Those who belong to the older generation had to put up with severe social restrictions in their youth. My own mother, for instance, who suffers from crippling arthritis, was unable to continue her teaching career after her wedding. In those days married women were not employed as teachers because it was considered that they were taking away men's jobs. Despite far greater freedom today, women can still readily copy their mothers and fall into the trap of giving up their own talents and ambitions in favour of their man's. The kind of inner discontent that follows does not lead to good health and happiness.

Ulcerative colitis, another auto-immune disease, also has a personality profile. In this disease, antibodies attack the colon. Studies have shown that, in addition to sitting on anger, patients characteristically have obsessive-compulsive traits of neatness, suffer from worrying and indecision, conscientiousness, rigid morality and conformity. Here again, the evidence is that people with this disease are in some way not being true to themselves, but put other people's standards and opinions first.

An acquaintance of mine with ulcerative colitis, in this case a man, is convinced that his psychological state brought the disease on, and is now finding that group therapy helps to modify his behaviour and so relieves the ill-effects of his disease. His fastidiousness ensures that he does his job well as a dentist, but he admits that he is too obsessed with perfectionism as well as personal neatness. One thing he has agreed with the group to do recently is to make a mess once a day until he no longer feels bad or guilty in any way! He is also learning to free up repressed anger by looking at his past and discovering what this is about. One safe technique he adopts is to beat a large pile of cushions supported by group members and let the rage out with movement, sound and words. His worries he is able to share with the group and, while no one gives him direct advice, the leader and members help him to find his own solutions. Through honest feedback, he is also learning to place greater value on his own opinions and judgment, rather than always going along with what others expect of him. He is gradually discovering that inner harmony leads to better physical health and he now has the colitis well under control.

Dr Solomon also provides a personality profile for another auto-immune disease – lupus erythematosus. Again, perfectionism features, together with independence, often expressed through excessive activity such as a highly competitive sport. Acute stress or serious loss of some kind triggers off depression, later followed by the disease. As for multiple sclerotics, they seem to have an excessive need for love and affection, which was not gratified in childhood.

It is not known exactly how these personality traits affect immune functioning, but the theory is that, among other causes, emotional distress results in an imbalance of T-suppressor cells. In the case of cancer, an excessive production allows tumours to develop; in an auto-immune disease, the opposite happens and there are too few T-suppressor cells. As you will recall from the first chapter, the correct balance of different kinds of white cells in the lymph is vital, and even though T-suppressor cells slow down immune response, too few nevertheless result in immune deficiency.

THE HARDY PERSONALITY

While some individuals appear to be more prone to serious illness, others evidently have an inborn resistance to disease supported by a highly efficient immune system. Three words beginning with 'c' describe these naturally hardy people: commitment, control and challenge. If, for example, a person is committed to relationships, then s/he will find support when stressful times or other problems occur. Long-term commitments also mean that events are kept in perspective. If people feel in control of life's events, then they are more likely to take direct action to remedy any problems, rather than allowing themselves to become submerged in the way that helpless victims do. Action and clear decisions point to solutions and reduce needless worrying. Thus, there is less chance of a build-up of damaging negative emotions inside the body. Hardy people are good copers. Any changes in circumstances are considered to be normal and are seen as a challenge rather than a threat to security. For instance, a person made redundant can either slide into feelings of worthlessness and depression or else see the situation as an opportunity to try something new. Hardy people view themselves as basically OK and have an optimistic outlook. They are likely to be cheerful and good-humoured and are not easily upset by criticism.

Dr George Solomon and John Morlem of America's UCLA tested the blood of elderly people and compared the white cells with those of people half their age. They discovered that the immune systems of the elderly who were in good health were as competent as, and in some ways even superior to, those of the younger people. Their conclusions were that the effectiveness of people's natural killer cells was associated with emotional hardiness and with a positive response to life's events.

An elderly relative of mine, now in his late eighties and still full of life, conforms very much to this naturally hardy type. He worked in the same bank all his life and never had a day's illness. The routine fulfilled his security needs and he enjoyed the company and friendship of his colleagues. He was totally contented with his lot, accepting promotion as it came, but not ambitious for a top job, which would mean less time at home with his wife, to whom he was devoted, and less time for his favourite hobby, painting. At weekends they would walk for miles with their dog to find a new beauty spot, setting up their easels and capturing the view in watercolours. The paintings were either given to friends or sold in aid of charities. They have lived in the same house for many, many years, moving only once since their marriage, to a slightly more comfortable residence within the same area. Long-term friendships they consider to be very important, and they maintain close contact with their daughter and grandchildren. Above all, their house is always filled with smiles and laughter, and the funny side of even difficult situations is readily appreciated.

ARE YOU AN IMMUNE-EFFICIENT PERSON?

Now it is your turn to find out whether you have an immune-efficient or immune-deficient personality. Answer either 'yes' or 'no'.

A

1 Do you belong to a close-knit community or group?

2 Do you have friends and/or relatives you are able to share with intimately?

3 If you get angry are you able to say so immediately and deal with the rage effectively?

4 If you are sad, do you allow yourself to express your grief through tears?

5 What do you do about your fear? Do you acknowledge it and release it through physical action?

6 Are you self-assertive and do you feel able to ask directly for what you want?

7 Are you willing to take risks in order to change things for the better?

8 Are you optimistic about your own future and that of the world in general?

9 Are you confident of your own abilities?

10 Do you feel satisfied with your work and home life?

11 Do you have clearly defined, achievable goals?

12 Do you have a good sense of humour?

13 Do you allow yourself to have fun?

14 Do you pursue interesting hobbies?

15 Do you take regular physical exercise?

16 Are you an individual, preferring to follow your own code for living, rather than other people's?

17 Are you good at making decisions?

18 Are you easy-going and unruffled?

19 Are you able to ask for help when you need it, without feeling apologetic?

20 If you score badly in this questionnaire, will you see this as a challenge to do something about yourself?

B

1 Are you very sensitive to criticism and do you easily feel hurt by other people's remarks?

2 Do you consider that other people's needs are more important than your own?

3 Do you often feel powerless or victimized by the world, or helpless or hopeless?

4 Do you feel trapped – that whatever you do there is no way out?

5 Are you frequently depressed?

6 Do you find your job and/or home life disappointing?

7 Do you feel that everything you do is pointless?

8 Are you often anxious and afraid?

9 Do you consider that it is wrong to express anger and generally bottle it up instead?

10 Are you apparently calm on the surface, but churning away underneath?

11 Do you feel guilty when you relax or do nothing?

12 Are you a perfectionist to the point where you give something up before you even start it, because you feel you will never be good enough?

13 Are you constantly worried about social behaviour and that you should be seen to be doing the 'right thing'?

14 Are you excessively conscientious?

15 Are you compulsively neat?

16 Did you learn your moral code from someone else and do you stick to it unquestioningly?

17 Do you feel that you are in some way sacrificing yourself for your family or employers?

18 Do you take work home at the weekend and in the evenings?

19 Do you believe that no one else can do a job as well as you?

20 If you score badly in this questionnaire will you believe that you are heading for a terrible illness and become depressed?

Scoring

a) If you answered 'yes' 15 – 20 times under A, and 'no' 15 – 20 times under B, then you have an immune-efficient personality and are likely to have high resistance to disease.

b) If you answered 'yes' 10 – 14 times under A and 'no' 10 – 14 times under B, then you have reasonably good tolerance to disease as far as your personality is concerned.

c) If you answered 'yes' 5 – 9 times under A, and 'no' 5 – 9 times under B, then you have little natural hardiness and your core personality will not help you to resist disease. Changes in attitude are therefore strongly recommended.

d) If you answered 'yes' 0 – 4 times under A and 'no' 0 – 4 times under B, then you have a severely immune-deficient personality. You have the opportunity to take the first step in the right direction at this very moment by deciding to do something to help yourself. Consulting a skilled counsellor would be a good start, and there are plenty of suggestions in this book.

Remember that personality is only a part of the holistic approach. You may be naturally blessed with a strong physical constitution and a healthy genetic inheritance. It takes several factors to produce serious degenerative disease. So, if your personality score is poor, don't panic. The good news is that you can learn to modify your behaviour to increase your resistance to disease. If you are already ill, personal improvements will help you a great deal.

You may be feeling perplexed and thinking, 'How can I possibly change who I am?' It really is feasible. I have done it and so have many thousands of others. It is not easy, and it takes perseverance and time. Readers with low scores will almost certainly need professional help. Sometimes it is very hard to see one's own behaviour patterns, and even harder to replace them with something more constructive, because there are very good reasons why we are the way we are. More of this later.

BECOMING AN IMMUNE-EFFICIENT PERSON

Look again at the questionnaire and, taking you 'nos' under A and 'yeses' under B, mark with an asterisk those that you feel you can remedy without too much effort. You can only make changes gradually, so choose the easiest things first, then write down in your notebook a list of aims. For example, if you have put an asterisk by A2, then you might write 'Would like to know Anna B. better. Will arrange to meet her for lunch within the next two weeks.' Or perhaps you marked A6. Think of a way in which you can be self-assertive during the next three days. Perhaps something has been niggling for a long time, but you have been putting up with it. For instance, you are fed up with your partner reading the newspaper over dinner. Say so. Say you want to have a conversation, that you need to communicate. Share your feelings.

Keep your changes simple and readily achievable. Little successes will help you to build up your confidence. And keep practising. The more you do so, the more the new behaviours will become established.

Needs
Why is it that so many of us have enough to eat and drink, good jobs and a reasonable standard of living, yet underneath we have a deep yearning, an all-pervasive feeling of discontent? What is it that needs to be satisfied? The psychologist Abraham Maslow did some pioneer work in the 1940s and '50s by studying not sick people, but healthy ones – people he called 'self-actualized'. If he could set down what made them so happy and well, then perhaps the not-so-well could learn something from them. One result of his observations was a 'hierarchy of needs'. The theory behind this is that when one need is satisfied, a higher one emerges and asks to be fulfilled. The five main needs are shown below.

Maslow's hierarchy of needs

5 SELF-ACTUALIZATION
4 ESTEEM
3 LOVE AND BELONGING
2 SAFETY AND SECURITY
1 FOOD AND DRINK

Our most basic need is for food and drink to ensure our survival.

If we have insufficient our lives become dominated by our hunger and thirst, and all our energies will go into satisfying these cravings. We will think of little else.

When we have a steady supply of nourishment, however, we then seek security in a home where we will be safe from dangers. We will tend to avoid the unfamiliar and will concentrate our energies on nest-making and on creating order in our universe.

The next need to emerge is for love. Human beings are social creatures who enjoy both giving and receiving affection. We hunger for intimacy. We need to belong to a social group of some kind, our neighbourhood or clan. If our love needs are not met we suffer terrible pangs of loneliness, and the search for a mate or friends can become desperate. One problem with modern Western society is mobility. Too much moving around makes permanent relationships and belonging very difficult, and a feeling of alienation can quickly overtake us.

If our love needs are satisfied, the next need to present itself is for esteem. This includes respect for oneself as well as for others. We want to demonstrate our competence, our skills, and be appreciated for what we do in the world. Satisfaction of this need leads to increased self-confidence and feelings of self-worth. If it is not satisfied, helplessness and inferiority can dominate our lives.

Supposing that all four needs are met, we still have an inner craving for something more. Maslow calls this a need for self-actualization. He means by this, being true to our real selves, and not spending our whole lives living up to others' expectations or pretending to be the sort of person our parents wanted us to be. How many of us 'follow in father's/mother's footsteps' because that is what is expected of us, rather than being true to our real, inner selves? The relationships of self-actualized people are marked by a free-flowing spontaneity and an absence of fear; they are not afraid to let go, to express themselves fully and to experience both the heights and depths of being human. They are true individuals, original in their approach to people and events. To be self-actualized means fulfilling one's true potential in every way – to be fully one's real self, whoever that may be. Surprisingly few people ever discover who they really are and they fail to understand why they feel so unhappy and unfulfilled.

Lawrence LeShan gives a classic example of this in *You Can Fight For Your Life*. A client of his, called John, had developed severe headaches. He was thirty-five years old, a successful lawyer in his father's firm, lived in a splendid house with an attractive wife and had three beautiful children. What more could he possibly want? During therapy, it emerged that his father had put pressure on him to become a lawyer like himself, and his mother had decided which girl he should marry. Being a dutiful son and somewhat timid, he had done what was expected of him, despite the fact that he had shown outstanding talent as a musician during his adolescence. He once attempted to leave his wife to follow his own dreams, but, being unable to earn enough money as a musician to support his family, he was forced to return and continue with his former profession. Shortly afterwards he was diagnosed as having an inoperable brain tumour. The prospect of imminent death gave him the courage to explore his true self once again by returning to his music, and he eventually gained a position with a symphony orchestra. For the first time in his life he began to experience true fulfilment, and the effect on his health was dramatic. The tumour gradually diminished in size until he was in complete remission.

We have already seen that the brain can influence immunity via neurotransmitters, the chemical messengers. So it is not at all fanciful to believe that our mood can affect our state of health.

Maslow's hierarchy of needs can help us to see what might be missing in our lives. Most of us are fairly good at providing ourselves with nourishment and security. In fact, much of our time is spent doing this. But how rewarding are our relationships? If you are without a partner at present, it is very important to have at least one friend with whom you can share intimately, and freely pour out your thoughts and feelings, as well as listening to theirs. Cultivate friendships. Make time for them and you will feel nourished and enriched by your closeness.

Do you feel you belong somewhere? Or do you live on your own in a bedsitting room in a city, unattached to any social group? In several studies it has been shown that lonely and unhappy people are more susceptible to infections. On both the T- and B-cells there are receptors for the hormones nor-adrenalin and adrenalin, responsible for feelings of well-being and alertness. If the impulse to survive is lowered because of a depressed mood, the immune system is more sluggish about responding to alarm calls. If you live and work alone it is essential that you join a group of some kind. Perhaps a hobby will point you in the right direction, or maybe a social club or religious group will fulfil your need to belong.

Humans are sociable by nature and are nourished by tender loving care. Child development researchers have recently discovered the disturbing fact that children can become physically stunted in growth if there is a hostile atmosphere in the home. The child's emotional centre in the brain, the limbic system, receives the message that life is intolerable, and acts upon the hypothalamus which reduces the pituitary gland's supply of growth hormone. This is a prime example of how the human body responds to the state of emotions.

The fourth need, esteem, is also of vital importance. This of course includes gaining recognition and respect for achievements in the world, but we also need to feel good about ourselves deep inside – we need self-esteem, we need to love and respect ourselves. Do you truly love yourself? Many, many people find this a difficult sticking point. We have mostly been brought up not to be vain and conceited, not to be 'big-headed'. However, the truth is that it is possible to have a deep regard for oneself without resorting to arrogance or narcissism. If we think unwell of ourselves, how can we heal ourselves? People who feel unworthy of love often feel unworthy of glowing health also. How can you heal yourself and have alert immune defences if you are constantly criticising yourself and making yourself feel bad? Healing flows out of love. It took me a good two and a half years fully to accept and appreciate myself – yes (dare I say it?), even to love myself. The peace and contentment that ensues is deliciously warming – an inner glow, a radiance. What follows from this is a zest for life that surely keeps the immune defences vigilant. So how did I arrive at this delightful state? Truthfully, I could not have done this on my own. I had such a poor opinion of myself that only a very experienced and exceptionally caring guide could show me the route to self-understanding and self-love. I was lucky enough to find this special kind of person; there is more about this under 'Counselling and psychotherapy' later in the chapter. For readers who suffer from poor self-esteem, I can wholeheartedly recommend that you seek help in this way.

Meanwhile, there is something you can do to feel better about yourself right now by affirming your own worth.

Self-affirmations

By making positive statements about yourself in a variety of ways it is possible to counteract those negative messages you may have received in the past which have contributed to your feelings of worthlessness. Where did these come from? What impressions did you gain about yourself from the people around you during your early years? Make some notes. My life as a child was dominated by religion, and I have vivid memories of kneeling in church and saying such things as: 'I am not worthy so much as to gather up the crumbs under Thy table . . .'. Unfortunately, I believed all of it.

Here are some suggestions for self-affirmations, but it is even better to make up your own. First of all, sit comfortably in front of a mirror, preferably a full-length one. You need to be very relaxed, so follow the instructions under 'Deep muscular relaxation' in chapter 3, and do the exercise keeping your eyes closed. (Alternatively, do the 'Quick relaxation'.) Now think of a time when you felt truly loving. Recall the situation in every detail, who you were with, where you were, what had just happened and so on. Re-evoke the feelings of love in yourself now and experience the quality of it – its tenderness, its joy, its warmth, or whatever is true for you. Remember that the quality of love is timeless and that you can re-evoke it whenever you wish. As you open your eyes to see the image of yourself before you, stay in touch with your feelings of love. Look at your image as if you have never seen this person before, through the eyes of this loving person within you. Appreciate everything about yourself that you truly admire, including personal qualities as well as physical characteristics. Then make statements to yourself, preferably out loud, using your own name, for example:

'Susan, you are an intelligent human being, you are tender and loving and you have an unusual strength of character marked by perseverance and courage. You are tall and graceful, Susan, with glossy black hair and deep brown eyes. You have a sense of mystery about you, which is intriguing. You have artistic hands, capable of creating the most beautiful things. Your voice is soft and low. I care about you deeply, Susan. I will love you always.'

Make sure you end with a loving statement. Then close your eyes again and repeat the affirmations, saying 'I', for example: 'I am an intelligent human being. I am tender and loving . . .' and so on. If you feel embarrassed, just notice the feeling and allow it to be present. Then continue with the affirmations. Other feelings may suddenly come rushing to the surface, perhaps sadness. This may be to do with all the love you have yearned for, but have never received. This is a natural feeling, so, again, accept it and stay with it. Remember that you are now learning to love and care for yourself and that you have all the resources within you that you need.

Practise the above exercise with a friend, each making positive statements about the other while making eye contact. You will find this deeply affirming.

The next stage is to imagine your ideal self. How would you most like to be – more loving, perhaps, or serene rather than wound up, more successful, thinner, full of energy? Close your eyes, relax as before, and see your ideal self, including as many details as possible. For example, if you are ill, then see yourself in perfect radiant health, enjoying a favourite pastime such as cycling. Then speak in the present: 'I am glowing with health and vitality. My limbs feel strong as I pedal up the hill. My heart pumps with vigour and the blood races through my veins, filling my muscles with energy . . .' and so on. If you affirm how you would like to be often enough, your body is likely to follow suit. You will also develop more positive and optimistic feelings about yourself.

Some people have a lot of fun making up little rhymes and songs about themselves: 'I am happy and alive, On my diet I will thrive . . .' They don't have to be inspired poetic works! Sing them aloud when driving the car or washing up.

In your notebook write down a list of all your accomplishments and talents. Include achievements at work, in your leisure time, at home, however small or large they may be. Go back to your childhood and remember everything you did well at that time, and all your successes since. Reminding yourself of your abilities in this way will give you added impetus to achieve more.

Another list can include everything that you have, or have had, that you can be thankful for. So often we take things for granted and forget how rich our lives are. Such reminders can help to keep our thinking positive.

Spend time with people who appreciate you and whose company you really enjoy. You will feel affirmed by them and will experience a boost of energy. Conversely, avoid the moaners and those who make you feel bad. There are far more constructive ways of passing the time than playing negative psychological games such as 'Ain't it awful . . .?'

Counselling and psychotherapy
At the end of my first session with the doctor at the Cancer Help Centre, he had talked about completing the mourning process over my brother's death, to achieve inner healing. Many people carry around with them a great burden of pain and guilt from the past. One thing that psychotherapy can help you to do is to let go of this burden, so that your energy is available for more healthy and creative purposes. I took the doctor's advice and presented my feelings concerning my brother to Christoph, my counsellor at the Centre. As we worked around the issue, I began to understand that Nigel's death was more bound up with my illness than I could possibly have imagined.

'After he died', I said, 'I felt I wanted to live his life for him – even to take up rock climbing and learn about medicine. It seems crazy now, but I remember how strong this feeling was. I wanted him to live on through me. I also felt that I hadn't just lost him, I'd actually lost half of myself.'

'It sounds as if you made an inner promise to live his life for him. This is really important', said Christoph. 'So you live out the "masculine" part of yourself for him; you've become a successful career woman, for him. And you've denied your own womanhood.' I stared at the floor, trying to keep control of myself. 'What would happen if you were to let go of him – to bury him?'

I felt a searing pain across my heart. 'I would be totally alone', I whispered.

'You may have to be alone, before taking on your womanhood. You may have to risk losing yourself also,' he said gently. I knew he was right, that I must let my brother be, let him rest in peace, so that I could fully own myself as a woman.

The issue of my womanhood had come up in my previous session. Somehow I had a vague notion that my cancer was partly the result of unresolved feelings about myself as a woman. During my adolescence I felt very uneasy in my ripening body, and had never wholly recovered from that. The breast clearly defines a person as female, more than anything else. Bernie Siegel, an American surgeon, suggests in his book *Love, Medicine and Miracles* that people develop 'target organs' during their lives, which become sensitised and therefore more vulnerable to illness.

Christoph proved to be an ideal person to discuss the feminine with, despite the fact that he was a man. His own recovery from cancer had also included the search for the feminine principle within himself, the caring, intuitive, expressive parts which had long been repressed. He had had a tumour near his spine, which had resulted in temporary paralysis from the waist down, yet to look at him now – alert brown eyes, tall, energetic frame – no one would know that he had been so ill. Radiotherapy had burnt out part of his left lung, so he had taken singing lessons to improve its capacity – such is the power of the human spirit. He was a real inspiration to all of us at the Cancer Centre.

I explained that my late marriage had provided a last-minute opportunity for motherhood. In my twenties I had stood on the sidelines, watching my friends marry and produce children, yet all the while knowing I was different. That wasn't for me. Inside, I felt a total failure as a woman. How could any man want me to be his wife? As the second daughter, I had been subtly encouraged to be a tomboy, especially by my mother, who had 'expected' me to be her son. My tree-climbing and other outdoor escapades generally received approval. But no encouragement was given to the growing woman inside me and I regarded childbirth with dread and terror. Being born female seemed like the worst fate that could have befallen me. Each month was beset by severe dysmenorrhoea, which sometimes left me rolling on the floor in agony. I instinctively felt that this had something to do with the conflict within me, but doctors seemed ill-equipped to help me. It was only in my late thirties, after a stint of group therapy, that I finally got in touch with tender feelings inside myself that I never knew were there. Suddenly the idea of having my own baby seemed enormously exciting. Then I found myself with cancer.

I recalled my first meeting with the oncologist. It was only a week after my operation, which luckily had not been too drastic, but I had a large 'pressure' dressing across my chest which prevented me from lifting my arms. I felt awkward. She fluttered into the consulting booth in high-heeled sandals and bright floral sundress, and perched elegantly on the couch. She joked about my distorted shape caused by the dressing, but soon started to explain that because of my relative youth there was a slightly higher risk of the cancer recurring. Putting her hand on my arm, she then said that I should have my ovaries irradiated to improve my prognosis. A chill swept over me as the meaning of this sank in. I stared at her red varnished nails and the huge diamond that glittered on her finger. Her gaudy outfit seemed strangely inappropriate. She chattered on, explaining that the resulting drop in oestrogen would be beneficial, that post-menopausal women do better than those who are younger.

'You mean, you would bring on the menopause artificially?' I asked, appalled.

'Yes.'

The tears started to rise in my throat.

'We haven't been married long. We were hoping for a child', I stammered.

'That is quite out of the question', she assured me. 'The change in hormone levels would reactivate the cancer. It would mean giving up your own life for a new one.'

Having just got in touch with my womanhood, it was now being snatched away from me. How could fate be so cruel?

Christoph had been listening carefully to this tale of woe. He asked me if there was any other way in which I could express myself as a woman, but there seemed to be no answer.

'Do you have an image of an ideal woman?' he queried. I looked blank. I had no models to emulate. My mother, a university gradu-ate, had always seemed resentful about her role as housewife. There was a pause. Then he said, 'How do you feel about me?' I was astonished.

'Do you mean personally?'

He nodded. I gulped.

'Make eye contact with me', he invited. This was difficult. His eyes bored into my soul, soft as they were. I wasn't used to such a penetrating gaze – in fact I wasn't used to anyone really looking at me at all. I felt exposed, ashamed of what he might see. I plucked up courage and took him in. Bearded. Tousled brown hair going grey. Despite his relaxed posture I found him a charismatic person. He was probably only a few years older than myself, but I felt slightly in awe of him. He was rather grand, with expansive gestures and a beautiful voice, but with diction that was almost too perfect.

'I like you and I trust you – as a therapist, I mean', I said. This seemed safe enough. He waited, holding my gaze. Clearly, there could be no concealment from this man.

Slowly I added, 'I'm afraid of you.'

'What of?' he inquired, as if he already knew the answer.

'Of your sexuality', I faltered, feeling slightly foolish. As I said this, I realised that I found him attractive. He had a frame to match his personality – large – with long limbs and expressive hands.

'Will you own that for yourself and say you are afraid of your own sexuality?'

The truth of the statement flashed through my mind as I pronounced it: 'Yes, I'm afraid of my own sexuality.'

'In what way?'

'I'm afraid of the power of my own passion.'

'Suppose you let it out, what's the worst thing that could happen?'

'Of going over the top, being out of control. The truth is, I have done that in the past.'

'Were you promiscuous?'

'Not exactly, but I had a number of lovers – not all at once!' I added hastily.

The scrutiny intensified and I sank more deeply into the armchair, heartily wishing it might swallow me up altogether, to spare me the discomfort of being so glaringly revealed.

'I see in front of me a very beautiful woman with a lovely figure. What do you make of that?'

I half looked round, expecting to see this beautiful woman he was describing somewhere behind me. No. He really meant me.

'Disconnected. I feel disconnected from my own body, as if it didn't belong to me. I don't think of myself as a woman. Mostly, I feel like a little girl still waiting to grow up.'

'As I look at this beautiful woman in front of me', he continued, 'I don't sense any feeling in her.'

'That's it!' I exclaimed. 'I'm in my head all the time. I've grown accustomed to using my intellect and nothing else. That's where I feel safe.' As I said these words, I realised how terrified I was to reveal myself truly as a woman, to own my femininity.

'When I was recovering from cancer', said Christoph, 'I discovered that my own sexuality could be used as a powerful healing force. The point is, it's a natural source of energy and we have a choice about how to use it. But first we need to own it, rather than repress it. You could use it for playing your cello – an instrument that vibrates between your legs!' I laughed. 'It's good to see you laugh. Or you can save it for your husband. It's entirely up to you.'

My burden of fear and guilt began to feel considerably lighter as he pronounced these words of wisdom. How truly human this man was! The notion of sexual energy as a force for good sent a warm wave of relief flowing through me and my skin started to tingle. Suddenly I realised how many different meanings can be attached to ideas, but we don't have to hold on to the old ones after they've outlived their usefulness. No, of course not! We can scrap them and take on new ones.

He looked at me warmly. 'A new woman is about to be born!' he uttered. I felt deeply touched. This was only my second session and this amazing man had put his finger right on the key issue. I remembered how I had fought the hospital authorities and finally refused to have my ovaries irradiated. I was glad. I needed my womanhood intact. I felt a rush of elation as a fresh vision of myself appeared before me.

We talked again about my brother, the youngest in the family. His birth gave me psychological permission to be female, as he could now take on the masculine role. But since his death it seemed that I had shifted back into the original position, not allowing myself to acknowledge my own femininity. Christoph suggested, as a piece of 'homework', that I write a fairy story about my family, with kings, queens, princesses, wizards and witches. It sounded fun and I promised to do it. 'Portraying the members of your family symbolically will help you to stand back, to disidentify from them and see them more objectively.' I could appreciate the point of this. At the end of the session he wrapped his long arms around me and gave me a delicious, all-embracing hug. How did he dare to be so open and loving? 'You're trembling,' he said. I was.

It took me several weeks to complete the story, which I entitled 'Princess Angelina's Journey'. I was astonished at how it suddenly became possible to tap my unconscious mind for creative images, which seemed to flow out of me. It was exciting. I had never experienced this before, never believed I could produce such imaginative work. I was allowing my subconscious mind to speak to me. In my story the princess goes in search of her brother, Prince Leopold, who disappeared after having a curse cast upon him for killing a great monster in the mountains. This creature had been threatening the safety of Angelina and her sister. After many adventures involving crystal palaces, a band of strolling players and a magic carpet, she finally arrives in a distant country. There she finds a note from Leopold hidden in a bell-flower tree. He says he is in a place where he always wanted to be, so there is no need to grieve.

Working through my own story symbolically like this spoke strongly to my subconscious, and I was able to achieve a real healing through it in relation to my brother. I was more able to accept that his life had ended and now I should continue with my own journey – a very different one from his. In our culture symbolism, myth and ritual have all but vanished, and with these have gone a creative and healthy means of releasing emotion.

After the session described above, I felt as if doors and windows had suddenly been opened on to my soul. Fresh air was blowing in. At last I was truly perceived, perhaps for the first time ever. Although it was uncomfortable and even painful at times, I had to go on. I had to know, to understand. Now, after two and a half years of therapy, my feelings towards myself have totally changed. Being a woman is now simply wonderful! There is no longer any need to feel inadequate or second-rate; on the contrary, my inner strength lies in expressing my warm, feminine qualities. And, incidentally, my dysmenorrhoea has disappeared. So how did this happen?

Counsellors are trained to offer their clients 'unconditional positive regard'. Whatever the client may bring to the session, the counsellor will not pass judgment, but will accept the person fully. Thus it becomes possible for the client not only to divulge the darkest of secrets, but also to acknowledge and accept this 'shadow' side of the personality, as Jung called it. The relief at being able to talk about submerged aspects of oneself is enormous. As we have seen, long-term repression can lead to illness; conversely, consciously to recognise the things we dislike or find difficult about ourselves reduces inner conflict and restores balance within the personality.

In life, not only do we push down strong emotions, we feel embarrassed if others display them. When friends or relatives are upset, our culture teaches us to dry their tears and cheer them up. In therapy the reverse happens; free expression of emotion is encouraged. The counsellor enters the client's world fully and stands alongside the person whatever s/he may be experiencing. After my session described above, I began to realise how much I had lost touch with my feelings. With time I learnt to be open to them, to welcome them. I also learnt to listen to my intuition and to hear what my body had to tell me. These are all important sources of information.

As trust is built up between the client and therapist, so the relationship deepens and intimacy develops. Most people have never been loved unconditionally. We all long for it, but rarely receive it – and indeed rarely offer it. Our parents generally give us only conditional love; they will approve of us if we are quiet children and behave ourselves, if we do well in exams at school, and so on. By experiencing unconditional love in a therapeutic setting, the client feels worthy to be loved and therefore begins to have a better opinion of him- or herself. The realisation eventually dawns that s/he has free choice about who to be. There is no longer any need to behave in a way that seeks parental approval.

Love is a great healer. Two Harvard psychologists, David McClelland and Carol Kirshnit, conducted an experiment in 1982. They tested the saliva of people who watched movies about love, and discovered that the levels of their immunoglobulin-A (specialised antibodies) increased significantly for up to an hour after each film was finished. The effect was extended if the subjects recalled times when they had received tender loving care from someone. A documentary on the work of Mother Teresa produced a similar effect. It is worth asking yourself, therefore, 'How loving am I? How open am I to receiving love?'

Many people have never, or rarely, experienced a deeply intimate relationship. Discovering how nourishing and rewarding this is can be a real revelation. The client can then be encouraged to take this rich experience into the outside world, where personal relationships take on a new meaning.

Careful listening and questioning draw the client out and open channels for flashes of insight about past behaviour. The developing relationship can also be examined. Is the client coy, domineering, manipulative, open, withdrawn – or what? Still no judgment is passed, but the question may be put: 'Is this a rewarding way for you to be?' or 'Do you want to carry on in this manner?' The next step for the client is consciously to choose to change. The therapeutic setting provides a safe place in which to test out new ways of being. For instance, I have always had problems with self-assertion. One week I was annoyed with my counsellor for not starting on time and keeping me waiting. As always, I pretended it didn't matter. But it did matter. I missed my usual train home and was very late. It took me three weeks to state my irritation about this and some other minor grumbles. It was important to practise sticking up for myself.

A good therapist holds in mind an image of the client's potential, so that s/he always has something higher to aim for. Little by little, the distorted ideas that the person carries begin to change until they concur with the image held by the therapist. Somehow from that scrapheap of misery that presented itself to him two and a half years previously, Christoph managed to envisage me as a ravishingly beautiful woman. With time, the ideas I held about myself began to improve.

Sometimes we project on to other people characteristics that we refuse to acknowledge in ourselves. Rather than owning my own sexuality and being in charge of it, I was projecting my fear of it on to men. Thus, they could be to blame for this dark secret within me, while I could remain pure and innocent! In such ways do we attempt to defend our egos, and in such ways do we become alienated from our true selves. Acceptance of everything that lies within is essential if we are to become whole, healthy people.

You may wonder what the difference is between counselling and psychotherapy. Counselling can be quite short-term and will probably deal with specific issues. Psychotherapy probes much more deeply into the psyche and explores all aspects of the personality over a period of time. Equally, a therapist's training is much more thorough than a counsellor's and very often lasts for five years or longer. It always involves an honest exploration and understanding of one's own self, for without this it is impossible fully to comprehend and accept others.

The effect of counselling on the immune system was recently put to the test at UCLA in America. Dr Fawzey, a psychiatrist, together with Norman Cousins (author of *Anatomy of an Illness*), divided malignant melanoma patients into two groups: one was formed into a support group and received therapy each week; the other was just used as a control. Members of the support group were able to discuss and resolve personal conflicts and problems, which resulted in lower anxiety levels and improved lifestyle, and after six months despair and helplessness had significantly diminished. Blood samples were taken at intervals and these showed an increase in the number of cancer-fighting immune cells as confidence improved. The control group, on the other hand, who had received no therapy, showed no such increase. Clearly, emotional support helps our bodies to fight illness.

Moving out of victim

The helpless and hopeless characters who often succumb to cancer see themselves as victims. Of course it is far easier to blame outside circumstances or other people for one's lot, rather than be responsible for oneself and begin to make changes. True victims will always manage to end up feeling bad whatever they do. Generally, people have no idea that it is possible to behave differently. All they are aware of is their misery. So how do you know if you are stuck in this victim position? There are some useful guidelines. For instance, if others make helpful suggestions and you find yourself repeatedly making excuses and saying 'I can't because . . .', then you could well be 'in victim'. Other pointers are phrases such as: 'Poor me, I'm always the one who . . .', or 'If it weren't for him, I could . . .', or 'You've made me feel bad about . . .'.

Usually the pattern has been a life-long one, learnt in early childhood. There is of course a difference between a genuine victim and someone who takes this position in a distorted way. For example, if a woman is refused employment on account of race or gender, then she is a genuine victim. If, however, she is refused a job because her qualifications are not suitable and she then goes round complaining to everyone that she didn't get the job because she wasn't a man, then she is putting herself in a distorted victim position. This is a truly unhappy and unhealthy place to be; nothing ever seems right and the person feels hopeless, unable to act, to make any decisions or improvements. I know. I was in it for years!

I also know how hard it is to chuck this habit and you may need skilled help. There are so many benefits of staying in victim. It is safe and known. Other people's reactions are predictable. You also gain a lot of attention (in a negative way). Friends are endlessly trying to haul you out of your stuck and helpless position by making useful suggestions: 'Why don't you . . .?' and you counter with 'Yes, but . . .' or 'I can't because . . .'. Paradoxically, you are now the one with the power! People have been rushing round trying to help you, but by refusing their help you are in fact the 'winner'. Just imagine how the others feel – put down, ineffective; however good their suggestions are, you never take them on board! Sadly, they are likely to become fed up with you and you may lose their friendship. Now you can reinforce your victim position with 'Poor me, I'm all alone.' And so it goes on.

How is it possible to move out of this unrewarding role? First of all, try replacing 'I can't because . . .' with 'I need help . . .'.

You have spent most of your life refusing help. Try asking for it instead. This will be difficult at first, but keep practising and it will gradually become easier. Then when help or suggestions are offered, show your gratitude and appreciation. You will instinctively find yourself wanting to give a list of reasons why it isn't possible to do as suggested, but resist this. Listen carefully and say, 'That is a really good idea. Next time, I'll do that' (or whatever is appropriate). The other person now feels useful and appreciated, and you will feel better because of this little gift of gratitude you have offered. If you are ill, then you really do need help – lots of it. The truth is that other people enjoy being useful, so take advantage of this and allow yourself to be cosseted. You are now gaining attention in a straightforward rather than a distorted way. You may worry that you will lose your independence by asking for help, but this is not the case; you can always return to your independent mode whenever you wish.

Victims always feel as if they have no choice, no free will. But the truth is, you do have a choice. The problem is that it takes courage to exercise free will; it means being totally responsible for yourself, standing on your own feet and taking the consequences for your own decisions. Victims manage to evade responsibility, and that of course is the main reason why they stay where they are.

Affirmations will help you to shift out of your stuck place. Tell yourself often that you are strong and courageous, and that you are able to exercise your will. Set yourself goals and work towards them gradually, starting with small, easily achievable ones. There is more advice about this a few pages further on. You will begin to feel much better about yourself as you take your life into your own hands. Remember, each time you make a choice, however small it may be, you are out of the victim position, so congratulate yourself and appreciate yourself for your good progress.

Another way to help yourself is to ask, 'What am I avoiding by staying in victim?' Yes, you are avoiding responsibility, but you may also be evading close human contact and warmth. Victim behaviour tends to keep people at arm's length. At one time you may have had a good reason for this. People who acknowledge that they need love also acknowledge their vulnerability, because they run the risk of rebuff or refusal. So perhaps your victim position is a roundabout way of protecting yourself from being hurt. It is true that some people may not be very good at providing love; others, however, are very generous with it. Learn to discriminate between loving and unloving people, and make sure you ask for warmth from those who enjoy providing it. Otherwise you may find yourself saying, 'Poor me, no one loves me.'

The more you are loving towards others, the more love you will receive. So think of ways in which you can be genuinely caring and make a list in your notebook. Include only the things that you will find fun or rewarding to do. Get in touch with all the warmth and joy inside you and start to put it out into the world. Affirmations will help you here also. You will be surprised how you will start to shift out of victim.

Don't be disappointed if you find yourself repeatedly sliding back, just when you thought you were making real progress. This is bound to happen. It takes a great deal of perseverance to break a life-time's behaviour pattern. After years of persistent effort, I finally managed to ditch my victim, and felt ecstatically happy and proud of myself. I can now recognise all the sure signs and nip them in the bud. For example, I had arranged to go to a concert with a friend the other evening. I was really looking forward to it. At the last minute, her cat was ill and she decided to opt out. No one else was free to go at such short notice. I nearly cancelled the event, but instead of saying, 'Poor me, no one wants to go to the concert with me', I told myself I was going to have a wonderful evening all by myself! So I bought the most expensive ticket for the front row. I arrived early and sat down. For a few minutes I began to feel nervous about all the empty places around me. 'What if no one comes to sit next to me?' I thought. 'Everyone in the hall will be able to see that I am all on my own.' I began to feel panic-stricken and thoroughly sorry for myself. Then I realised I was playing my old victim trick again, so I switched my thoughts to my beautiful surroundings. Just as I was appreciating the glorious flower arrangement in front of me, an interesting-looking man sat down next to me. I smiled and soon we were in the midst of a fascinating conversation. He had been to college with one of my heroes – a famous concert pianist – and was a well-known musicologist himself! We discussed the performance avidly in the interval, with whispered comments in between pieces. Afterwards he shook my hand warmly, saying how much he had enjoyed meeting me. He then went off to talk to my hero who was sitting anonymously in the back row. What a fabulous evening I had

had! I sang to myself loudly as I drove home. Life is much more fun now I am no longer a victim.

Giving up martyrdom

Martyrs are also unable to receive help, because they spend their lives 'sacrificing' themselves. Unfortunately, many of us have been brought up to believe that selflessness is 'good for the soul', but the truth is that it is good for neither the body nor the soul. As we have seen, self-respect is essential for well-being and health. If we don't care for ourselves, how can we genuinely care for others? Long-suffering martyrs are encouraged by the Christian tradition with the promise that their rewards are in heaven. The reality is that they can be a real pain to live with. There is little joy in their lives. They consistently reject both fun and love, because they are too busy working hard and sacrificing themselves. Their psychological suffering is also likely to appear as physical symptoms. They now have the opportunity to reinforce their martyrdom: despite their aching limbs, they will still be scrubbing the floor at eleven in the evening and saying in effect, 'Look what I do for you.'

Like the victim, they are avoiding true intimacy and warmth. So, similarly, one remedy is to start asking for help and learning to enjoy receiving it. You deserve to be cared for! A new problem now emerges. The martyr will find that there is extra time to fill and may feel at a loose end. Make a list of all the things you have always wanted to do but have never allowed yourself time for. Consciously start to bring these things into your life. Remember, you will be a much nicer person to know if you feel happy and fulfilled. So give yourself permission to have some fun. Decide how you can enjoy yourself at least once every other day and stick to it.

Martyrs may consciously restrict themselves from real achievement. Their energies are usually totally absorbed by unrewarding routine tasks. Many housewives find themselves in this role. Being out there in the big wide world is a scary prospect and martyrdom is a useful way of protecting themselves. They may say, 'I gave up a successful career for you' and hold a lot of inner resentment, blaming their lack of achievement on their spouse. As we have seen, long-held bitterness of this kind can lead to disease. If you find yourself in this position, acknowledge your fear. It is natural to feel afraid of the unknown. Make a list of some little responsibilities you can take on in the outside world – a contribution you would genuinely like to make. Consider your aptitudes and talents. Perhaps you can offer to run an evening class or maybe you would like to be a school governor. Meanwhile, give those tedious tasks at home to other members of the family, or hire a home help for a few hours. Remember, other people like to help. Don't worry if they can't do them as well or as quickly as you. It doesn't matter. What really counts is that you are making an inner shift towards finding life truly rewarding. As a result, you will be far healthier and happier, and so will everyone around you.

Your Wise Being

Inside each of us there is a source of wisdom that we can call upon. Part of our unconscious mind knows absolutely everything about us, who we are, where we have been and where we are going. All of those feelings, thoughts and memories that we have banished from consciousness are hidden within us and hold the truth about us. This source of truth can now be used to our advantage. It has our very best interests at heart and is able to give us guidance.

You can contact your Wise Being through meditation. It may not appear as a person; it may be a star, an angel or a dove, for example. Mine is a wise old blackbird who hops on to my shoulder and chatters into my ear. Your questions may not be answered in words. Sometimes an image will appear that will hold some special meaning for you. So, whenever you have an important decision to make, or if you are facing a crisis, need to understand yourself or others better, or are just feeling lonely, find a quiet place, sit comfortably and relax your body completely (see 'Quick relaxation' in chapter 3). Take three deep, slow breaths, then meditate on the word 'peace' (see 'Meditation', also in chapter 3). Think only of this for about five minutes, or until you feel totally relaxed and calm. Now visualise a lighted candle. See the flame flicker and sway until it becomes still. As you look into the flame, your Wise Being emerges from it. You know that this Being truly loves you and wants only the very best for you. Now ask it whatever you need to know and see what happens. Allow as much time as necessary, then thank it and say goodbye.

Remember that your Wise Being loves you. If a critical or authoritarian figure appears, this is a projection of your superego and does not represent the source of your inner wisdom.

Knowing that we have all we need to make the right choices for ourselves gives us a real sense of inner strength, even when faced with a seemingly intolerable crisis. It is a sure way of pulling us out of feelings of helplessness and hopelessness, and in turn contributes to our future well-being.

Setting goals

While recovering from cancer, I tried to work out whether there were any psychological 'advantages' in being ill. If so, how could I meet these needs without resorting to disease? What healthy goals could I then set myself? I came up with quite a list.

First of all, I noticed how much attention I was receiving. Suddenly, sympathy and understanding were poured out in my direction from friends and relatives. Then there was professional care from doctors and nurses, and loving support from my counsellor and therapy group. The shock of my illness seemed to have nudged the lid off my cauldron of feelings, and the contents were spilling themselves out. I was no longer the reserved, quiet person of my pre-cancer days. Most important of all, I was feeling nourished and enriched by so much sharing. So one new goal was to make sure that this quality of exchange, this loving closeness with people, should become a permanent feature of my life.

Next, I had been under appalling stress for far too long. There was no way that I could continue to carry such a workload and stay alive. The illness had given me an excuse to take two months off work and I began to realise how quickly my health began to improve once the pressure was off me. The goal that followed from this, therefore, was to find a way of working part-time only. I was eventually able to do this by selling my Finchley house and investing half the proceeds. I also learnt to ask for help and not to take so much on. This sometimes involved saying 'no', which I found very difficult. But knowing that I might die if I again put myself under so much stress gave me the courage.

My third goal followed from the second: to have more time and space for myself. For years I had done virtually nothing but work, and what had it all added up to? Very little. I had suffered some kind of spiritual death and now felt an urge to search for wisdom and truth. This meant looking inside myself, finding a way of growing as a person and of expressing who I really am. It also eventually led to the study of psychology and psychotherapy, the most rewarding things I have ever done.

Part of the work stress consisted of a dreary boredom, which meant that I was constantly forcing myself to do something that my heart was never in. In fact I never realised how much I disliked my work until cancer forced me to re-evaluate it. A new goal, therefore, was to move into a more creative sphere, initially to switch from editing to writing. After finding myself a literary agent, who was both encouraging and businesslike, I was gradually able to achieve this.

Taking time off work gave me the opportunity to play my cello again. How much I had missed the joy of artistic interpretation and expression! Yet another goal was to organise chamber music sessions with my friends, to go on musical holidays and also to find myself an inspiring teacher.

Recuperation gave me a wonderful excuse to be in the country where the air was fresh. How free and happy I felt there! I was determined that one day I would live in a place that was peaceful and beautiful. Eventually I was able to do just that. Hopefully, I will never need to suffer from serious disease again.

If you are, or have been, ill, then examine what you 'gained', and set goals that will fulfil your deepest needs. Readers who have not been ill can do the same exercise by imagining how they would benefit if they were to become unwell. Additionally, look back at the section covering 'Needs', earlier in this chapter, and work out what is missing from your life. Find ways of filling these gaps.

The overall aim should be balance within your personality. Do you remember the opening exercise that involved being aware of your body, your feelings and your mind? Make sure that your goals satisfy each part of yourself in a harmonious way.

Anyone who has goals to aim for has positive expectations about life. When we look to the future with hope, then we send an 'I want to live' message to our bodies. We are also taking a self-assertive stance and moving out of the helpless victim position. There are many stories of terminal cancer patients who have far outlived their prognoses simply because they had something special to look forward to: a daughter's marriage, a journey to make, or a book to write. Ask yourself what you truly want to do before you die. Have you left anything unfinished that is really important to you? How can you make your life complete and meaningful? Setting goals for yourself will give you a sense of direction. Remember that it is not so much the achievement of goals that is the main thing, but rather the process of working towards them. So, however long or short your life may be, this is something well worth doing.

Self-assertiveness

Assertiveness is not the same as aggression. It means calmly and firmly sticking up for yourself at the appropriate moments, without resorting to rage or violence. The problem with non-assertive, 'helpless' people is that they do not express their needs or their point of view, but allow others to take advantage of them. This leads to a build-up of inner resentment, which, as we have seen, can be extremely damaging to health. By asserting ourselves we are practising positive, coping behaviour that dispels anxiety as well as anger and therefore allows immunity to function normally.

Many of us were brought up on a diet of self-effacing politeness and were never taught how to assert ourselves effectively. Happily, this is something that can be learned later in life and it improves with practice. If you find that your wishes are never taken seriously and you are being repeatedly walked over, then take yourself to an assertiveness training course. Meanwhile, use every opportunity that life presents to practise being firm and positive, and make sure you are listened to. For example, you may be standing in a check-out queue, and a man pushes in front of you. Don't let him get away with it. Point out that you were there first and ask him to move behind you. There is no need to be aggressive; you can say this in a friendly way. Or maybe your boss has a habit of criticising you unjustly. Next time stick up for yourself and make sure s/he understands that s/he has made an error of judgment. A friend may ask you to do something you really do not wish to do. Say so in a tactful way. If you go ahead and do it, you will only feel resentful about it. Real, lasting friendships are based on openness and honesty. Saying 'no' is particularly important for cancer patients, since we have a life-time's habit of pleasing others. It also reduces stress, by cutting down the burden of endless, sometimes unnecessary tasks.

If you are inexperienced at getting you own way, assertiveness will seem very difficult at first. However, knowing that it is good for your health will spur you on. You may also experience some pleasant surprises. A few weeks ago I ate a meal at a so-called healthfood restaurant and suffered severe food poisoning, with stomach cramps and sickness half the night. When next in the area, I called in, asked for the manager and told him in a matter-of-fact way what had occurred, stressing that I was sure he would not wish the reputation of his restaurant to suffer. As a result, I was offered thanks, humble apologies and a free meal, freshly cooked. It is in the interests of business people to keep their clients happy, so there is no need to feel apologetic about making justifiable complaints.

The way in which you hold yourself and the tone of your voice are just as important as the words you say. Stand upright in an open way, arms preferably not crossed in front of you but by your sides, and speak pleasantly but firmly. You will be amazed at how much better you feel once people are really taking notice of you and respecting your wishes.

Dealing with anger and resentment

Have you ever been to a fair and paid your 50p to smash crockery? Most cultures have invented safe, ritualised ways of getting rid of surplus aggression. Sport is an obvious example. A good hard game of squash can be very cathartic, or even energetic digging in the garden will release pent-up tension.

How do you know if you have repressed anger? If you find yourself over-reacting to a relatively harmless situation, the chances are that you have been storing up rage. We often see examples of this in the street. For instance, a driver may be a little slow about pulling away when the traffic lights change to green. This then becomes an excuse for vigorous horn-blowing and even verbal insults which are far more abusive than the situation calls for.

It really is important to get the anger out of your body physically so that it doesn't build up and fester inside you, eventually causing a life-threatening illness. Instead of tearing yourself to bits inside, tear a newspaper into little pieces. As you tear, say aloud the words you would most like to say to whoever provoked your anger. Alternatively, wring a towel. Twist the towel so that you can spare your own insides from being twisted into knots. Cushion bashing has already been mentioned. Pile them up on the floor, kneel beside them and beat them vigorously with your fists. Choose a time when everyone is out of the house so that you can have a good yell too. You will feel much better for it. Another powerful means of venting your fury safely is to write a letter to the person you hate, putting everything in it that you most detest about him or her. You do not, of course, post it, but the very act of expressing your rage on paper reduces the intensity of the feeling inside you.

All these techniques act as safety valves, allowing pent-up anger to be released in a harmless way. You then feel cool enough to be self-assertive and deal with your persecutor tactfully but firmly.

This is far more effective than shrieking at someone in an irrational manner.

There is no need to feel guilty about your anger. We all have it. Think of it as a force, as a stream of energy that, if well directed, can be extremely productive. Remember Florence Nightingale who, when asked why she was doing such difficult work, replied simply, 'Rage.'

Forgiveness

I alway imagined that this was to do with feeling smug and virtuous and getting sore knees in church. I now realise that, in essence, it has nothing at all to do with religion, but is simply a way of letting go of inner hurt. To carry hatred and bitterness around with us is very, very bad for the health. If you lust after revenge, then remember that this emotion is eating you up inside. If you let it go, then you will be doing yourself a favour; you will be healing yourself.

This letting go often involves sadness – a mourning of some kind – together with fully being open to what it was that you needed from this person, but never obtained. Having realised your need, find another way of meeting it, because it is extremely unlikely that the person you resent will ever be able to fulfil this for you. When you have completed this process you may discover that the resentment has dissolved, that you now accept the person for who s/he is, and that there is no longer anything to forgive.

For example, at one of the firms where I worked, a woman who had been there for a very long time was promoted to director of my division. At first I respected her for her efficiency and we got along quite well. After a while, however, she began to veto my best ideas. These projects were put together with great care, but she always managed to pick holes in them. At first I thought it was simply because she was lacking in flair and vision, but the situation deteriorated after she began to compare my work unfavourably with a colleague's. I began to doubt my worth. Perhaps I really was no good. I slid into a combination of depression and rage. Then someone said, to my astonishment, 'Perhaps she feels threatened by you.' Could that be the reason? I remembered a meeting some months previously when she had made a financial forecast which had seemed to me to be totally unrealistic. I had asked some very probing questions. Perhaps she had taken that as implied criticism. Whatever the reason, her treatment of me seemed totally unfair and resentment began to build. I tried to tackle her about it, but she had a brilliant way of diminishing me and I was no match for her. Two options remained: either I could stick it out and hope that one day she would be given the push, or else I could hand in my notice. In the end, the situation became unbearable and I took the latter course of action, knowing that she had won.

It was years before the time came when forgiveness was possible. There had been much to mourn: in addition to loss of my job and the security that went with it, there was loss of self-esteem, loss of the companionship of my colleagues, loss of the dream of being a success at that firm. Gradually I was able to open to what I had needed from her – appreciation, encouragement and support. Happily, my current situation was satisfying all three needs and I felt much valued by the people around me. It was no longer necessary to hold on to my hatred for her, and finally I was able fully to see her with all her limitations, to realise that she could never have given me what I needed, and at last I was able to let her go.

Joy and laughter

Norman Cousins, editor of an American medical journal, lay dangerously ill in hospital. He was suffering from an incurable illness, a disease of the connective tissue, and was in chronic pain in every part of his body. The large doses of aspirin administered had caused irritating rashes to appear everywhere. He had worked out that his illness had probably been triggered by adrenal exhaustion, caused by stress, frustration and suppressed rage. Clearly his endocrine system (consisting of the ductless glands that secrete hormones into the bloodstream) had become disrupted. If negative emotions could affect his body in this way, what effect could positive emotions have? Perhaps, he reasoned, love, hope, faith, confidence and laughter could help restore his endocrine system to balanced functioning, which in turn would help fight his disease. That left the problem of inflammation, which the aspirin had controlled. Perhaps huge doses of ascorbic acid would relieve this. He had nothing to lose, so, enlisting the help of his friendly doctor, they planned their campaign. Cousins already had faith and love, but what about laughter? There is nothing remotely funny about lying on your back in agony with a death sentence hanging over you. So he managed to borrow some amusing 'Candid Camera' films and a projector. He then made the amazing discovery that ten minutes of real belly laughter gave him two glorious hours of pain-free sleep. In addition, the nurse read him extracts from humorous books. His blood was tested after each episode of laughter, showing that there was a slight reduction in inflammation. After eight days of this treatment there was noticeable improvement, and eventually Cousins completely recovered. He became known as the man who laughed his way back to health.

It has recently been discovered that laughter releases hormones in the brain called endorphins. These are opiate-like substances which actively relieve pain and inhibit the emotional response to it, thus helping to relieve suffering also. Even more fascinating is the realisation that cells of the immune system have minute receptors for hormones. Dr Nicholas D. Plotnikoff of the University of Illinois has found that if the level of enkephalins (similar to endorphins) is altered in cancer and Aids patients, then their immune responses are simultaneously enhanced or decreased. The therapeutic effects of natural opioids, and thus of laughter, are therefore well proven.

If your medical condition prevents you from taking normal physical exercise, then there is no better way of compensating than by having a good belly laugh, for it provides a kind of 'internal jogging'. Your vital organs, including your lungs and heart, also the pancreas, liver, spleen, stomach and intestines are all stimulated by the action of laughing, which in turn heightens your resistance to illness. Dr William Fry, Jr, of the Department of Psychiatry at the Stanford Medical School, has made a direct comparison with sport: the puffing speeds up your heart rate, raises blood pressure, quickens breathing and thoroughly oxygenates you. He says that twenty seconds of hearty laughter is equivalent to three minutes of strenuous rowing.

It is also a wonderful way of alleviating emotional tension, such as frustration and annoyance. I find I achieve the greatest relief by laughing at things that have caused me much pain in the past. My childhood was severely restricted by a large overdose of religion, often doled out by petty-minded people who had no understanding whatever of true spirituality. Any send-ups of religion I therefore find simply hilarious. Dave Allen was always a favourite of mine, and whenever his shows are repeated I am glued to the television. One sketch I loved was set in a Roman Catholic cathedral. The priests had spent several arduous hours in their confessional boxes listening to the guilt-ridden mumblings of their parishioners. Afterwards, they locked up the cathedral and then indulged in their chosen sport – playing dodgems with their confessional boxes!

If you have ever been in hospital, then the film *Carry on Doctor* is compulsive viewing. It is a most marvellous antidote to all those ill-feelings that build up towards the medical profession. The patients rebel against the staff for the undignified treatment they have had to put up with. The women capture Matron, hold her down and give her the routine hospital torture – the blanket bath. The men capture the Chief Physician, who has brought about the dismissal of their favourite doctor (to cover his own tracks) and bundle him into the operating theatre. There they threaten him with the surgeon's instruments to extract a confession from him and eventually succeed in giving him an enema. The patients also delight in outwitting Matron. There is a hilarious scene in which the hero dresses up as a nurse to chat up the girl he fancies in the next ward.

Never despise anything that makes you laugh or dismiss it as 'silly rubbish'. Indulge in silly rubbish as often as possible. It does you good! Dr Kathleen M. Dillon of Western New England College in America carried out an experiment with ten students. She asked them to view thirty-minute videos, some of which were very funny and others were serious. After each one she took samples of their saliva and measured the concentrations of immunoglobulin A (specialised antibodies that protect against some viruses). After the humorous videos, these levels had increased significantly, but after the serious ones, they remained unchanged. There is no doubt, therefore, that if you approach life with cheerful good humour, your disease-fighting forces will receive a worthwhile boost.

Your laughter quotient

	OFTEN	OCCASIONALLY	NEVER
Do you share jokes, puns, amusing anecdotes with friends or relatives?			
Do you browse through books of cartoons?			
Do you read humorous books?			
Do you go to hilarious feature films?			
Do you hire funny videos?			
Do you go to amusing revues or plays?			

Do you watch funny programmes
on TV?
With what frequency do you
have a good belly laugh?

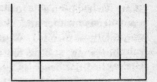

Scoring
Count up the number of ticks in each column. If you have only, or
mainly marked 'never', then make a special effort to build laughter
into your life in one of the above ways. You can only do yourself
good! Make it one of your goals to start off by having a good
laugh once a week, then gradually increase the frequency. If you
have mainly ticked the 'occasionally' column, then there is plenty
of room for improvement here also. Explore your own humour.
Discover what you find really funny, then indulge yourself, often.
Perhaps you have scored well in this questionnaire: congratulate
yourself and keep it up.

Creativity
Concentration was intense in the Art Room at the Cancer Help
Centre. Four of us, clad in plastic aprons, were bent over a huge
sheet of paper. We were creating a finger painting. After a good
deal of embarrassed giggling from us, the art therapist had finally
cajoled us into dipping our fingers into the colours. In no time at all
we were deeply involved. Black arrows and red darts shot across my
corner of the painting. At last I was able to work through some of the
rage that had been stored up for many years. Opposite me, a patient
who ran a chain of flower shops was experimenting with elaborate
spirals and sprays of colours. Someone else was creating a fountain of
greens and blues, while the fourth person depicted a solitary man in a
prison cell. After a while, we were invited to swap places and add to
another person's area. It was interesting to take on different feelings
and shapes in this way. A decorative border eventually emerged and
finally our creation was complete. It was hung up on the wall and
then we shared our experiences. Everyone spoke enthusiastically and
many feelings were expressed. Even abstract shapes had meaning for
the person who created them. The fountain had been a healing place,
the man in a prison cell represented gloom and depression for that
person, while the spirals and sprays indicated a search for gaiety and
adventure. None of us had any idea how to paint, but this was not the

point. We had been able to investigate a part of ourselves in a free and spontaneous manner and, during this period, critical judgment had been totally suspended. We all agreed that the experience had been truly liberating, and we felt much better, much happier for it.

If we had not been cancer patients undergoing therapeutic treatment, none of us would have experimented with this kind of creativity. Rather, we would have dismissed it as 'a waste of time', yet it proved to be quite the reverse. Human beings have a natural tendency to play, but our culture generally allows only children to indulge in this kind of spontaneous free expression. So our natural creativity becomes pushed down, repressed, and a very important part of ourselves is denied.

When I found myself with cancer, I realised instinctively that I had become totally out of balance with myself. The only part that was regularly in use was my intellect. Spontaneity, fun and free expression had all got lost somewhere, and along with those had vanished my natural delight in living. My music, too, had become submerged. W.H. Auden wrote a moving poem about cancer in which he describes it as 'foiled creative fire'. The analytical psychologist Carl Jung expressed a similar idea when he talked of cancer as unlived life.

Since time immemorial, music has been used to restore the health. The Ancient Greeks believed that illness was the result of disorder between body and soul, and that harmony was needed. Music, considered to be a gift from the gods, was a means by which this could be achieved. It is significant that Apollo, the god of medicine, also presided over music. Some physicians considered that the vibrations produced by the flute actually had the power 'to make the flesh palpitate and revive'. Democritus, for example, in a treatise on 'Deadly Infections' prescribed this instrument as a medicine for many ills of the flesh.

Modern research in this area is still in its infancy, but there is now enough evidence to indicate that the Ancient Greeks were on the right track. Hans Jenny, a Swiss engineer and doctor, has carried out pioneering work to show the effect of sound on matter. He has demonstrated that liquids, pastes and fine powders, when treated with sound, form themselves into the most exquisite patterns. If the sound changes, so does the pattern. In France a musician, Fabien Maman, has joined forces with biologists and physicists to research the therapeutic effects of sound on the body, and results prove that sound waves can affect the behaviour of individual cells. In the 1950s, Allen Winold tested the electrical skin resistance of people listening to music, through electrodes registering on a galvanometer. His experiments demonstrated that music can affect the electrical conductivity of the body.

There is general agreement that the emotional impact of music provokes involuntary physiological responses, such as changes in the breathing rate and blood circulation. Do certain passages of favourite music send cold shivers down your spine? They do to mine. Bernie Siegel, the American surgeon and author of *Love, Medicine and Miracles*, uses baroque largo movements to soothe himself, his colleagues and his patients while performing intricate operations. The rhythmical bass line of about sixty beats per minute slows the heart rate of the listener, inducing deep relaxation.

I remember seeing the great cellist, Pierre Fournier, holding a masterclass shortly before his death. He appeared to have suffered a stroke and had to be helped on to the stage, each step clearly needing an enormous effort of will. He was lowered into his chair, his cello placed between his legs, and his bow handed to him. It was a sorrowful sight. I imagined that playing would be virtually impossible for such a crippled man. The first pupil performed the unaccompanied Suite in G by Bach and Fournier's concentration was complete. After she had finished, he described how his own interpretation differed, and, despite the awkwardness of his bow hold, gave a demonstration, creating a gloriously rich and flowing sound. I was both astonished and thrilled. How could this be explained?

Norman Cousins relates a similar experience in his book *Anatomy of an Illness*, when he was invited to the house of Pablo Casals. The eighty-nine-year-old cellist was suffering from severe rheumatoid arthritis, and his hands were badly swollen and clenched. Yet when he sat down to play Bach a miracle happened. His fingers slowly unlocked, his badly stooped back straightened and soon he was totally immersed in the music. This was followed by a dazzling performance of a concerto. Cousins concluded that creativity for Casals was the source of his own cortisone and that no other medication could have been as effective as that of his mind and emotions on his body.

After reading about stress in chapter 3, you will understand that chemical reactions occur in the body as the result of anxiety and fear. These can eventually lead to serious illnesses. Equally, beneficial chemical reactions are brought about by creativity and the will to live. Lawrence LeShan in his book *You Can Fight For Your Life* observes the effect that this has on terminal cancer patients. By being true to themselves, by discovering their own creativity and 'singing their own song' as he puts it, several patients have gone into complete remission. Many others improved their prognoses and the quality of their lives was greatly enhanced.

A leading endocrinologist in Roumania, Ana Aslan, has concluded that creativity produces brain impulses that stimulate the pituitary gland, which in turn triggers the pineal gland and the whole of the endocrine system, which controls the flow of hormones. As we have seen, this system is closely related to immunity. We are all capable of creativity, but so often we ignore these inborn talents, believing that we are not 'good enough'. As far as healing is concerned, it is the process that counts; whether or not we produce a work of art is insignificant. It is generally thought that creativity is a right-brain activity, and this is where the natural function of healing is set in motion.

Your natural joy and creativity may be expressed in many ways, perhaps in taking a guitar out of a dusty case, knitting a jacket for a grandson, or in the natural rhythm of horse riding. I remember how passionately my brother talked of rock-climbing. To him it wasn't just a sport, but an aesthetic experience of the highest order. Whatever makes you come alive, do it – and do it regularly. This is a way of sending 'I want to live' messages to your body.

My poor old cello was neglected for ten years. Now I play it enthusiastically. If I am feeling wound up at the end of the day, just half an hour with my instrument releases all tensions, as I allow the music to vibrate through me. The thrill of just closing my eyes and letting my fingers improvise and explore, of becoming one with those deep velvety tones, is indescribable. It doesn't matter that I am not a Jacqueline du Pré and never will be. All that matters is that I am expressing something of the real me.

3 Letting go of stress

The underground train came to a halt in the tunnel. It was the rush hour and the occupants of our carriage were packed together uncomfortably close. No doubt the signals were against us. Several trains rumbled by on an adjacent track as the minutes ticked on. People began to sigh loudly and look impatient. It was stiflingly hot and I could feel the perspiration drip down the back of my neck as I shifted my position in an attempt to retreat from the soggy armpit on one side and the overweight thigh on the other. My shoulder ached with hanging on to the strap. Soon there were several loud comments: 'It's disgusting.' 'These trains never run on time.' 'I waited nearly twenty minutes to get on this one.' 'It's about time London Transport sorted itself out, considering the amount we have to pay for tickets.' And so on. More minutes ticked by. 'Oh hell. I'm going to be late for work again,' said a young woman looking anxiously at her watch. I began to rehearse my own excuses for arriving late at the office, and could already see the disapproving faces. Those who could, buried themselves more deeply in their books or newspapers. Alas, my paperback was at the bottom of my bag, which was jammed between my feet, and it was impossible to bend down and retrieve it. One of the strap-hangers cracked a joke: 'Cuddly, isn't it?' and several passengers sniggered. The tension eased a little.

Then all of a sudden the lights went out. Everyone groaned loudly. I began to feel panic-stricken. We were in the second to last carriage and it was all too easy to imagine that one of those rumbling trains might hurtle into the back of us. My heart started to thump loudly, my mouth felt dry, my stomach churned and the sweat was now running off my forehead. I was overwhelmed with a desire to fight my way out and escape, but too many bodies were pressed up against me. My head swam and I thought I was going to faint. I desperately

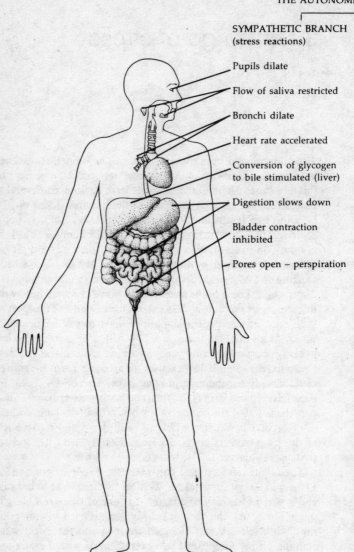

THE AUTONOMIC

SYMPATHETIC BRANCH
(stress reactions)

Pupils dilate

Flow of saliva restricted

Bronchi dilate

Heart rate accelerated

Conversion of glycogen
to bile stimulated (liver)

Digestion slows down

Bladder contraction
inhibited

Pores open – perspiration

ERVOUS SYSTEM

PARASYMPATHETIC BRANCH
(during quiescence)

Pupils contract

Flow of saliva stimulated

Bronchi contract

Heart rate slows

Release of bile stimulated

Digestion stimulated

Bladder contracts

Pores close

INTERACTIONS BETWEEN THE ENDOCRINE AND NERVOUS SYSTEMS

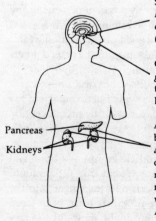

Pancreas

Kidneys

Stress causes neurons in the *hypothalamus* to secrete corticotropine-release factor (CRF).

CRF travels to the *pituitary gland* and stimulates it to release adrenocorticotrophic hormone (ACTH).

ACTH is carried by the bloodstream to the *adrenal glands* and other organs, causing the release of about 30 more hormones to deal with emergency. Adrenal glands secrete adrenalin and noradrenalin.

tried to steady my breathing and to fix my mind on something far away and soothing – a field full of wild flowers and the hum of bees. After a while the lights came on again, much to our relief, and those who could, resigned themselves to their reading. Eventually the guard came to tell us that the signals had failed and that we would have to be patient a while longer.

This scene will be familiar enough to many readers as one that is clearly fraught with stress. Just pause for a moment in your reading and consider whether you identified with anyone in particular in the carriage. Would you have cracked a joke, felt frightened, switched off, read a book, or worried about being late for work? How would you have responded to this situation? Make some notes.

Behavioural psychologists have listed six types of stress, four of which can be recognised here. People who felt panic-stricken or frightened, such as myself, saw the potential danger in the situation and were responding to the *threat stressor*. Those who diverted themselves by reading were attempting to avoid the *boredom stressor*, whereas those who sighed and groaned and worried about being late for work were reacting to the *frustration stressor*; there was nothing they could do about the situation. Additionally, many of us felt uncomfortable because of the heat, lack of space and the fact that we were standing for a long time, and were suffering from the *physical stressor*.

Interestingly, although the situation was exactly the same for everyone in the carriage, each person had their own way of perceiving and responding to it. This is a key factor in determining personal stress levels. The joker was instinctively taking good care of himself by finding a way of relieving the tension. At the same time he helped others to relax. I, on the other hand, being prone to claustrophobia, felt panic-stricken and suffered from pronounced physical symptoms.

What had happened to me was that the sympathetic branch of my autonomic nervous system had been triggered off by my perception of the situation as threatening and fearful. My body was thus prepared to deal with the emergency by running away or by fighting. Blood was being pumped to my large muscle groups and brain and my heart was beating faster. My cooling system (the perspiration) had been activated and my liver had been releasing sugar into the blood to produce a spurt of energy (see p. 88). If I had been faced by a rhinoceros in the African bush, no doubt these involuntary reactions (known as the 'fight or flight response') would have been extremely useful. Our man-made jungles, however, rarely provide opportunities for physical expression, either to fight our way out of a threatening situation, or to run for it. Very often the culprit is invisible – like the signalman in our little drama – and all one can do is suppress feelings of frustration and rage. As we have already seen, strong feelings repressed over a long period can lead to compromised immunity and increased risk of disease.

My body, then, had been geared up for action, but no action had resulted. Instead, the hormones – namely adrenalin and a group known as the corticosteroids – which had been behaving as the chemical 'messengers' to the various parts of my body were coursing uselessly around in my bloodstream (see p. 89). Adrenalin is something we are all familiar with, because its effect can be easily felt in the body. For instance, if you step off the kerb and suddenly see a vehicle heading straight for you, you can instantly feel the rush of adrenalin which prompts you to leap smartly out of the way. The corticosteroids, however, cannot be sensed like this, and these are the ones that can have a damaging effect on the immune system. One of them in particular, cortisol, has been proved to be a virulent immunosuppressant. Indeed, a high level in the bloodstream is known to be closely connected with stress-related diseases, such as skin disorders, ulcers, diabetes and heart attacks.

THE GENERAL ADAPTATION SYNDROME

Experiments with rats have shown that if they are subjected to a stressor (such as cold, heat or mild electric shock) over a long period of time they go through three distinct phases. After the initial alarm reaction, in which the animal mobilises its defences, a stage of resistance sets in. During this period hormones continue to be secreted into the bloodstream, the adrenal glands expand in size and the animal copes well. If the stressor continues for longer, the rat eventually appears to adapt and the adrenal glands return to normal size. Appearances are deceptive, though, for if a second stressor is introduced at this time the animal is totally unable to resist it and may die. If the first stressor alone continues for even longer, a point of exhaustion and collapse will be reached. This may be accompanied by the re-occurrence of alarm symptoms. Examination of laboratory animals after this kind of prolonged exposure to stress shows damaged adrenal glands, shrunken lymph nodes and thymuses (both basic to healthy immunity) and bleeding stomach ulcers.

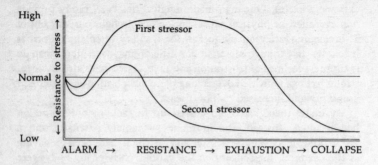

General adaptation syndrome (GAS)

Although these reactions can be tempered in humans by mental attitude and by the nature of the stressor, the physiological processes remain similar, as do the three stages of alarm reaction, resistance and exhaustion; these were identified by Hans Selye, and are known as the General Adaptation Syndrome. Clearly, important conclusions can be drawn from animal experiments concerning the damaging nature of prolonged stress.

The implications are obvious. If we are to remain in the best of health it is vital to learn how to control unwanted stress, and if necessary, avoid it, so that this physiological reaction is triggered off only when we really need it.

BEING IN CONTROL

Another classical experiment, conducted in 1985 and also involving animals, examines the question of control. Two groups of rats were exposed to mild electric shocks of the same intensity, but only one group was able to control these shocks by turning a wheel, which they soon learned to do. A third group was placed in the same kind of box, but no shocks were given at all. The aim was to study the tumour-killing ability of the T-cells called natural killer (NK) cells, which play a prime role in tumour surveillance. The NK cells of the rats which received shocks but were able to exert some control over them were as effective at killing cancer cells as those of the rats which received no shocks at all. The NK cells of the rats which had no control over the shocks, however, were less able to kill tumour cells.

The conclusion drawn from this is that people who respond to negative life events with feelings of depression, hopelessness and loss of control have lowered ability to fight off malignancies. Indeed, one study with humans in 1984 had already shown this to be true. It also showed that people who coped extremely well with stressors had even higher levels of NK cell activity than people who had suffered very few negative life events. Being in control of events therefore has a positive effect on the immune system; conversely, loss of control has a detrimental effect.

ASSESSING YOUR STRESS LEVELS

Not all stress is bad; in fact a modest amount is beneficial because it keeps us alert and helps us to operate to our full potential. So we need to distinguish between the sources of stress that actually enhance the quality of our lives and those that are damaging. Then we can consider how we can cut out, or at any rate alter, the effects of harmful stress.

Before we can make these decisions, we need to be aware of all types of stressors and how they affect us individually. We also need to appreciate that stress is cumulative and that we can cope with only so much. Beyond that point, we enter the danger zone.

But how do we know whether our stress levels are getting too high? It isn't always so obvious. If we are lucky, friends or relatives may notice a change in our behaviour and gently suggest that something is amiss. These signals are usually fairly obvious to others, though not at all apparent to ourselves.

A little while ago, as I lay on the couch in the hospital undergoing a routine ultra-sound scan, I occupied myself by observing the doctor. First of all I was impressed with his good looks, but then I noticed the worry lines along his forehead and the tension around his mouth. He snapped at the orderly who was tidying up, telling him, not very politely, to leave the room. 'Let's have a look, then', he said somewhat abruptly to me, and squirted me with jelly. He switched on the machine and rattled away at the keyboard. I noticed the frequent sighs and the way he ran his fingers impatiently through his hair. Every so often he leapt up to do something else – always at a fast pace. As the probe slid around my skin, he rubbed his eyes in an effort to concentrate on the screen. I engaged him in conversation about the dots (my cells) coming into view, hoping to focus his attention and interest. The consultant made an unexpected appearance and asked him if he could discuss a pancreas operation as a matter of urgency. I held my breath, expecting an outburst, but the doctor kept his temper with difficulty, saying the scan was nearly finished. My tissue then had his total concentration for two minutes until he was finally satisfied with the image. He took a picture and left the consulting room at a run, shouting, 'That's fine.' As I calmly put on my robe, I thought to myself: if he doesn't slow down soon, he will be a victim of an early coronary or of the very disease he is trying to cure. So, watch out for irritability and rapid swings of mood, as well as excessive hurrying. These are common stress signals, as are an increase in smoking and drinking.

However, unless we are suffering from physical symptoms, we may not be aware of how hard we are pushing ourselves. We accept that this is how life has to be. We have to get to work, to earn our living, to pay the mortgage, to look after our partners and children, and so on. This is what our lives consist of. How can we change any of it? Many of us feel stuck within the system. Yet it is possible to make changes, as we have seen, and you will find some more ways of doing this later in the chapter.

Physical symptoms
First, let us deal with the most obvious symptoms of stress – the physical warning signs.

When faced with situations that you perceive to be stressful, such as meeting strangers, sitting an examination, being late for an important appointment and so on, do you suffer from any of the symptoms indicated in the chart opposite? If your answer is 'yes', tick the box which indicates whether this response is occasional or frequent.

These are all indications that your sympathetic nervous system has been triggered and your body is preparing itself for fight or flight. If this happens occasionally, when the situation is particularly demanding or threatening, and the rush of adrenalin helps you to feel more alert, give a better performance – or whatever is demanded of you – and if the symptoms immediately subside after the task is completed, this is fine. If, however, the symptoms are severe, for instance your mouth is too dry to speak or you feel too faint to stand up, then, clearly, your body's response is excessive and is hindering rather than helping you. In this case something has to be done to prevent

	YES	NO	OCCASIONALLY	OFTEN
Churning stomach				
Nausea or even vomiting				
Racing heart or palpitations				
Trembling				
Diarrhoea				
Dry mouth				
Sweatiness				
Breathlessness				
Aching head				
Aching or stiff neck				
Clenched jaw or fists				
Dizziness				
Confused thoughts				

this happening. Regular practice of physical relaxation will certainly become important to you, because after a while you will be able to switch off the activities of the sympathetic nervous system when not needed (see 'Deep muscular relaxation' and 'Quick relaxation' later in this chapter). You will also find other useful hints here.

If you are suffering from persistent symptoms that seem to have no obvious cause, then it could be that your general state of arousal is so high that you are entering the danger zone and are suffering from chronic stress.

Do you additionally frequently suffer from any of the following?

Chest pains	Loss of appetite
High blood pressure	Indigestion
Abdominal pain	Colds and 'flu
Migraine	Overeating
Insomnia and/or tiredness	Loss of libido
Wheezing	Phobias or obsessions
Dermatitis or eczema	Depression
Pre-menstrual tension	Accidents

Alcoholism   Low back pain
Excessive smoking

Do check with your doctor first to ensure that there is no other identifiable cause of your symptoms. Chest pains can be either the result of tension in the chest wall, or else the serious sign of coronary artery disease. Perhaps you already have a tendency towards a certain physical weakness, and if so this is where strain will manifest itself. For instance, asthmatics are liable to more severe attacks if they have a sudden emotional upset.

Dealing with anxiety symptoms

Physical symptoms of anxiety can be very alarming, but it is possible to learn to control them. If you feel nervous before a stressful event, such as an interview, or before making a speech, you can calm yourself by taking slow, deep breaths from the diaphragm. Shallow breathing from the chest is characteristic of anxiety and can make you feel dizzy. This symptom will go when you change the way you breathe. Full yoga breathing, described in chapter 5, will slow your pulse rate and calm a racing heart.

Meditating on a single object is very soothing if you have to undergo something fearful, such as dental treatment or a hospital examination. I used this technique while having a needle biopsy performed under local anaesthetic and found it very helpful. All you have to do is relax physically (see 'Quick relaxation' later in this chapter) and then focus on a single object. It makes no difference what it is; just pick anything around you and then lose yourself completely in its details. Notice its colour, shape, texture, the way the light catches it, and so on. Carry on until you feel more balanced. This simple technique can be useful in many unpleasant or difficult situations, such as a crowded lift if you are feeling claustrophobic, or at a funeral, when you need to keep control.

The symptoms of panic attacks are very frightening indeed. In my case, my chest pains were so severe that I thought my heart would stop and that I would collapse and die. I had no idea that such sensations are the natural result of an over-aroused nervous system. Some people have a palpitating heart or legs that go to jelly, while others suffer from confusion or feelings of unreality. In all cases, there is an overwhelming dread that something terrible is about to happen. A build-up of stress from several sources has created sensitisation to such a degree that the sympathetic nervous system goes into overload and reactions can become extreme. Although the symptoms appear so frightening they are not in fact a warning of impending heart failure; they are simply the result of excessive tension. Part of the terror is fear of the symptoms themselves. Therefore, when the sufferer realises that these can be brought under control and that they will naturally pass with time, this part of the fear recedes. I have successfully relieved my own chest tension by doing vigorous exercise, such as press-ups, jogging and cushion-bashing. Pressing very hard against a wall also provides relief. Physical exhaustion quickly sets in and the chest wall naturally relaxes. Knowing that I can alleviate this symptom with such straightforward techniques definitely cures my fear of an impending panic attack.

The main thing is not to fight the panic itself. Relax yourself physically by going completely limp, then accept the nervous feelings and go along with them, knowing that you are not going to collapse and that they will pass. This stops the panic from escalating. Gradually, you will lose the fear of the symptoms and then they will begin to recede.

Acceptance and inclusion of nervous feelings is extremely important. A former colleague of mine had to make a speech at a sales conference. When the moment arrived, her legs were shaking so much she could scarcely stand, and then, horror of horrors, she felt her jaw seize up so that she was unable to open her mouth. It was only when she decided to admit to the five hundred people present how nervous she was that she found her mouth opening quite naturally, and the words flowed out.

Fear of one's own reactions actually hinders many people from living life to the full. Agoraphobics are mostly afraid to go out because they fear having a nervous attack while away from home. Knowing that the symptoms are not at all life-threatening, and that they are simply the result of an over-sensitised nervous system, helps many agoraphobics to cope. Behavioural psychotherapists treat all kinds of phobias with desensitisation techniques, with considerable success. The principle is that the sufferer, after relaxing, is exposed to the feared object or situation in a sequence of graduated steps, until the fright eventually diminishes. For example, someone who is afraid of spiders may first be asked to imagine one, then to look at a photograph of one, to see one in a jar, and finally to hold one. All of these techniques are valuable, but none involves treating the original causes of the anxiety. Many people do not consider themselves cured until they understand and have dealt with the underlying problems.

Finding the causes
Look back again under 'physical symptoms' at whatever you have ticked on the first list and recall as many situations as possible that have triggered off your sympathetic nervous system, causing these unpleasant effects. Describe the scene exactly in your notebook, adding where you were, which people were present, what they said and did, how you responded and how you felt. Do you wish you could have responded differently? Did the symptoms prevent you from making the best impression? Are there any similarities in the situations – or in the type of people present? What exactly is it that causes you so much anxiety? There may be several things. Whatever they are, write them down and add any insights you may have. Continue to keep a record in your notebook of any recurrences of these stress-provoking situations.

Now look at the second list and think carefully about whatever you have ticked. What is this symptom telling you about yourself? If you have no idea, record-keeping will help you discover its source. Welcome it as a useful piece of information. As with the other list, whenever your symptom or symptoms occur make a note of the day and time, where you are, what you are doing, how you are feeling, and record exactly the events immediately preceding the onset. Also note how you react to the situation and what happens afterwards. If any symptom is persistent, try and discover what makes it worse or, equally, what makes it better. In a few weeks, you will be able to see a pattern emerging which should help you to identify the cause of the stress. Then you can decide what to do about it. Either you can use avoidance tactics if possible or appropriate, or else you can learn new behaviour patterns – more of this later. Again, physical relaxation techniques, such as those described in this chapter, will help you greatly.

Workaholics may already have thrown up their hands in despair, complaining that they have no time to stop and think about themselves, let alone keep a diary. So let me say again, if you have ticked 'yes' and 'often' more than once in the first list and have also ticked several symptoms on the second list, your stress level is almost certainly too high and your immune system correspondingly depleted.

It may not be long before serious illness strikes. So please take care of yourself, and – however difficult this may be – give yourself time, time to do a little work on yourself until your symptoms are under control. Just ten minutes at the end of the day to review its events, your reactions and feelings, is a first important step towards taking control of your stress levels.

LIFESTYLE STRESSORS

By now you will already have come up with several personal causes of stress and recorded them in your notebook. Many people, however, are not fully aware of what can be stressful. Boredom, for instance, is not generally viewed as a prime source, but it is worth remembering that there is a very high rate of heart disease among the unemployed. Perhaps consideration of the six main stressors may help to jog your memory. We discovered four in the scene on the underground train, and the other two major ones recognised by behaviourists are the *performance stressor* and when one suffers a serious loss and finds oneself in a state of *bereavement*. 'Performance' does not necessarily mean getting up on a stage and singing a song; it can, for example, include an everyday event such as attendance at a meeting at which you may wish to make a contribution.

Equally, 'bereavement' has a wide meaning and can include a loss of, say, self-esteem, if you are demoted in your job. It has been recognised for a long time that recently bereaved people are far more likely than normal to become ill or even die. A study in Australia found that lymphocytes from the bereaved were significantly less responsive two months after their loss than those of other people matched for age, sex and ethnic origins.

The following questionnaires are designed to assist you with the discovery of other sources of strain that have not been immediately obvious. They are divided into the two life areas of work and home. It is not so much the stressors themselves, however, that can be damaging, but your response to them and your ability to cope. Promotion at work may be met with enthusiasm by one person, or dread by another, depending on whether the employee feels that s/he can rise to the occasion. Look at each question. If your answer is 'no', score 0; if 'yes', ring the figure that best represents the amount of strain you suffer from, with 5 as the most stressful. Insert this figure in the 'yes' column.

Stressors at work

	YES	NO	STRESS RATING				

Threat

	YES	NO	STRESS RATING
Are you under threat of redundancy?		0	1 2 3 4 5
Is your boss abrasive or uncommunicative?		0	1 2 3 4 5
Do you have to deal with hostile customers?		0	1 2 3 4 5
Are those in power untrustworthy?		0	1 2 3 4 5
Do you suffer from sexual harassment?		0	1 2 3 4 5
Are you the victim of 'office politics'?		0	1 2 3 4 5
Are your workmates untrustworthy?		0	1 2 3 4 5
Do you have to cope with difficult juniors?		0	1 2 3 4 5
Does anyone under you consider they could do your job better than you?		0	1 2 3 4 5

Frustration

	YES	NO	STRESS RATING
Does the workplace equipment frequently break down?		0	1 2 3 4 5
Are your co-workers incompetent?		0	1 2 3 4 5
Is your immediate superior incompetent?		0	1 2 3 4 5
Are too many meetings held at your workplace?		0	1 2 3 4 5
Are you poorly rewarded for your work in terms of salary and prospects?		0	1 2 3 4 5
Are you excluded from decision-making?		0	1 2 3 4 5
Are your goals unclear?		0	1 2 3 4 5
Are your values incompatible with those of your employers?		0	1 2 3 4 5

Bereavement/loss

	YES	NO	STRESS RATING
Have you recently been demoted?		0	1 2 3 4 5
Have you been given notice or made redundant within the last eighteen months?		0	1 2 3 4 5
Have you just retired?		0	1 2 3 4 5
Have you been transferred to a different area?		0	1 2 3 4 5
Do you have new managers?		0	1 2 3 4 5
Are you having to adjust to technological change?		0	1 2 3 4 5
Have you recently lost a lot of money?		0	1 2 3 4 5

Boredom

	YES	NO	STRESS RATING
Is your work dull or repetitive?		0	1 2 3 4 5
Is there a lack of opportunity for learning new things?		0	1 2 3 4 5
Is there too much futile paper-pushing?		0	1 2 3 4 5
Are your workmates poor company?		0	1 2 3 4 5

Physical

	YES	NO	STRESS RATING
Do you work in shifts?		0	1 2 3 4 5
Do you work long hours?		0	1 2 3 4 5

Do you have a long journey to work?	0	1 2 3 4 5
Have your work conditions recently changed?	0	1 2 3 4 5
Is there a lot of noise?	0	1 2 3 4 5
Are you frequently interrupted by telephones etc?	0	1 2 3 4 5
Is the lighting, heating or ventilation poor?	0	1 2 3 4 5
Do you wear an uncomfortable uniform?	0	1 2 3 4 5

Performance

Have you recently been promoted?	0	1 2 3 4 5
Have you recently changed jobs?	0	1 2 3 4 5
Do you have too much work to do?	0	1 2 3 4 5
Are you constantly working to deadlines?	0	1 2 3 4 5
Is there fierce competition with other companies?	0	1 2 3 4 5
Do you have heavy responsibilities?	0	1 2 3 4 5
Have you achieved something outstanding?	0	1 2 3 4 5
Do you have high expectations of yourself?	0	1 2 3 4 5
Does your boss have high expectations of you?	0	1 2 3 4 5

SCORE

Stressors at home

Threat	YES	NO	STRESS RATING
Is your partner having an affair?		0	1 2 3 4 5
Are you having more arguments than usual with your partner, or suddenly far fewer?		0	1 2 3 4 5
Is your partner an alcoholic?		0	1 2 3 4 5
Are you financially insecure?		0	1 2 3 4 5
Does your spouse have a more interesting or rewarding career than you?		0	1 2 3 4 5
Are your in-laws causing problems at home?		0	1 2 3 4 5
Do you live in a high-crime area?		0	1 2 3 4 5
Do you suffer from racial tension?		0	1 2 3 4 5
Are you subject to class discrimination?		0	1 2 3 4 5
Are you under threat of physical violence?		0	1 2 3 4 5
Do you have rows with the neighbours?		0	1 2 3 4 5
Are you or is a member of your family in trouble with the police?		0	1 2 3 4 5
Do you have a new family member?		0	1 2 3 4 5

Frustration

Are you and your partner sexually incompatible?	0	1 2 3 4 5
Are you without a suitable partner?	0	1 2 3 4 5
Do you have no time for hobbies?	0	1 2 3 4 5
Are your interests and talents unappreciated by others?	0	1 2 3 4 5
Are your children ill-behaved?	0	1 2 3 4 5

Bereavement/loss

Has your partner or close family member recently died?	0	1 2 3 4 5
Has a friend recently died?	0	1 2 3 4 5
Has a pet recently died?	0	1 2 3 4 5
Have you just been divorced or separated?	0	1 2 3 4 5
Have you just moved house?	0	1 2 3 4 5
Have friends or kind neighbours moved away?	0	1 2 3 4 5
Have your offspring recently left home?	0	1 2 3 4 5
Has your child just started school?	0	1 2 3 4 5
Has your partner or family member become uncommunicative?	0	1 2 3 4 5
Do you frequently have to give way to another's priorities?	0	1 2 3 4 5
Has a family member been imprisoned?	0	1 2 3 4 5
Has your spouse ceased work?	0	1 2 3 4 5
Has your mortgage (or large loan) been foreclosed?	0	1 2 3 4 5

Boredom

Does your partner work very long hours?	0	1 2 3 4 5
Are the domestic chores mainly your responsibility?	0	1 2 3 4 5
Do you follow the interests of family members rather than your own?	0	1 2 3 4 5
Do you live in an isolated area?	0	1 2 3 4 5
Are you lonely?	0	1 2 3 4 5
Do you have to transport your children for long distances?	0	1 2 3 4 5
Does your partner dislike socialising?	0	1 2 3 4 5

Physical

Do you have a serious injury or illness, or have you recently undergone surgery?	0	1 2 3 4 5
Is there injury or illness in the family?	0	1 2 3 4 5
Is a member of your family handicapped?	0	1 2 3 4 5
Are you a single parent?	0	1 2 3 4 5
Do you have a dependent parent?	0	1 2 3 4 5
Are you or a family member unexpectedly pregnant?	0	1 2 3 4 5
Does your baby frequently cry?	0	1 2 3 4 5
Do you live in overcrowded conditions?	0	1 2 3 4 5

Are your partner's sleeping habits different from yours?	0	1 2 3 4 5
Does your spouse snore?	0	1 2 3 4 5
Are you a non-smoker who has a smoking partner?	0	1 2 3 4 5
Are you or your partner overweight?	0	1 2 3 4 5
Have you changed to a new diet?	0	1 2 3 4 5
Are you subject to loud music or other noise from neighbours or children?	0	1 2 3 4 5

Performance

Are you newly married?	0	1 2 3 4 5
Have you taken up a competitive hobby?	0	1 2 3 4 5
Are you socialising more than usual?	0	1 2 3 4 5
Is your child doing poorly at school?	0	1 2 3 4 5
Do your relatives or partner have high expectations of you?	0	1 2 3 4 5
Are you the sole breadwinner?	0	1 2 3 4 5
Do you have a large mortgage or loan?	0	1 2 3 4 5
SCORE		

Your scores should give you a clear picture of your major sources of strain. Add up the points to make a total under each life area and compare these to see which is most stressful. Then add the two together for your overall score, and plot this on the scale below:

Minimal stress	Moderate stress	Stress too high
1	50	100

You may be astonished at how high this is. We often pretend to ourselves that we are coping splendidly, unaware of the accumulation of stressors. We tell ourselves that we have to make the best of things, however bad they may be. But do we?

Reducing lifestyle stressors

Before I became ill with cancer, my experience of stress was extremely high, with 48 points for work and 45 for home. The total of 93 was clearly far too much for me and I was well in the danger zone. Changing my career enabled me to reduce my work stressors dramatically, and my score is now down to 21, with 35 for home stressors. Yet there is still some scope for improvement. Only you can know if your stress levels are too high. If they are, what can you do to cut down?

Take a look at your work stressors first. Are other people causing you problems? You can help yourself greatly by being self-assertive (discussed in chapter 2). For instance, an uncommunicative boss can be plainly and politely asked to provide more information. Or, if you are frequently left out of decision-making, go to your superior, explaining that you feel your opinions are valuable and that you would be able to do your job more effectively and enthusiastically if you could make a direct contribution to decisions. Write a report to support your views. Even if this has no immediate effect, you will have taken some positive action, which is far better for you than harbouring frustrations or resentments. When did you last ask for a salary rise? Don't be shy. You are valuable, so go ahead.

The same principles apply at home. Being assertive by stating your feelings can often clear the air and help release tension. Suppose you are secretly aware, or fear, that your partner is having an affair. Take your fury out on a few harmless cushions first (see 'Dealing with anger and resentment' in chapter 2), then declare your grief and hurt plainly and clearly. Don't let this kind of upset fester; it is unlikely to go away and can only grow worse. Similarly, sexual difficulties can often be overcome by stating your own needs openly and asking your partner to express his or hers. If you are not used to being assertive, such new behaviour can seem very risky at first. But with practice, you will improve. You will also be encouraged by the positive response you receive in return.

If you continually have to face onerous tasks at work, such as dealing with hostile customers, consider whether you can offload any of this on to someone else who doesn't take the rejections so personally. Alternatively, tackle the unpleasant jobs first thing in the day. This will leave the rest of your time relatively stress-free. If you have heavy responsibilities, can you share them with a colleague? Similarly, can anyone else help with your work load if it is too great? Delegation eases strain considerably. Perhaps you are the sort of person who believes that no one else can do the work as well as you, in which case you are heading for trouble. It is essential (for your health) to allow others to be imperfect and make the occasional mistake. The same goes for you.

There may not be much you can do about an incompetent superior, apart from waiting for the time when s/he makes an expensive mistake, which alerts the management to his or her ineffectiveness. Should this person cause you undue stress, you may have to consider applying for a different position. The same holds true if you find that your values conflict with company policy.

Perhaps you are bored, in which case look for a new job or an absorbing hobby. One tax specialist I heard of took up the breeding of rare and exotic insects, winning prizes and acclaim at national shows. Be open to possibilities. Allow yourself to dream. What really makes you come alive? What would you most like to do with your life? You only have one!

There may be practical ways of reducing or even eliminating physical stressors. If they are really getting you down, a move to a quieter area or more convenient location could be well worth considering. Can you use your assertiveness to improve conditions? Smoking can be limited to certain areas where others are not troubled by the fumes. Neighbours can be asked to restrict their rowdiness to reasonable hours. Make your home environment less cluttered by creating more storage space, and by maximising natural daylight. This is important physiologically, as light regulates the levels of the hormone melanonin; a build-up of this in your body can cause depression and lethargy. So work near a window and take a walk outside as often as possible. Another good tip is to stick a green dot onto the face of your watch, so that every time you see it it will remind you to relax!

Some stressors are unavoidable, such as the death of someone close, but the way you deal with a crisis like this can significantly affect your well-being. It is important to express your grief and not bottle it up, and to give yourself time to recover from such a serious loss. Don't be afraid to ask for support at a time like this. If your friends and relatives are unable to provide what you need, then consider joining a support group or seek bereavement counselling. Equally, people who are suffering from serious illnesses such as cancer or multiple sclerosis, or those with handicapped children, will benefit from joining a group. I know from experience how much my own burden has been alleviated by sharing my fears with others.

As you go through your list of stressors, you will come up with ideas of your own about how to deal with them. Write them down in your notebook, formulate a plan of action, then tackle them one by one. Avoid allowing things to drag on until your health deteriorates. An acquaintance of mine, called Barry, did just this. He evaluated his own stressors as follows.

Having been unemployed for several months, Barry eventually found work as a salesman with a window company, and represented this firm for a number of years. He got along with his immediate colleagues quite well, but his boss was aggressive and demanding (threat 3) and Barry, although a conscientious person, found it increasingly impossible to satisfy his high expectations (performance 4). The number of his sales was sometimes unfavourably compared with his colleagues' (threat 3). He worked on commission, so, while it was feasible to make a good living, in fact Barry's record had been uneven and he suffered from some financial insecurity (threat 4). One problem was that he had a particular regard for old houses and he hated to see them ruined with modern aluminium frames (frustration 3). He found the endless travelling stressful (physical 3) and, because he could not always succeed in making the sales he needed, he had to put in extra hours (physical 3) to ensure adequate commission to meet his many bills at home (performance 3). Then there was the paperwork, which he did immaculately, but he found it tedious (boredom 2). One part of his job he disliked intensely was ringing up potential customers 'cold'. He found frequent refusals hard to take (threat 2) and competition with other companies was fierce (performance 3). Another difficulty was that, being a straightforward, honest person, he was worried by the white lies that found their way into the sales talk (frustration 4).

Barry's mother had died recently (loss 5) which had left him greatly saddened, but he had to keep going; there was no time to grieve. How he longed for some space for himself and a few hours each week to devote to his hobbies (frustration 4)! At one time, he had enjoyed the company of his neighbours who lived in the semi next door, but they had recently moved away (loss 2). The new neighbours were rowdy and played loud pop music late at night (physical 2). The home he shared with his wife and family was pleasant enough, but they lived in a high-crime area (threat 2), and then there were other minor aggravations such as his wife's insomnia (physical 2), and her smoking (physical 1), and of course he was the sole breadwinner (performance 3). But as long as everything seemed normal at home he managed to get by. Unfortunately, because of his irregular earnings, Barry started to lag behind with his mortgage repayments (performance 3), and a letter arrived from the building society threatening to claim the house unless the amount he owed was paid within one month (threat 4). The strain was becoming severe. Then on top of all this, his wife admitted one day that she had been having an affair (threat 5) and Barry was devastated. She accused him of ignoring her and the children (threat 4), one of whom is handicapped (physical 3), and Barry had to admit that his long working hours and the amount of travelling he had to do were keeping him away from home (loss 3).

At this juncture, Barry moved into serious overload (with a total of 80 stress points). He went to his doctor with abdominal cramps and diarrhoea and was eventually diagnosed as suffering from ulcerative colitis (physical 5).

During his extended sick leave, Barry had the opportunity to review his life and to spend time with his family. While doing some DIY jobs around the house he realised how much he enjoyed working with his hands. After discussions with his personnel officer and recommendations from his doctor, he was transferred to the carpentry section of his company, starting, initially, at a fairly low level, assisting with the making and installation of wooden frames. He was quickly promoted. Meanwhile, his wife had found a place in a special school for their handicapped child, which enabled her to take a part-time job. The financial burden was now at least partly shared and they were able to catch up with the mortgage repayments. Barry's new position allowed him to spend more time at home and his relationship with his wife improved steadily.

No longer in the front line of the aggressive world of sales, Barry is much happier and more relaxed. He has discovered that his true nature is that of a craftsman, and working with his hands gives him great satisfaction. This is totally contrary to his father's view, which is that in order to get on in the world you have to be a hard-headed businessman. By changing his job Barry has cut down significantly on threat, performance, frustration, physical and loss stressors. At the same time the quality of his home life has become enriched. Eventually he plans to set up on his own as a carpenter.

All too often, it takes a major crisis to jolt people out of unrewarding, stressful and destructive situations. If you are in touch with your real feelings and are able to express them and ask for what you want, and if you know what you find most fulfilling and stay true to yourself, the chances are that you will be able to adjust to any changes creatively and will avoid hitting major crises that bring disease in their wake.

So many people come towards the end of their lives and say, 'If only . . .'. 'If only I had been an apple farmer instead of an accountant. Growing food is so satisfying,' said my uncle as he lay ill with pneumonia. 'If only I had worked in a hospital instead of running a business. Caring for people is so much more worthwhile,' said a friend in a cancer support group. And so on. Being true to yourself means lower stress levels and healthier immunity. But we are already entering the realms of the next section.

INTERNAL STRESSORS

So far, you have looked at your physical symptoms and identified the stressors that result from your style of living, mainly at work or with your family. These are stressors which are fairly easy to pinpoint, given a little time and thought, although intensity of response to each will vary according to the individual.

Far more elusive are those inner conflicts that operate mostly at an unconscious level and result in a general feeling of nervousness, anxiety or depression. These involve our feelings about ourselves, probably originating long ago in childhood, and beliefs that we have held for many years. Usually they are central to the way in which we perceive ourselves; or, to put this the other way, if we no longer experienced those familiar feelings or carried on believing what we always have, then we might find it difficult to recognise ourselves any more. This is why we are so reluctant to challenge old beliefs or investigate the origin of feelings, because the secure knowledge of who we are is then threatened. Indeed, it takes great courage to make changes to oneself, but if glowing health and happiness are to be achieved, then some changes will almost certainly be necessary.

Repressed feelings

When you were small you learnt to behave in certain ways, so that you could win your parents' approval and ensure your own survival. You learnt that it was all right to express some feelings, but not others, and you gradually developed various ideas about yourself and your environment which were the best for you at that time. As an adult, however, many of those childhood feelings, beliefs and behaviour patterns are no longer so valuable to you; indeed some may be positively damaging and causing unnecessary stress. For instance, if you learnt when you were a child that every time you tried to assert yourself and express your own feelings and wishes you were punished, then it is likely that now, as an adult, you will feel extremely anxious whenever you try to be assertive. Happily, it is possible to relearn a behaviour pattern such as this, as we have already seen. So it is time to review yourself, keeping those aspects that are still very valuable and replacing those that are not with something more appropriate.

Sigmund Freud was the first psychologist to realise that anxiety neuroses (that is, feelings of anxiety not resulting from objective dangers) were caused by strong instinctual urges which were severely repressed in childhood, especially sex and aggression. Was sexuality freely mentioned in your family when you were a child, or was it a taboo subject? And how about anger? Were you allowed to express this safely, or were you forced to hide your rage and suppress it? If you had to repress these strong feelings when you were small, it is likely that you will still have difficulty being open about your own sexuality and in expressing your anger effectively. As we saw when discussing personality and illness, repressed rage and resentment over long periods of time can contribute to such serious diseases as cancer and ulcerative colitis.

Write down in your notebook what happened to you as a child whenever you tried to express anger. Did your parents laugh at you, ignore you, take you seriously, punish you? Unless you were taken seriously, then it is likely that feelings of anger for you will be accompanied by considerable stress.

And what about your sexuality? Were you allowed to discuss this freely or were you made to feel guilty about your own body? Write this down, too, because your discoveries may throw considerable light on your behaviour today. Do you find it easy to express your needs to your partner? Can you say openly when you want to make love? It could be that you have a lot of anxiety surrounding this issue. If you have no partner at present, how do you deal with your sexual energy? Is it pushed under, or are you able to divert it into, say, a creative outlet?

Anger can also be the reaction to a stressful situation – which, again, you may feel you have to repress. Studies with animals have shown that they will start fighting if they are suffering from stressors such as overcrowding, mild electric shocks or if their food supply is unexpectedly cut off. Levels of anger can be very high in overcrowded inner cities, as we are often aware by the aggressive horn blowing, or the sudden outbursts of rage from people sitting in a traffic jam. I was startled the other day to see two people racing across a crowded street, the one in pursuit of the other. 'Help, call the police!' screeched the one in front, a rather portly gentleman with gold-rimmed spectacles. The younger man behind, who was dressed in slim racing pants, soon caught up with him and started to push him around and punch him. 'You bastard. You pulled me off my bike. You pulled me off my bike,' he yelled, while the older chap beat on a shop window appealing for help. Passers-by scuttled out of the way. Fortunately the cyclist calmed down before doing too much damage. But such scenes are common in cities. How do you feel in a crowded, noisy street? Next time, be aware of your feelings and acknowledge them, rather than letting them lie buried. Just think how much energy it takes to keep these powerful feelings submerged! Look back again at 'Dealing with anger and resentment' in chapter 2 for safe ways of coping.

If you were never allowed to express your anger as a child what did you do with it? Many adolescents who have learnt that it is inadvisable to express feelings become withdrawn and depressed, and a feeling of helplessness sets in. Whatever they do seems wrong. If you suffer from depression, consider what may be beneath it. Is it really unexpressed anger accompanied by a feeling of helplessness?

Inner conflict
'There are times', said Somerset Maugham, 'when I look over the various parts of my character with perplexity. I recognise that I am made up of several persons and that the person that at the moment has the upper hand will inevitably give place to another.' Most psychotherapists today recognise that the human personality consists of different parts, often expressed through the interminable chatter that goes on inside our heads. Freud identified three main areas: the id (basic biological drives), the ego (the rational part) and the superego (in charge of values and morals). The ego develops as it confronts reality; gratification of the id has to be delayed until an appropriate moment when circumstances are right. The superego is learnt from authority figures, such as parents and teachers, until their rules for behaviour are internalised inside oneself.

Modern psychotherapists have developed this basic idea of the multiplicity of personality, dividing it up in various ways. Perhaps the most flexible and accessible of approaches is provided by psychosynthesis, which calls these divided parts 'subpersonalities'. To put it simply, we play different roles according to the circumstances we find ourselves in. For instance, a young nurse, while on duty, will most likely be in her role of Carer. Suppose she has arranged to go out to a dinner and dance with her boyfriend one evening. She takes off her uniform, puts on a stunning, revealing dress and may find herself stepping into the role of Seductress. The next morning, she oversleeps and arrives late to work. She is faced with an angry matron who reprimands her severely and she immediately feels extremely small. She has become the Naughty Little Girl – and so on. Most people play out the same roles over and over again, revealing different aspects of their core personality. Other characteristics lie half hidden, only occasionally coming out to express themselves.

As long as the subpersonalities get along with each other and serve the central personality effectively, all is well. Frequently, however, they are at war, resulting in tension, frustration, anxiety and depression. To give you a simple example, one of my subpersonalities is called Ragamuffin, derived from a childhood nickname, 'Rag'. I was quite a wild kid, always outside, climbing trees, riding my bike – a real tomboy. This part of me has tremendous energy and is full of fun, but is rarely allowed to express herself. As I sit here at my desk, writing and doing research for my book, my Earnest Student is feeling thoroughly virtuous. But Ragamuffin is restless. The sun is shining outside. It is a beautiful autumn day and she wants to go and play in the garden, plant the bulbs I have bought and dream about how pretty and colourful it will look next spring. A third voice joins the dialogue in my head. It is Miss Whip. She frowns disapprovingly: 'How dare you waste so much time? Just stop all this day-dreaming and get on with your work. Don't you realise that you're falling behind schedule?' She is nasty and threatening, but she has her uses: she always makes sure I get things done in good time. Yet she can make me feel extremely anxious. Meanwhile, Ragamuffin has to wait, and wait, becoming ever more frustrated and miserable. I can only placate her by making a bargain between her and Miss Whip: after I have written 500 words, then I can go and plant a dozen bulbs. Now everyone inside is happy! I have learnt that it is very important to allow Ragamuffin to have plenty of fun, otherwise I can easily slip into depression. Also, any schedules must be manageable, preferably with plenty of leeway, so that Miss Whip has little opportunity to plague me. She is capable of driving me to panic and despair.

Regarding one's own character as a collection of subpersonalities can be a very useful aid towards self-knowledge. It may seem a bit zany at first, but giving each of them a name and a clear identity is the first step towards accepting them as important parts of you. Self-acceptance is crucial if you are to reduce inner stress levels. Also, by naming the subpersonalities, you are able to stand outside them, in the position of a non-critical Impartial Observer. You are then able to appreciate what the drives are that motivate them, and their good as well as their awkward qualities. Rather than being at their mercy, you now have the choice, the free will to decide which parts are really valuable, which need greater expression, and how to resolve their conflicts. By recognising and meeting their collective needs, you will find yourself living a much more harmonious existence. You will also find that you suddenly have available an enormous amount of untapped energy. It is exciting to experience this release!

So now it is your turn to get to know some of the crowd inside you. Your subpersonalities may not necessarily reveal themselves to you as people. They might be disguised as animals or even objects. Allow your subconscious to speak to you in the following meditative exercise. Since it is more effective to close your eyes, you may wish to record the instructions on to a tape to guide yourself through the daydream.

Beyond your mask

Sit in a quiet and comfortable place where you will not be disturbed, place two other chairs a little apart facing you, and close your eyes. Take a few deep, slow breaths and relax your body completely. Now turn your mind to your customary persona. Which part of your character do you normally present to the world? How do people usually see you? What aspects do you feel safe to show? Allow your body to take up the posture that goes with this part of your character. Exaggerate it a bit. Really get into the part. Become familiar with the facial expressions, the gestures, and the clothes. Now open your eyes, stand up and move about as this person. Again, overdo it.

Now sit down in the second chair, maintaining the character, and talk to yourself still sitting opposite you. Speak in the first person and tell yourself who you are, how you behave, how others react, what you want them to see, how you want them to feel, and what your immediate wants and deepest needs are. When you have finished, give this person a name. For example: 'I am a workaholic. I can't sit still for a minute. As I talk to you I feel agitated. I feel as if I ought to be doing something useful. I want you to see how hard I work. I need your approval. I drive fast. I can never get where I want to go quickly enough. I name myself "Driver".' Then return to the first chair as yourself and speak to your persona, acknowledging what you have heard and saying that you understand her or his needs. For example: 'I see how hard you need to work and how agitated you become. I understand that what you really need is attention and approval.'

Close your eyes and relax again. Now consider which aspects of your personality you very rarely reveal. Who is the secret you? As before, adopt the posture that goes with this hidden subpersonality and imagine clearly the gestures, expressions, clothes, age and so on. Open your eyes and, moving in character, sit in the third chair. Again, tell yourself who you are. Say as much as you can and get in touch with your deepest needs as this person. Find a suitable name. Return to the first chair and acknowledge your secret subpersonality. Say you understand and welcome her or him.

Very often, the secret subpersonality is the opposite of the revealed persona. For instance, the words might be: 'I'm a lazy good-for-nothing. All I ever want to do is lounge around in the sun. I am not a person, I'm an animal. My fur is soft and golden and I love to be petted and stroked. I need warmth and attention. I am sensuous and sinuous and I move with a feline grace. I'm a marmalade pussycat named Ginger.' If a subpersonality such as this emerges, then explore your sensuality through movement. If it feels right, stretch out on the floor or curl up in a chair. You may want to make some sounds. Experience fully what it is like to immerse yourself in this part of your character. Don't censor!

Acceptance and integration

It is likely that your outer persona was the part of your personality that received approval from authority figures when you were a child. To continue with our example, the workaholic probably earned a lot of attention and praise for high marks in examinations, while the lazy sensuous creature may have earned disapproval and become submerged. It is extremely important to accept fully your secret side. If it is not allowed expression, it will cause you great inner conflict and pain. Give it appreciation and love. Consider how it can enrich the quality of your life. Does this sensuous side of you enjoy listening to music by candlelight, say? If so, give it what it needs on a regular basis, even if it is only for half an hour twice a week.

Set up a dialogue between your persona and secret self, using the chairs as before, and sitting in the relevant one when you take on that subpersonality. You may be astonished at how much you hate yourself! Can you just hear Driver saying to Ginger: 'You lazy good-for-nothing! You're stupid, idiotic and vain. What use is it lounging around all day?' – and so on? While Ginger retorts: 'Get off my back, you bastard. I'm just going to lie here and do nothing at all . . .' The truth is that Ginger has a glowing warmth and beauty that, if allowed expression, can greatly enrich the whole personality.

Continue the dialogue, but this time let each subpersonality see and appreciate the qualities of the other, and find a way in which they can agree to get along with each other better. If necessary, use your Impartial Observer as arbitrator, to help sort out the conflicts. Ginger might say to Driver: 'OK, I know you earn me my living, and you're very good at that, but you would do it even better if you took some time off and allowed me to listen to my music.' Driver might reply: 'You've got a good point there. It's true that I'm overtired. The fact is, I'm rather envious of you. I wish I could lounge around without feeling guilty. I've got an idea – how about a week's holiday in the South of France, doing absolutely nothing at all?' Ginger: 'Wow!'

All parts of yourself are valuable. Give them the attention and time that they deserve. Even if your secret subpersonality appears threatening or nasty (like my Miss Whip), discover the useful and creative qualities and consciously express these in your life. This is the road to self-fulfilment and lower stress levels.

Another source of pain

Inner pain is not always the result of conflict between two or more subpersonalities; it can also be a persistent emotion strongly felt by one subpersonality. Your tendency may be to identify very closely with that one subpersonality, generally your persona, believing that that is who you are. You will realise by now that this is not the case; you are more than any one part of your personality and it is always possible to stand back in the role of Impartial Observer and view that part objectively.

Emotions associated with chronic stress are as follows: feeling panic-stricken, oppressed or confused; insignificant or undervalued; helpless; at a dead end, stuck or trapped; defeated; manipulated; hopeless or lacking in purpose. If you are suffering from any of these, urgent action is necessary, because your immune system is likely to be depressed.

To contact the prevailing subpersonality, relax and close your eyes in a quiet place, as before, and experience the painful emotion. Allow the feeling to rise in you. Then let an image emerge from that feeling. Don't rush. Just let it appear in its own time. See it clearly in every detail. Engage it in dialogue, using the following questions as a guide. Is there anything it wants to tell you? How do you feel about its response? Is there anything you want from this supersonality? Is there anything it needs from you? Probe as deeply as you can. Find out if it wants to give you something. Can you offer it anything? Try and reach its deepest needs.

Open your eyes and write down everything you can remember. Draw a picture of the subpersonality if you like. If you have managed to identify its need, then make a plan for meeting that need, even if it seems unreasonable. For instance, if your original feeling was of helplessness, you might have met in your fantasy a three-year-old infant whose need is to be cuddled eight hours a day! Clearly, this cannot be fulfilled, but you might make a deal with it and agree to give it undivided attention for one hour every other day. If you have a partner, ask for what you need. If not, arrange to have a massage or find ways of pampering yourself. You will discover that if you consciously meet this deep-seated need, even for a short time, feelings of helplessness will gradually recede and energy will be released.

Emergency action
If you are already suffering from a stress-induced disease, you will know that taking better care of yourself is a matter of urgency. The following is a summary of what you need to do right away.
1 Time is of the utmost importance. Somehow you must find a way of giving yourself this gift. If necessary, take sick leave – as much as possible. I took two months off work. If you are seriously ill or distressed you will need this much. At the very least, unless of course you are suffering from the boredom stressor, you must *do less*. Cut down on commitments. Get other people to do things for you. You will be amazed at how willing they are to help. Don't be diffident about asking.
2 Learn how to do physical relaxation and then progress to meditation also (described later). Gradually your anxiety levels will drop and you will discover how to control the action of the sympathetic nervous system, so that overdoses of hormones are no longer circulating uselessly in your veins, threatening the effectiveness of your immune system.
3 Know thyself. Learn to understand your inner needs through self-analysis, employing any of the methods suggested in this book.

Practise being assertive, expressing your feelings openly and asking for what you need. If you feel really stuck, go and see a counsellor. Many specialise in helping people to lower their stress levels.

4 Keep a sense of proportion about your work. Consider living more simply. You don't have to impress others by making lots of money or being perfect. You are quite all right just as you are. I sold my house in a trendy London suburb and bought another elsewhere for only half the price. By doing this, not only did I provide myself with a private income, enabling me to halve my workload, but also with clean air and country walks.

5 Get in the habit of making lists! This may seem an obvious piece of advice, but it is surprising how many people increase their burden of stress by living in an appalling state of muddle and confusion. Plan your days by writing down everything that you want to or have to do. Allow plenty of leeway. Remember to build in time for relaxation and for healing and renewal.

6 Release physical tension with exercise. After reading chapter 5 – 'Moving for Immunity' – plan a daily programme. Choose something that you enjoy.

7 Deep, restful sleep is vital. Make sure you have enough.

LETTING GO

At the beginning of the chapter you learnt what happens to your body when you are under various sorts of stress, and you will almost certainly have ticked off some of the physical symptoms on one of the lists. Stress is cumulative. If you are already in a high state of arousal something quite small may trigger off your sympathetic nervous system, causing pronounced symptoms. Conversely, the more relaxed you are in general the less likely you are to suffer from these, even when presented with similar stressors. This means that when you are relaxed, your immune system can function to maximum effect.

The importance of physical relaxation cannot be over-emphasised. If you practise this regularly you will gradually become so used to that feeling of looseness and freedom in your muscles that you will notice any tension in your body immediately. Then you can use this as a stress gauge. In my case, although I have banished virtually for ever those persistent pains in my chest, through a combination of relaxation techniques and a change of lifestyle, I just occasionally feel a slight twinge. I know instantly that a stressor is hovering around me, event though I may not be consciously aware of its origin. I use this as a signal to discover what is going on, before the situation can deteriorate.

To begin with, practise the full physical relaxation (see below) three times a day and follow it with meditation and visualisation. If you are genuinely short of time spend five minutes doing a complete relaxation just before you get up and again before going to sleep; try and fit in another session during the lunch hour. When you are sure that you can easily achieve complete relaxation you can speed up the process until you can switch it on almost instantly (see 'Quick relaxation' on p.119). Wherever you are – standing in a bus queue, talking on the telephone, in your car waiting for the traffic lights to change, and so on – and whenever you feel yourself clench your jaw, or start to wheeze or hear your heart race, then tell yourself to let go.

Remember, each time you relax groups of muscles you are also resting nerve endings and their corresponding brain function. You are also reducing your pulse rate and lowering your blood pressure, as well as slowing down your metabolic rate. In other words, the parasympathetic branch of your autonomic nervous system is taking over.

Deep muscular relaxation

You may find it best to record these instructions on a tape and talk yourself through the exercise. Alternatively, a variety of ready-made tapes on relaxation techniques can be purchased. To begin with, allow about twenty minutes to complete the exercise. You can reduce the time as you become more competent. It really is essential that you should not be disturbed, so take the phone off the hook, put a notice on the door, or just explain to everyone that you need to be quiet for a little while. Lower the light or close the curtains. Loosen any tight clothing and take off your shoes.

Sit comfortably in a chair in an upright position, making sure that your spine is straight. Place your feet flat on the floor, a little apart, and rest your hands on your lap, palms up, your fingers gently curled. Close your eyes. Make a statement to yourself such as, 'This is a time to relax and let go.' Be aware that you are giving yourself up totally to the chair and the floor. Keep your breathing calm and regular.

Now direct your attention to your feet. That is, drop your focus of awareness (which is usually in the centre of the forehead just above the eyes) right down into your feet. Become totally aware of them and feel their weight on the floor. Tense them completely by drawing the toes up and back (keep the balls of the feet where they are). Hold for a few seconds, then on an outward breath let the muscles go and drop the toes. Become conscious of how your feet feel now that they are relaxed.

Shift your attention to your calves. Tighten them by flexing your feet upwards from the ankles, keeping the heels on the floor. Focus on the tension. Then, on an out-breath, let the muscles relax. A pleasant sensation of warmth will begin to flow up your legs.

Now move to the thigh muscles and tense these by making an effort to lift your feet off the floor (without actually doing so). Hold and relax as before. Then tighten your buttock muscles by squeezing them. Hold, and relax. Become aware of the physical feeling of deep relaxation in your legs.

Turn your focus of attention to your stomach. Contract the muscles tightly, as if resisting a blow. Let go as before. Feel the relaxation spread through the whole abdominal and lower back regions.

Move to your chest. Contract the muscles here until the area feels rigid. Let go on an out-breath.

Tighten your fists, as if about to punch someone, and tense the muscles up the arms. Hold, then relax completely. (There are innumerable nerve-endings in the hands, so relaxing these is especially important.)

Raise the shoulders and pull the head down until they feel quite uncomfortable. Then enjoy the pleasurable sensation of letting go.

Clench the jaw and tighten the face muscles around the mouth, lips and lower cheeks. When you let go, allow the jaw to drop and the lips to part slightly. The tongue will fall to the floor of the mouth.

Screw up the eyes and forehead. Then relax on an out-breath as before. Allow the frown lines to melt away. (Again, there are many, many nerve endings here. Heavy lines in this area are a real sign of ongoing stress and tension.)

Keep your eyes closed for a little while longer and feel the weight of your body in the chair and on the floor. Surrender yourself. Enjoy the pleasant warmth that is flowing through your muscles.

Before continuing with your daily tasks have a good yawn and stretch. Stay calm and relaxed! If you are truly relaxed you will be able to release energy when needed, without becoming tense and anxious. The state of your body has a direct effect on your mind and psyche, as well as vice-versa.

Quick relaxation

Tense your whole body deliberately. Feel all the muscles straining. Then let them go on an outward breath, concentrating particularly on areas prone to tension. Take a couple of deep breaths.

Practise this regularly whenever you feel the tension build, whether washing up or in a crowded store. Gradually, you will gain control over your sympathetic nervous system until you can switch it off at will. The more often you practise, the more relaxed you will become and the more control you will have over your response to stress.

To test whether you are truly expert at instant relaxation, ask someone to lift your arm and then let it go; it should drop like a stone. This is a useful way to find out if you are truly letting go.

I am now so addicted to the warm, glowing sensation that relaxation gives me that I cannot do without my regular practice.

Meditation

Many people imagine that this is something mystical and peculiar and therefore not for them. Although meditation is a technique used by mystics to achieve enlightenment, it can also be employed for the more straightforward purpose of self-healing. By consciously stopping that endless chatter in your head and achieving an inner stillness, important physiological changes take place. Brain waves gradually slow down from their usual beta rhythms of conscious awareness, to the longer alpha rhythms. This is the state in which healing most naturally occurs.

Before trying meditation I was full of reservations. A voice in my head (my Critic subpersonality) kept saying, 'How boring – just sitting and doing nothing. What a waste of time!' If you have such a voice, let it have its say, then make a deal between that subpersonality and the part of you that wants to give it a go. For example: 'OK. We'll try it for ten minutes a day for five days and see what happens. But during each of those ten minutes, I am allowed to give the exercise my total concentration, unimpeded by you.'

Some people ask, 'How do I know if I am doing it correctly?' There is no right or wrong way to meditate, since it is a process, rather than a goal to be quickly achieved. However, signs that alpha waves are taking over are a floating sensation or a light pressure-band across the forehead.

The practice is very simple: you keep your thoughts on one thing only. This can be a repeated word or phrase, an object, a sound or a quality. If thoughts intrude, let them gently float away. I imagine them being captured in a bubble and wafting away over distant hills.

How to meditate

In a quiet place, take up the posture for deep muscular relaxation and let your body go totally, as described. Keeping your eyes closed, make a statement to yourself such as: 'This is a time to be still.' Now go on to practise one of the three methods suggested below.

1 Meditating on the breath

Focus your thoughts on to your breath. Go with its rhythm. Feel its rise and fall. Think of nothing but the way the air enters and leaves your body. Become at one with it.

If thoughts enter, let them float away on an out-breath. Watch them go and think of nothing but your breathing.

Maintain your concentration for ten minutes.

If you wish to continue, imagine that the rise and fall is like the sea. Picture yourself floating on the waves, rising and falling, gently moving up and down, to and fro. Feel the sensation in your body. Let the sea hold you, and surrender yourself totally to the rhythm.

Your breathing may become quite slow and shallow – a normal state during meditation.

2 Meditating with a candle

Light a candle in a darkened room and take up your position for relaxation, making sure that your spine is straight. Let your muscles go limp.

Look at the flame of the candle. Think only of this flame and nothing else. Look at its shape, its colours, the halo of light around it. Watch how it sways and flickers.

Hold your attention on the flame for five minutes.

Imagine that the flame is drawing you towards itself. You move closer and closer until finally you are absorbed by the light. The healing glow radiates through every part of your body.

Stay with this experience for as long as you wish.

3 Meditating with a word

With your eyes closed, allow a word to come into your mind; its quality should be peaceful. On every outward breath say the word, either silently to yourself, or aloud. Try 'calm', 'peace', 'stillness', 'tranquillity' or 'letting go'.

Repeat for ten minutes or longer.

The staff at the Bristol Cancer Help Centre were so positive about the beneficial effects of meditation that I found myself joining in their sessions for half an hour each morning. A counsellor led us through these. My first experience was a revelation. When I opened my eyes at the end, the room in which we sat looked dazzlingly beautiful. The large houseplant near the opposite wall was no longer just a static object; I could 'see' the energy with which it climbed and twisted itself around its supporting pole. The surface of its leaves shimmered. The carpet, which I had taken to be beige, was now filled with innumerable tiny blobs of colour, never noticed before. Paintings had a new richness and feeling of movement, and shafts of sunlight coming through the windows gave an extra intensity to the shapes of the furniture. I felt awe-struck and a little frightened. I was worried about having hallucinations or strange visions. Clearly, I was in a state of heightened awareness. Now I recognise the experience for what it is, and know that it is entirely enjoyable and completely harmless.

You may or may not have similar experiences. Unless you want to explore altered states of consciousness, then, for our purposes, it really doesn't matter. What does matter, however, is the achievement of inner calm combined with mental alertness – both highly desirable qualities if we are to function with optimum immunity.

Dr Ainslie Meares, a well-known Australian psychiatrist who has written several books on meditational techniques, has had remarkable results working with cancer patients. Intensive meditation of three hours a day or more has helped even terminal patients to go into remission.

Healing visualisation

Psychotherapists have known for some time that mental imagery can influence healing. The pioneers in this field were Carl Simonton (a radiotherapist) and his wife Stephanie, a psychotherapist, who set up the Cancer Counseling and Research Center in Dallas, Texas. They discovered that cancer patients did significantly better if their treatment was supported by images of their immune systems fighting the cancerous tumour. Patients conjured up their own protagonists, using whatever symbols worked for them. It seems that the processes of healing respond best to images straight from the unconscious, rather than to logical thought.

Since then Dr Barry L. Gruber of the Medical Illness Counseling Center in Chevy Chase, Maryland, USA, has collaborated with Dr Nicholas R. Hall of the University of Florida to evaluate the benefits of relaxation combined with imagery. For one year they tested the immune systems of adults with cancer who were regularly using these mental techniques. They were asked to create their own images of their white cells conquering the cancer. Throughout the year the doctors found that the action of the patients' lymphocytes became enhanced, that antibody production increased, that NK cells could more effectively discharge their cell poisons and that the manufacture of interleukin 2 improved (these regulate the growth of immune cells). Interestingly, if the quality and quantity of relaxation and imagery were heightened, so were the immune changes, and if they were lessened, the alterations in immunity followed suit. There is no longer any doubt that these natural therapies can be remarkably beneficial.

I quickly latched on to the technique. My T-cells were knights in gleaming silver armour with white plumes in their helmets who charged around on beautiful white mares with flowing manes and tails. They patrolled a grass-covered hill (my breast) and all the surrounding countryside, on the look-out for any wild cucumbers (cancer cells – it's best to imagine something inert than can easily be captured!). These they speared and carried off to the Queen (me), who ordered that they should be fed to the herd of white goats (my macrophages) who devoured them greedily.

To help protect my bones from secondary spread, I imagined that my skeleton was a tall tree and that my white cells were a flock of doves. They investigated every branch for little black grubs (malignant cells) and pecked up any that they found. Their droppings fell to the earth and fertilised the tree, which grew big and strong.

The best time to do these visualisations was directly after my relaxation sessions, when I felt completely calm and receptive. To reinforce their potency I also made drawings of them. The technique helped me to feel much more positive about my prognosis and I began to believe that I really could influence my own healing process – that I was the one in charge.

So, take a few minutes to go through the 'Deep muscular relaxation' (or 'Quick relaxation'), then allow your mind to come up with some healing images. Don't worry if they seem a bit bizarre at first – subconscious imagery often is. If you are suffering from an auto-immune disease, encourage your immune system to make a clear distinction between self and non-self. Perhaps your white cells are students in a classroom who are being re-educated by a very learned teacher.

Alternatively, you may prefer to use a more general healing visualisation, such as the one that is included in the meditation with a candle. Recently, I led my cancer support group through the following imaginary journey and they all found it very soothing. Record it on a tape so that you can relax and listen to it with your eyes closed.

A healing journey

Imagine you are in the country in a beautiful meadow. It may be a place that you know, or just somewhere in your imagination. The sky is a perfect blue, apart from one dark cloud that hovers above you. You know this cloud. It is a cloud of little resentments, of anger, of fears and regrets. Now you are aware that a gentle breeze is blowing. It blows towards your cloud and drives it away. You watch as your cloud becomes smaller and smaller, until it is only a tiny blob. Finally it disappears completely over the horizon.

You realize how light and free you feel, how warm the sun is on your skin, and that the meadow is filled with wild flowers. You turn around to walk to the other side, where there is a river flowing by. The water is so clear that you can see fish darting around between the stones. You decide to follow the river to its source, and take the path running along its bank. After a while you realise that you are in a valley, with hills sloping away on either side, and that the path is climbing upwards. The river narrows to a stream. You pass through a cool pine forest, where it is so quiet that all you can hear is the splashing of the stream and the sound of the gentle breeze rustling through the branches.

When you emerge on the far side you can at last see what you have been looking for – the source of the river – a spring of pure water pouring from a crevice in some granite rock. You know that this is a special place, a place of healing, where everything is clear, pure and more essential. You walk up to the spring and drink the sparkling water. You feel its energy pervading every part of your being, and you are filled with lightness and joy.

Just by the spring is a deep, clear pool. The sun is hot and you long for a swim. So you take off your clothes and step into the pool. You allow the water to flow gently over you. You know that it has the power to heal you. As you float in the pool, you imagine that the water flows through each one of your body cells and in between them. As it does this it cleanses and heals every one of them. You experience the purity of the refreshing spring water; its purity becomes your purity, its energy becomes your energy. Finally you seem to become one with the flowing spring, you are the fount itself, where all is possible and life is forever new.

You gently float across to the other side of the pool, and as you climb out the golden sunlight warms and heals you. You see a beautiful robe lying on a grassy bank. You put it on, and as you do this you know that you bring with you into the world a new resource: the power of the healing spring.

Biofeedback

Half a dozen of us sat around the large polished table in the Committee Room at the Cancer Help Centre. We were each presented with a small black box, from which extended two thin wires. At the end of these were a couple of round flat electrodes and we were invited to strap these tightly to the palm of our left hand with the elastic supplied. The metal box had two scales on the front, with a needle that swung in an arc across these when the machine was switched on. We were asked to allow the needle to settle, and then were invited to take an initial reading from one of the scales. This recorded our present state of arousal and would be compared with a similar reading at the end of the session. The second scale gave a more sensitive reading, measuring emotional state or degree of relaxation from moment to moment. The further the needle dropped to the left, the deeper our state of calm.

At first we had some fun experimenting with different thoughts. Our leader suggested that we should sit still but imagine something exciting and watch what happened to the needle. 'Sex!' shouted one young man. We all laughed aloud as our needles careered frantically to the right. 'Mother' said another, and the effect was almost as dramatic. I found this simply staggering. Here was proof indeed of the instantaneous effect that the mind has on the body. How does this happen? When we are in a state of arousal the tiny sweat glands in the skin open, causing dampness and therefore increased electrical conductivity. When we relax and become calm the opposite happens, with glands closing and the skin becoming drier, resulting in reduced conductivity. The battery-operated machine (called an ESR or Electrical Skin Resistance meter) is able to measure these subtle changes, so that the needle responds immediately to any alteration in the intensity of the emotions. I was impressed.

We were then asked to relax physically and led through a healing visualisation, such as the one described earlier. Although we were supposed to have our eyes closed, I couldn't resist peeping at the meter in front of me to see how it was responding. Yes, the needle was gradually dropping to the left as my body and mind became more deeply relaxed. Just opening my eyes caused it to jerk a little to the right. Curiosity satisfied, I allowed myself to go as deep as I could into a meditative trance, knowing that our leader was recording the meter readings for us. I began to feel light and peaceful as my brain ticked over into the slow alpha rhythms, a state of relaxed awareness.

Afterwards I was pleased with the result. My needle had dropped rapidly to a low reading, indicating an ability to relax easily at will. Clearly, this machine was a useful teaching aid. By watching the needle as I changed my thoughts, I could quickly learn which were stressful and which peaceful. By concentrating on one thing only, as in meditation, the needle always gradually dropped to a low reading. It was easy then to see how relaxed I was.

If blood pressure is taken at this point, it is found to be lower than usual, and the pulse rate is slower. It was once considered that these automatic responses were beyond conscious control and the name 'autonomic functions' was applied to them. Biofeedback proves, however, that anyone can learn to slow down the heart rate – a valuable tool for those with high blood pressure. It also proves that we can moderate the physiological effects of the fight or flight mechanism. As you will remember, a stressful situation prepares the body for action, the perspiration being the body's cooling mechanism – essential while physically exerting ourselves. Much of modern stress demands no such exertion, so it is extremely beneficial to our health to bring this response under conscious control. Thus, we do not allow damaging hormones to course uselessly around in our bloodstream, possibly preparing the way for disease.

There are other types of biofeedback machine. Some make bleeping noises when you are aroused, gradually becoming silent as you relax. The most convenient is the Healthwatch, designed at the Aston University Science Park. The watch displays numbers between zero and 99 on its small screen. High numbers indicate activity and tension, whereas lower numbers indicate relaxation and poise. A simple gauge is a special thermometer that you can tape to your finger to measure the temperature of your skin. Stress causes the blood to drain away from the skin, making it available for the big muscles in case they need it for running or fighting. Relaxation allows the blood to fill the small capillaries again, so the skin becomes warmer. You may be aware of the tingling in your fingers when you do your relaxation. Equally, you can raise the temperature simply by imagining the hands becoming warmer. This may sound like an odd sort of a party trick, but you will find it quite easy. Children are particularly good at this because they are less sceptical than adults. The remarkable things that yogis can do in the way of mind over matter, such as walking on burning coals without hurting their feet, or stopping their heart and re-starting it, come within the realms of possibility once we have had a few sessions with a biofeedback machine.

The following chart on the wall of the Committee Room encouraged us all at the Cancer Help Centre:

Tension and relaxation
Body function

Effects of tension	Body function	Effects of relaxation
up	heart rate	down
up	blood flow to muscles	down
up	oxygen usage	down
up	blood pressure	down
up	muscle tension	down
up	cortisone output	stabilised
down	blood flow to skin	up
down	blood flow to organs	up
down	food and energy reserves	up
Result		**Result**
Action of disease		Proper function of organs Healing

4 Man-made threats

WORK-PLACE HAZARDS

Shortly before finding myself with cancer, I was working in a large open-plan office, along with other editors, a couple of secretaries and several designers. It was a happy enough place and my colleagues were cheerful and friendly, but some of us suffered from a number of persistent symptoms: swollen glands, sore throats and headaches. At first we thought these were due to general tiredness, until gradually the causes became clear. Whenever designers were pasting up pages of books the lids were removed from their tins of 'COW' gum and the air became filled with a heavy vapour. Added to this were fumes from the photocopiers, which were frequently in use for long periods. The secretaries and editors contributed further to the cocktail of chemicals in the air by their lavish use of Tipp-Ex correction fluid. Here then was the source of the swollen glands and sore throats. There was a frequent plea to open windows, followed by groans from editors who found it hard to concentrate on their work against the blare of pop music from the boutiques in the street below, plus the roar of traffic with its attendant fumes. The choice seemed to be between two different kinds of pollution. The headaches were found to come from eyestrain caused by rapid flickering of the fluorescent lighting.

A condition known as 'sick building syndrome' has become a feature of modern office life. Workers afflicted by symptoms similar to mine, who have been medically tested, have been found to have several poisonous chemicals in their bloodstream. In addition to the hazardous substances that we use consciously in the course of our work, many modern furnishings made from plastics, foam and chipboard give off vapours, such as formaldehyde which causes allergies, as do carpets which are moth-proofed with pesticides. The human detoxification system has never had a chance to evolve sufficiently to cope with chemical vapours of this kind, and the body simply goes into overload. The long-term effects of low-level chemical pollution are unknown.

In America, patients suffering from office allergies are treated in a stainless-steel building entirely devoid of pollutants. They are detoxified with vigorous workouts, which expel the chemicals through perspiration. A fresh, organic diet is also given. Tests are carried out to discover which chemicals are causing the reactions, so that patients can consciously avoid these in future. In extreme cases it may mean a change of job. Thankfully, alert managements are beginning to take the syndrome seriously, and to provide a working environment which is less toxic.

As we have seen, our respiratory passages are cleverly designed to trap small dust particles and other unwanted organisms, either in the hairs inside the nose, the cilia along the windpipe and bronchi, or on the sticky mucus. These defence mechanisms were entirely adequate protection for our ancestors living in a natural, pollution-free environment. Since the industrial revolution, however, people have been increasingly crammed into cities, and man-made toxic smoke and gases have belched out into the atmosphere, affecting not only workers but the general population also. The assault regularly made on some workers' lungs, for example miners who are constantly exposed to coal and silica dust, inevitably increases the likelihood of diseases such as bronchitis. Dust extraction is the obvious solution, but in Britain only one out of five faces has such a system.

Patterns of work-related disease have changed as industry has developed. For instance, during the heyday of the Lancashire cotton industry, cancers of the groin and skin were common. It was eventually discovered that they were caused by the mineral oil used to keep the spinning machines running smoothly. Today, people employed in the petro-chemical industry are at increased risk from cancer. Surveys in America show that the highest number of bladder cancers occur in Salem County, New Jersey, where one-quarter of the employed population works in the chemical industry. High rates of cancer are also found around oil refineries.

Solvents from paint have for a long time been associated with nervous disorders. In Denmark 1,400 workers have received a state pension over the last thirteen years for 'painters' dementia', and oil-based paints are being phased out. Yet, despite a warning from the World Health Organisation that painters in general have a 40 per cent higher than average chance of contracting lung cancer, with spray painters being prone to testicular cancer, other countries have failed to act. Even more worrying is the discovery that children of painters are at increased risk of leukaemia and brain tumours.

Employees in the chrome-plating industry are also at risk from both lung and bronchial cancers at twice the rate of workers in general, from exposure to chromic acid. These fumes affect welders, too, especially in the stainless-steel industry, yet managements still fail to recognise this hazard. Perhaps the new regulations issued by the Health and Safety Commission in the UK in 1988, entitled the Control of Substances Hazardous to Health, will give more effective protection to workers in future, at least in this country.

Sadly, many people have to become ill and die, before controls are eventually brought in. Even after safety standards have been improved this may be too late for many people. Some cancers can take between fifteen to thirty years to form, and meanwhile workers can appear to have normal good health. A few years ago we decided to have our kitchen improved, and a carpenter and plumber came along to give us an estimate. They had been partners for a long time, were clearly well qualified and skilled, and their quotation was fair, so we immediately booked them to start work as soon as possible. A couple of weeks later, Denis, the carpenter, rang to say that his mate, Bill, was in hospital. There seemed to be something wrong with his lungs. Since he was a non-smoker, the doctors were mystified. He would contact me again with further news.

The following week Denis sounded very upset. Could we please find another plumber, because his mate was very ill with cancer and would probably not survive. I was appalled. An energetic and apparently perfectly healthy man in his early fifties had walked into our house only three weeks before and now he was dying of cancer. When Denis finally came to fix our cupboards and shelves we heard the whole story. The cancer was called mesothelioma and was caused by asbestos fibre. Although Bill had never worked in an asbestos factory, he recalled having welded some pipes in his early twenties which had asbestos insulation. Internal laceration and scarring caused by the inhaled asbestos dust eventually produces either asbestosis, a crippling respiratory disease, or cancer. Mesothelioma lies dormant for up to thirty years and then the tumour finally becomes active, rapidly spreading to other parts of the body and causing death within six weeks.

As with many industrial diseases, the large asbestos companies suppressed information concerning health hazards for fear of being put out of business by enormous compensation claims. The dangers of asbestosis have been recognised by specialists since the 1920s, yet it was not until 1972 that warning labels on asbestos products became mandatory in America. Meanwhile, many thousands of people have died from asbestos-related diseases.

Similarly, the high incidence of leukaemia around nuclear power stations has been noticed for some time, especially among children, yet electricity generating boards have continued to deny the dangers. During the ten years after the Lingen reactor near Niedersachsen in West Germany began operation, the surrounding population suffered 230 leukaemia deaths, 170 of which were children under fifteen. Yet in the ten years prior to its opening, only 30 leukaemia deaths were recorded. Human beings are fallible, and, despite extreme precautions, accidents such as the one at Chernobyl do occur. Workers' clothes may become contaminated from small leakages and their families are then also at risk.

It was not until February 1990 that a definite link between leukaemia and nuclear plants was finally established by scientists in a study led by Professor Martin Gardner of Southampton University. They discovered that the fathers of four out of five victims of leukaemia and lymphoma in the region of Seascale in Cumbria were employed at Sellafield nuclear reprocessing plant. Immediately before their children's conception, the workers had received higher doses of external ionising radiation than their matched controls. The risk was greatest for fathers who had received total doses of more than 100 milliSieverts (approximately fifty times the level of natural background radiation). The conclusion is that the radiation causes a genetic mutation in the men's sperm.

I myself was brought up in the north-west of England, within striking distance of Sellafield, then Windscale. None of us knew that, in the fifties, local milk had become contaminated by radiation. The authorities were quick to hush up the affair. Perhaps that contributed to my susceptibility to cancer. Who knows?

In addition to the nuclear, chemical and pharmaceutical industries, the toxic-waste-disposal and the microwave and electricity industries also have poor safety records. In 1973 the medical journal the *Lancet* published an editorial which accused 'a sinister complex of big industrial manufacturing firms' of being mainly concerned with their own profits and 'indifferent to the health of exposed workers'. Apart from deliberately flouting health and safety regulations, they 'set up supposedly independent research institutes whose scientists seem always to find evidence to support the stance taken by the firm, despite massive contrary evidence'. Indeed, the vast majority of indictments brought against industrial companies are for breaking anti-pollution laws or for ignoring regulations concerning the safety and the health of their workers.

Some of the stories are hair-raising. At the Kerr-McGee Nuclear Facility in Cimarron, Oklahoma, where fuel rods were made for a 'fast' breeder reactor, many workers had no idea that plutonium causes cancer. There were incidents of pipes leaking, spilling plutonium solution on to the floor. Protective rubber gloves had holes in them. One teenager brought a popgun to work and fired uranium dioxide fuel pellets at his colleagues for fun. A bag of plutonium waste burst into flames and spewed radioactive dust into the air, contaminating workers. Uranium dust covered the floor of the plant. Yet the management was unwilling to stop production so that the place could be cleaned up. Plutonium, as it decays, emits 'alpha particles' which are charged nuclei of helium. These travel at thousands of miles per second. Any cell that is hit by an alpha particle is bound to suffer irreversible biological damage.

Millions of people worldwide are exposed to hazardous materials at their place of work. At the very least, it is estimated that 4 per cent of all cancers are caused by workplace exposure, mainly to chemicals, and that means 6,000 unnecessary deaths in Britain alone. Some experts put this figure a great deal higher. It isn't worth being blasé and hoping that nothing will happen to you. Make sure that health and safety regulations are carefully followed.

RADIATION

Much of the radiation we are subject to is natural and comes from the sun. There is also low-level radioactivity emanating from the earth and from cosmic rays. Small doses of sunlight are good for us and actually stimulate our immune systems, but too much – especially of ultraviolet radiation – has the reverse effect. The fragile ozone layer miles above us in the stratosphere acts as a shield against harmful UV radiation, but chlorine and bromine produced from gases such as CFCs (chlorofluorocarbons) which humans have recklessly released into the atmosphere, mainly from aerosol cans and refrigerators, are now causing holes to appear in it. A mere 1 per cent depletion of the ozone layer will lead to an extra 70,000 cases of skin cancer per year worldwide, yet losses are predicted to soar to 30 per cent by AD 2000. Tests carried out in 1992 already show a 15 per cent depletion over Europe in winter. The lowered efficiency of the human immune system that will occur as a result of increased UV exposure will also make people more susceptible to other skin disorders, parasite attacks and hepatitis, in addition to cataracts and other eye problems. Wild and domestic animals will suffer similarly.

While superficial skin cancers are curable, advanced malignant melanoma is not. The symptom of this disease is simply a mole that changes colour or size, or that bleeds. Shades of red, blue or white are colours to watch for. Fair people who live close to the equator are at particular risk. In Queensland, Australia, melanoma rates are particularly high. Even in Scotland, the disease has increased by 5 per cent each year over the last two decades. To preserve yourself from this fatal disease, always avoid going out in intense midday sun. Use screening lotions and expose yourself only very gradually to sunlight, especially if you are untanned. The sun itself does not cause the cancer, but acts rather as a 'cocarcinogen'. Added to other damage to the skin, the action of hormones, inherited factors, chemicals in the air and stress, malignant melanoma can take hold.

Radiation suppresses the immune system by destroying the B-cells, which, as you will remember from chapter 1, are responsible for antibody production. The extent of the damage depends on both the duration of exposure and its intensity. The horrifying after-effects of ionising radiation caused by the atomic bombs dropped on Nagasaki and Hiroshima in August 1945 have been well documented. At 500 rems most human beings die; at 300 rems the immune system is grossly impaired; at 100 rems severe radiation sickness is evident – vomiting and nosebleeds. Those who survive such doses initially usually die later from cancer and leukaemia. 'Safe' limits of radiation are still disputed. In the late 1920s it was 73 rems, but half a century later, it was down to 5. In 1987 the National Radiological Protection Board of the UK recommended that no worker should receive more than 15 milliSieverts (1½ rems) a year, yet the legal limit is still set much higher at 50 milliSieverts (5 rems). The maximum safe dose for a member of the public was put at only 5 milliSieverts (½ rem). During that year more than 1,100 workers at Sellafield nuclear reprocessing plant received annual doses above 15 milliSieverts. Some scientists maintain that there is no safe limit of exposure.

Why then is radiation used in the treatment of cancer? I received approximately 5,000 rads (a measurement of absorbed dose) over a six-week period, carefully calculated to cover only the affected area and nearby lymph nodes. Considering that a normal X-ray uses less than 1 rad, you can appreciate how much radiation I received. Indeed, if only a fraction had been given over my entire body, it would have killed me. Cancer cells divide more rapidly than healthy ones and are essentially weaker, so they are destroyed by the radiation, while many healthy ones can recover. Radiotherapy may not necessarily provide a total cure, but it does at least delay recurrence. On the other hand, there is some evidence to show that the treatment actually causes leukaemia at a later stage. I am well aware how damaging radiotherapy is. Doctors have to weigh up the risks of cancer treatment against the likely prognosis. My friend Jennifer postponed her radiotherapy out of sheer fright and the cancer spread into her lymphatic system. I stood by helplessly as the disease affected her bones and then her lungs. Within two and a half years she was dead.

Different kinds of radiation are gauged along the 'electromagnetic spectrum', starting with extremely low-frequency (ELF) waves which are generated, for instance, by high-voltage power lines. Then come microwaves, infra-red radiation, visible light, UV radiation and X-rays, with gamma rays (emitted after nuclear reactions) at the top end.

The term 'non-ionising' is used to describe sources of low-frequency radiation. This means that the waves are unable to create charged particles in the material through which they pass. They can cause electrical shocks or burning, but are otherwise considered to be harmless. Evidence has been accruing, however, to show that micro-wave exposure, even below the present 'safety' limit of 5 milliwatts per square centimetre of exposed flesh, can cause other kinds of long-term damage, including cataracts, decreased fertility, cancer, genetic damage and birth defects. The Russians have recognised the dangers of low-frequency radiation for a long time. Their safety limit for workers is 0.01 milliwatts per square centimetre, and is ten times stricter for civilians.

An extraordinary story emerged from the United States in 1972. The CIA had discovered in 1965 that the US embassy in Moscow was being irradiated at a level of 4 milliwatts. Since this was well within their own safety limits (at that time 10 milliwatts), nothing was done about it. However, in 1975, blood tests on staff revealed that the counts of white lymphocytes were 40 per cent higher than normal. Shortly afterwards the ambassador resigned, suffering from a rare blood disorder. Two of his predecessors had died of cancer and three embassy children were flown home to be treated for leukaemia-like conditions. The blood of four embassy officials showed chromosome changes, and babies born to embassy women suffered from unusually high rates of deformity.

A study in Alabama has also shown a link between microwaves and genetic damage. At Fort Rucker there is a US army base where helicopter pilots are trained, and there are forty-six radar installations within a thirty-mile radius. Radar generally uses ultra-high frequency pulsed signals from the microwave range of the electromagnetic spectrum. Because helicopter pilots fly at low altitudes, they are continually exposed to radar waves. Between July 1969 and November 1970 seventeen of their children were born with congenital clubfoot, well over four times the expected rate. Other children were born with abnormalities of the heart. After this, the army blocked further research, saying that radar levels to which pilots were exposed were a military secret.

Modern studies increasingly demonstrate that an illness such as cancer cannot be explained by chemistry alone, but that electrical fields within cells also play a role. Scientists have been aware for some years that minute electrical currents in the body help to control biological activities. If, then, this natural electrical microenvironment is interfered with from outside sources, inappropriate responses may be triggered. This explains how low-frequency electromagnetic radiation could lead to biological degradation and long-term genetic damage. Indeed, Russian surveys of electricity workers and experiments with mice substantiate this view.

'Electrical smog' is the term given to this invisible menace that we are all exposed to in the developed world. Television transmitters, radar installations, satellites, microwave ovens, CB radios and high-voltage power lines are all contributors. It has been calculated that the average American is subject to a daily dose of electromagnetic radiation that is 200 million times more powerful than that received from natural sources.

If we wish to keep our immune systems healthy, therefore, it is as well to avoid living near radar installations or overhead power lines, and not to spend too much time in front of the television. At any rate, sit well back from the screen. The safety of microwave ovens is still suspect. They have a history of leaking microwaves way above even American safety limits. Children should certainly never be allowed near them. Is it really worth risking possible long-term biological damage for the sake of speed and convenience of cooking?

CHEMICAL POLLUTION

If someone were to test your body fats right now, they would find traces of pesticide stored there – and not just one or two varieties, but several hundred. Each year, an estimated 2 billion tons of pesticides are sprayed on crops, as well as on forests and grasslands the world over. In our houses they are used to prevent woodworm and fungi, and they are in our carpets, clothes and upholstery to keep away the moths. Indeed, they are now global contaminants. They are found in human sperm, in fertilised eggs and in unborn foetuses. Even after babies are born, they drink their mothers' milk which is contaminated with pesticides. Dieldrin, known to cause cancer and for some time banned in the US, but on sale in Britain until March 1989, has been found in the milk of Western mothers at seven times the safety limit set by the World Health Organisation. Before banning dieldrin, the US Food and Drugs Administration carried out a survey on this pesticide: it was found in every human tested, in 96 per cent of all meat, fish and poultry, in 90 per cent of air samples, and in 85 per cent of dairy products. It is also found in rain and tap water. Rivers are badly polluted. A recent survey in south-west England showed that eels in the River Newlyn contain more than 200 times the amount of dieldrin thought to be safe for human consumption.

So where can we go to escape contamination? The answer is, nowhere. Traces of pesticide are even found in the bodies of Antarctic penguins. How can our livers and kidneys and poor beleaguered immune defences go on coping with such a barrage of poisonous, artificial substances? Of the pesticides currently in use

89 have been linked with allergies or skin irritation; more than 40 have been linked with cancer, 61 with mutagenic effects (alteration in hereditary material of cells), and 31 with teratogenicity (birth defects). In the Third World, at least 500,000 people suffer severe poisoning from pesticides every year and of these 5,000 actually die.

Between 1962 and 1970 the US air force sprayed 500,000 acres of crops and approximately 4.5 million acres of forest in Vietnam. This was intended to expose Viet Cong guerillas and ruin their food supplies. The spray was known as 'Agent Orange' and contained phenoxy-herbicides, 2,4,5-T and 2,4-D which had been developed during the Second World War. These powerful chemicals promote uncontrolled cell division – in other words, they give plants cancer. Despite assurances from the Pentagon that the spraying of Vietnamese land was 'not dangerous to man or animals', by 1969 birth defects were being recorded. In the Hue district of North Vietnam, stillbirth rates rose to almost 50 per cent and congenital abnormalities were found in 7.4 per cent of those born alive. Additionally, cases of Down's Syndrome increased. In Saigon, the incidence of spina bifida multiplied thirteenfold between 1966 and 1967, and cleft palates increased similarly. Teratogenicity has thus been established. Eventually, the US Environment Protection Agency placed a ban on the use of 2,4,5-T for spraying forests, roadside verges and public open spaces, after evidence from Alsea in Oregon suggested that it was causing miscarriages. Yet it is still used by the Forestry Commission in the UK. Additionally, tests on rats carried out by the US Food and Drugs Administration concluded that 2,4-D was a carcinogen. Today you can walk down to your local garden shop and buy any popular lawn herbicide and it will almost certainly contain 2,4–D. In Britain, most of the controls regarding the sale and use of pesticides are voluntary, surely an unacceptable system, considering the dangers involved.

Of the insecticides, the most persistent are those in the organochlorine group, including DDT, dieldrin and HCH. They are insoluble in water and slow to break down in the environment, and they build up in the fatty tissues of animals until such a high level is reached that death results. This happens especially in winter among certain species, when the fats – and the pesticides – are mobilised. The process continues for many years, even after spraying has stopped. Peregrine falcons were severely affected in the 1950s and '60s, and dieldrin has brought about the decline of the British otter. Paraquat, a highly toxic herbicide, has caused the deaths of thousands of hares eating treated stubble.

All insecticides kill indiscriminately, so that natural predators are destroyed along with the pests. When eventually the pests develop immunity to the chemicals – as is happening now – disease is of course rapid and widespread. And so the crops must be sprayed yet again, and our food becomes more and more contaminated. Some crops receive up to twelve treatments. It is likely that the fruit and vegetables that you eat over the next year will have had approximately one gallon of harmful pesticides and herbicides sprayed on them. And the effects on the body are cumulative.

If certain pesticides are banned in the West, they are simply exported to Third World countries, where controls are less stringent. Back it comes to us in food imported from those countries. The moral of all this is to eat organic food and, ideally, grow your own vegetables. We now know for sure that 1 per cent of all cancers are caused by chemicals in our food. Long-term use of pesticides will aggravate this situation and contribute to the number of stillbirths, genetic defects and the degradation of our environment.

You may have been persuaded by clever advertising that 'whiter than white' is synonymous with cleanliness and good hygiene. The truth is that the dioxins used in the bleaching process are seriously threatening our health. Since they are particularly used to turn wood pulp white for paper, they reach us directly from milk cartons, coffee filters, tea bags, sanitary towels and babies' nappies. In June 1989, a disturbing report was released by a UK government team set up to study the effects of dioxins on human health. The report revealed that levels in the breast milk of British mothers were 100 times the government's own guidelines. One dioxin, TCDD, is 70,000 times more poisonous than cyanide to some mammals. It is a potent carcinogen and severely affects the immune system, particularly while it is still developing in infants. It seems tragic that we can no longer guarantee our babies maximum immunity at the start of their lives.

DUMPING

During the summer of 1953, cats in the fishing town of Minamata, Japan, seemed to be suffering from a strange disease: they had difficulty in walking. A few months later, local residents were affected by convulsions, lack of coordination and blindness. In all, an estimated 6,000 people were affected; 43 residents subsequently died and 68 were incapacitated with cerebral palsy. Several years passed by before the cause was finally discovered: mercury poisoning from eating contaminated fish. Where was it coming from? Despite strenuous denials from the nearby chemical plant, part of the Chisso Corporation, investigators found out that the company had been discharging mercury in its effluent.

Every year Britain disgorges more than a million tonnes of domestic and industrial waste into the North Sea alone. We have heard in recent years of the disastrous effect on the immune systems of seals that this has had, with at least 17,000 dying from a vicious viral infection. Many of the chemicals discharged do not kill marine life outright but lead to disorientation, behavioural defects, reduced fertility and long-term genetic impairment. This kind of damage is impossible to assess. What we do know is that our seas are dying.

Some wastes decompose, but others, such as heavy metals and chlorinated chemicals like DDT, build up in the environment. Recently, in Wood Spring, North Devon, residents were warned not to eat more than four ounces of shellfish per week, or they would be exceeding the safety limit for the intake of cadmium set by the WHO. This metal is a powerful immunosuppressant. It impairs the response of B- and T-cells, of antibodies and phagocytes. Generally, shellfish and inshore flat-fish are the most likely to be polluted and therefore best avoided.

As far as dumping on land is concerned, not even Harwell, the principal UK Government research body dealing with hazardous wastes, knows exactly how much is disposed of, by whom, what it consists of or even where it has been buried, although a register of some suspect sites is currently being compiled. It is estimated that some 5 million tonnes per year are involved. Some wastes will eventually become harmless through natural biological processes, while others are excessively toxic and have to be specially isolated from the environment for very long periods. Unfortunately, it is impossible to guarantee absolute containment because there is always a chance that some chemicals and heavy metals will eventually leach from the site and find their way into water supplies.

One of the worst tragedies involving dumping took place at Love Canal near the Niagara Falls. A housing estate had been built on a former dump there, believed to be securely sealed with clay. Yet noxious fumes had been noticed in basements. Then, after prolonged snow falls in 1978, a thick black slime appeared over gardens and 235 families had to be evacuated. Analysis revealed that at least 10 per cent of the contaminating chemicals were carcinogenic, mutagenic or teratogenic. Indeed, between 1974 and 1978 almost half the children born in the worst-affected areas were deformed. By 1980, a report claimed that 30 per cent of the residents were suffering from rare chromosomal aberrations. America was shocked, especially when it was disclosed that 90 per cent of hazardous wastes were being disposed of 'improperly, unsafely and irresponsibly'. As many as 34,000 other sites could eventually cause significant environmental problems.

It is as well to know what your house has been built on before moving in to it. In Willow Tree Lane Estate, Ealing, West London, residents have complained of skin and stomach disorders, blaming them on chemicals previously dumped on the site. Yet the local authority refutes these charges and refuses to act.

THE NITRATE TIME BOMB

Nitrates are naturally occurring substances essential for the growth of plants. They can also be produced artificially as fertilisers and their use is now widespread, with some 1,200,000 tonnes applied to farmland each year in Britain alone. Compost and sewage sludge, also used as fertiliser, contribute even more nitrates. Added to this, they have been released in vast quantities through the ploughing up of grassland. Nitrates are thus finding their way into our drinking water in ever-increasing quantities, either from sewage effluents, from the run-off of fertilisers from agricultural land, or from their gradual seepage into underlying rock strata. When they reach the water table, the results on health could be very serious indeed. Nitrate levels in rivers are rising rapidly. In the ten years between 1965 and 1975 tests showed that they had more than doubled in the River Lea, which supplies water to North London.

One problem with nitrates is that they are believed to cause stomach cancer. When they are absorbed from drinking water, bacteria in the digestive tract convert them into a similar compound called nitrite. This can combine with chemicals in food to produce substances called N-nitrosamines, which cause stomach cancer in laboratory animals.

Nitrites also combine with haemoglobin, the chemical in the bloodstream that conveys oxygen from the lungs to other parts of the body. A serious condition called methaemoglobinaemia can follow, in which the person becomes starved of oxygen. In babies this can be fatal.

A healthy immune system depends on the cardiovascular system being in excellent condition. Anything that affects the blood adversely also affects immunity. It is known that malignant cells flourish in an environment low in oxygen, so nitrates are especially bad news for cancer patients.

You can test your own drinking water for nitrates very simply yourself. The appropriate tablets and instructions are available from shops that sell tropical aquaria.

ACID RAIN

There are two major components of acid rain: nitrogen oxide and sulphur dioxide. The first is steadily pumped out of the exhaust pipes of cars and lorries and is converted into nitric acid in the atmosphere. The second results from the burning of oil and coal, with power stations contributing the most from their tall chimney stacks. Sulphur dioxide forms into an acid when dissolved in water. We all know the disastrous effects that acid rain has on trees and buildings. Rather less publicity is given to the effect on our drinking water and to the pollution of fish.

Britain emits around 3.8 million tonnes of sulphur dioxide every year, more than any other country in Western Europe. Much of it is driven by prevailing winds over the North Sea to Scandinavia and the Netherlands. Here it falls into the lakes, making them so acid that they are no longer able to support life. Lakes in Norway and Sweden are particularly susceptible to damage as many of them have no limestone to act as a neutralising agent. The acid causes poisonous heavy metals to leach from the rocks, including lead, cadmium, zinc and mercury, and especially aluminium which is lethal to fish. In humans, heavy metals, when ingested, cause serious impairment of all aspects of immune functioning. The numbers of T-cells drop, the natural protection given by bodily fluids (humoral immunity) becomes less efficient and the ability of cells to gobble up invaders (phagocytosis) becomes depressed. We are thus left more vulnerable to infections, cancer and auto-immune diseases. Additionally, the brain and nervous system can be affected by heavy-metal pollution, especially in children, and aluminium is a known cause of Alzheimer's disease, resulting in disorientation and loss of memory. By 1982, the mercury levels in fish were so high in 100 Swedish lakes that fishing had to be banned.

Luckily it is possible to avoid serious damage to your own health. Filters help to remove heavy metals from drinking water, so do use them. It is best not to eat freshwater fish, since the chance of pollution is fairly high. Deep-sea fish are much less likely to be contaminated.

SMOKE AND EXHAUST FUMES

Sulphur dioxide was largely to blame for the deaths of 4,000 people in the terrible London smog of 1952. Since then, the Clean Air Act of 1956 has dramatically reduced the amount of coal smoke in the atmosphere, and hence the mortality rates from bronchitis and other respiratory diseases. Instead, our cities are now severely affected by traffic exhaust fumes, and the existing law in the UK covering this kind of pollution is laughable. In 1963 forty-eight observers were asked to sit by the roadside and decide how much smoke they found acceptable, and their subjective opinions became the basis for legislation. Health factors were given no consideration. By contrast, federal laws in the USA enforce stricter standards.

The sunshine state of California now leads the way, with tough new regulations to curb the gas-guzzlers, and the onus will be on employers to reduce the number of car journeys to work by organising car pools for four-day weeks. Special car-pool lanes are already being provided on major highways to encourage the sharing of vehicles, and the building of any new drive-in establishments is likely to be banned. Smog in southern California is so bad that 98 per cent of the population suffers from its ill-effects, ranging from stinging eyes and headaches to heart attacks and early death. Children brought up in the most polluted areas have a reduction in lung capacity of up to 15 per cent. In 1988 school children and those suffering from respiratory diseases were advised to stay indoors on a total of 75 days. On more than 200 days of 1990, people inhaled air that exceeded nationwide health standards, despite the fact that catalytic converters on car exhausts became compulsory in the 1970s. The Air Quality Management Plan aims to cut pollution five-fold over the next twenty years to protect human health.

After a long battle initiated by pressure groups and plenty of incriminating evidence, lead is at last being phased out of fuel in Europe, with unleaded petrol on sale in Britain at a lower price than leaded, as an extra incentive to have cars converted. For many people the damage has already been done, the average city-dweller containing 500 times more body lead than his or her ancestors. As we have seen, in addition to brain damage, high lead levels impair immunity by inhibiting B- and T-cell proliferation and reducing the effectiveness of phagocytes to gobble up invaders.

Even without lead, we are still left with several other noxious gases, namely carbon monoxide, nitrogen oxides and hydrocarbons. The faster the cars go, the more they spew out. It is calculated that between 2,000 and 3,000 city-dwellers die each year in England and Wales alone from lung cancer due to the inhalation of exhaust fumes. Many others suffer from asthma and bronchitis aggravated by the millions of minuscule particles that carry the toxic hydrocarbons. These cause damage to the membranes in the respiratory passages and the effectiveness of the mast cells which line their surfaces is reduced. Mast cells secrete vital immunoglobulins, specialised forms of antibody that fight specific pathogens. They also contain memory granules. Damage to the mast cells results in memory loss, so that more pathogens or pollutants are likely to gain a hold. One of the hydrocarbons is benz-a-pyrene, which is a carcinogen – the same one found in cigarette smoke. 'Lean burn' engines reduce the amounts of carbon monoxide and nitrogen oxide, but only three-way catalytic converters control hydrocarbons. Fumes from diesel engines are particularly high in hydrocarbons, resulting in an increased risk of bladder cancer to drivers of buses, taxis and lorries.

Carbon monoxide in the bloodstream damages its oxygen-carrying capacity. It is reckoned that an hour spent breathing in heavy city traffic fumes is as bad as smoking four cigarettes in the same time.

In fact cigarette smoke is very similar to traffic fumes in terms of damage to health. Rather than lead, cigarettes contain cadmium; both of these heavy metals are zinc antagonists and zinc, of course, is vital to healthy immunity. It is needed for tissue building and for the production of lymphocytes. Take zinc supplements, therefore, if you are exposed to pollution from either cigarette smoke or traffic fumes. Cadmium absorption increases the risk of vascular disease for both smokers and non-smokers alike.

Altogether there are more than 200 toxins in tobacco smoke. Apart from lung cancer, bronchitis, heart and circulatory diseases, it increases the risk of cancers of the liver, pancreas and cervix. It changes the balance of enzyme activity in the digestive tract and adversely affects the detoxification systems of the liver. The smoke causes excess mucus to form in the air passages and it paralyses the tiny cilia, which have a cleansing function. As with vehicle fumes, mast cells are damaged.

So, if you value your life, stay away from traffic fumes, don't smoke, and avoid other smokers like the plague.

Many people do not realise that smoke from neighbourhood bonfires can also harm the health, especially if plastics are involved. These should be specially incinerated at a high temperature, otherwise they emit dangerous dioxins, the same type of chemical that caused such an appalling disaster at Seveso in northern Italy, where there was an explosion at a chemical plant in 1976. Congenital abnormalities have been the result of that accident.

HOW POLLUTED IS YOUR ENVIRONMENT?

	YES	NO
A *Where do you live?*		
1 Near a chemical plant?		
2 Near a nuclear power station?		
3 In a city?		
4 In an intensively farmed area?		
5 On a former tip?		
6 On granite rock?		
7 Close to overhead power lines?		
B *How do you keep your home warm?*		
1 With untreated coal?		
2 Gas fires?		
3 Calor gas fires?		
4 Paraffin heaters?		
5 Formaldehyde cavity-wall insulation?		
C *What do you clean your home with?*		
1 Ammonia-based cleaners?		
2 Disinfectants?		

	YES	NO

3 Commercially produced oven cleaner?

4 Lavatory cleaner and/or block deodorant?

5 Drain cleaner?

6 Carpet and upholstery cleaners?

7 Furniture and floor polish?

8 Metal polishes?

9 Mothballs?

10 Room fresheners?

11 Washing powders, detergents and conditioners containing enzymes, optical whiteners, bleaches, or synthetic perfumes or colourings?

12 Fly killers?

13 Flea killers, including pet collars?

14 Dry cleaning of clothes and soft furnishings?

D *Do you beautify yourself with hazardous chemicals?*

1 Anti-perspirant?

2 Hair dye or bleach?

3 Permanent waving?

4 Hair sprays or mousses?

5 Soaps, shampoo or conditioner with synthetic colourings or perfumes?

E *Do you use toxic chemicals for DIY?*

1 Glues?

2 Paint stripper?

3 Brush cleaner?

4 Paint thinners?

5 Paints and varnishes, especially if they contain asbestos or lead?

6 Wood treatment?

F *How do you furnish your home?*

1 With vinyl, eg. for seat coverings?

2 Soft plastic tablecloths, shower curtains?

3 Are your carpets new?

G *How does your garden grow?*

1 With weedkillers?

2 Insecticides?

	YES	NO
3 Fungicides?		
H *Do you work with hazardous materials?*		
1 For instance in the petrochemical, pharmaceutical, nuclear, asbestos, electricity-supply, or waste-disposal industries?		
2 With radar?		
3 Down a mine, or in a dusty atmosphere?		
4 As a farmer, or forester?		
5 In damp proofing and insect control?		
6 Are you a taxi, bus, or lorry driver?		
7 Any other type of work that involves exposure to noxious fumes, dust, radiation or hazardous chemicals and waste?		
8 In a 'sick' office building?		
9 Do you drive to work, or on the job?		
10 Is your journey to work congested and fumy?		
SCORE		

Assessment

A All of these locations can be sources of pollution. In addition to the problems already discussed, granite can release an invisible inert gas called radon, thought to be responsible for up to 1,500 cases of lung cancer each year in the UK. You could have an impermeable floor installed to keep it out. If you have answered 'yes' to one of the others, then you will have to balance the advantages of the area against the health risks.

B 1 to 4 all emit smoke and/or fumes containing toxins. They also use up life-giving oxygen. Keep rooms well ventilated; preferably consider alternatives. Have you ticked 'yes' to 5? Formaldehyde gives off noxious fumes which can cause allergic reactions, so a good flow of fresh air is vital.

C Nearly all commercial cleaners, even some of those that claim to be 'environment friendly', are toxic and many are also irritants. Ecover products are not, so use these when practicable. Here are other harmless alternatives:

1 Use baking soda and water, or a mixture of vinegar, salt and water.

2 Dissolve a little borax in some water.

3 Baking soda and water.

4 Vinegar, baking soda, or mild detergent.

5 Use a plunger, then flush with a mixture of boiling water with 2 tbsp vinegar and the same amount of baking soda.

6 Rub salt into stains and use a mild detergent to clean up. For a general clean, sprinkle cornflour all over, then vacuum up.

7 Beeswax is the traditional furniture polish. Linseed oil gives a good finish too.

8 Silver can be cleaned by soaking in boiling water with baking soda, salt and some aluminium foil. Two tablespoons of vinegar and one of salt dissolved in 1 pint/570 ml warm water work well on brass. To shine, rub with vegetable oil.

9 Thyme or cedar chips are effective.

10 How about opening the windows?

11 Ecover washing powders are made from harmless ingredients. Other varieties can cause allergies, especially those with enzymes. Some perfumes and colourings are irritants. Detergents produce 'free radicals' that interfere with genes during cell division, so don't use for washing up. Soap flakes are much safer. Rinse well.

12 Dangerous to people as well as flies. Swat them instead, or shoo them outside. An obliging spider weaves a web near a light and catches most of mine for me!

13 Pet shops now sell non-toxic flea collars. Eucalyptus and mint are traditional repellants.

14 They will continue to give off noxious fumes for several weeks, so avoid drycleaning where possible.

D 1 to 4 often contain harmful chemicals which are absorbed into the system through the skin and hair follicles. Some are carcinogens, notably hair dyes, and others can cause allergic reactions. Anti-perspirants contain aluminium salts that clog the pores and interfere with the normal function of the sweat glands. As we have seen, this metal is a cause of Alzheimer's disease. As for aerosols, for example hair sprays, these give off halocarbon vapour, the same gas emitted by solvents. So stick to natural ways of cleaning and beautifying yourself. There's nothing to beat soap and water. Some make-ups are non-allergenic and are advertised as such.

E Solvents found in 1 to 5 give off heavy vapours that can irritate the throat and lungs. Memory loss can be another consequence. Do not leave tops off unnecessarily and make sure the area is well ventilated. Chemicals breathed in end up in the bloodstream.

5 Use emulsion paint in preference to gloss. It doesn't contain lead. Avoid using a blow lamp or power sander on old paintwork which will contain lead. If you inhale this it will adversely affect your immune system.

6 Particularly avoid any that contain the deadly chemical lindane, thought to have caused cancer and leukaemia in some workers. Permethrin is less hazardous. Follow safety instructions carefully.

F All of these give off noxious vapours. Very poisonous gases are released from PVC when it is attacked by a fungus that flourishes in warmth and moisture, a likely cause of cot deaths. Avoid 1 and 2.
Ventilate rooms that have new carpets, which will contain moth-proofing.

G None of these are necessary and all are extremely toxic, many being linked with cancer, damage to genetic material in cells, and birth defects. Some herbicides contain 2,4-D, now known to be the cause of higher than normal incidence of non-Hodgkin's lymphoma in farm workers. Switch to organic gardening and keep weeds down with mulching material such as straw or bark. Encourage pest predators, for example birds and frogs. Soapy water helps to control aphids. Otherwise pyrethrum and borax are acceptable pesticides in small amounts.

H These hazards are covered in the main text. Here again, especially if you have a history of immune-deficiency diseases in the family, weigh the advantages against the health risks. Even a drop in salary is worth considering for better health.

Scoring
Count up the number of times you have ticked 'yes' and assess your rating as follows:
26 and over Your environment is extensively contaminated and therefore immunity-depleting. There is no need to use so many chemicals in the home. Cut down wherever you can. This is particu-larly important if you are exposed to pollution for long periods, for

instance at work. Your body is likely to be suffering from overload, and if it isn't already complaining it soon will.

19 to 25 Exposure to pollution is still too high. See how quickly you can adjust your score to below 19.

10 to 18 You have a certain consciousness about the hazards of chemicals, but there is still room for improvement.

9 and below Well done! Your home is relatively pollution-free. If you have also ticked 'no' to **A** and **H**, then your environment is likely to be immunity-enhancing.

5 Moving for immunity

Among our group at the Cancer Help Centre was an energetic young woman who, despite her illness – or perhaps because of it – dressed herself in her track suit each morning and went for a jog before breakfast. I was much in awe of her self-discipline, especially as it was a cold December, and promised myself each day that I would join her. But when the moment came to climb out of bed half an hour earlier than absolutely necessary, my resolve faltered and I snuggled even deeper under my cosy duvet. So I am doubly proud of the fact that, while working on this book, not only do I spend ten minutes first thing in the morning on exercises for flexibility and strength, but I also set aside part of each afternoon to do something physical in the fresh air for at least an hour, perhaps energetic digging on my allotment, or a bike ride – making sure I stay in the saddle up every hill – or a combination of quick walking and jogging. (I have made it a rule never to go by car for journeys of less than three miles; either I walk or I cycle.) If I am short of time, I skip.

To help our immune systems do their job effectively it really is important to work the heart and lungs and get the circulation moving. You will know this is happening when you start to go pink in the face, to puff and pant, and perspire. But, please, take it easy if you are unfit. If necessary, check with your doctor before embarking on vigorous exercise, always start with a gentle warm-up and avoid being too ambitious at first. You can gradually increase the amount of energy you expend and the length of time that you exercise.

This 'aerobic' exercise, as it is called, is the best way of sending fresh oxygen to the body's tissues. It also increases the efficiency of the lymphatic drainage system, so that toxins are less likely to collect and create a suitable breeding ground for invading pathogens. Many organisms that cause disease characteristically thrive in a stagnant environment that is lacking in oxygen. Conversely, a good supply of fresh air boosts our immune defences. It is now established that cancer cells are less likely to survive in well-oxygenated tissues.

Oxygen is vital to our survival. The air that we breathe in comes into close contact with the bloodstream in the lungs. Here the blood vessels are so thin that the haemoglobin within the red cells is able to attach to the oxygen chemically, and then transports it to every part of the body. Humans can survive for only a very short time without oxygen. If someone suffers a cardiac arrest there are only three minutes in which to get the heart going again by applying mouth-to-mouth resuscitation and cardiac massage. Otherwise the patient will die. The same applies to a drowning person. During a stroke, part of the brain is deprived of blood and therefore of oxygen. The cells quickly die, or are so badly damaged that the result is often paralysis.

Oxygen is also needed to create energy from the food we eat. As much as half our energy supply keeps our body just ticking over, and is used for breathing, for the pumping of the heart, for metabolism and for the health of our muscles and other tissues. The red, oxygen-rich blood travels from the lungs via the arteries, which form a network of smaller arterioles, and these in turn subdivide into minute capillaries. The walls of the capillaries are permeable, and the oxygen and nutrients from the blood are able to pass through them to feed the hungry tissues. In turn, the cells relinquish their waste products, including carbon dioxide, which are carried away in the blood, first in the tiny capillaries, then the small venules and finally the larger veins. These have valves in them to prevent the blood from flowing backwards. This bluish blood is carried back to the heart. From there it is returned to the lungs and once more replenished with vital oxygen. And so the process repeats itself.

If our lifestyles are sedentary and we make no effort at all to give our bodies the oxygen they so badly need, a gradual decline in health sets in and we become more vulnerable to infection. Equally, waste products accumulate in the tissues and aggravate the situation. Exercise is therefore physiologically truly essential.It is not merely a gimmick for health freaks! Another benefit results from exercise: all those nutrients that have been taken in in the form of food can be quickly carried in the bloodstream to the places where they are most needed to keep the body in top working order. Human beings were never intended to spend most of the day sitting about.

Our ancestors, as hunter-gatherers, were on the move every day, to ensure an adequate food supply. Physical activity is thus part of our evolutionary heritage.

Exciting new research carried out by Dr George Solomon at UCLA in America now shows that the activity of natural killer cells (the ones that kill invaders directly with a cell poison and help to fight off cancer) is considerably enhanced after a bout of vigorous exercise. Dr Solomon believes that the endorphins (the hormones that give us a feeling of euphoria) which are released during exercise are in some way involved in bringing about these changes in immunity. Indeed, it is now known that immune cells carry tiny receptors for hormones, a means of direct communication between the two systems. It is becoming increasingly clear that the brain, the endocrine system (which releases hormones) and immunity are all linked together. At last, the intuitive wisdom of psychotherapists, Oriental healers and philosophers is being proved by scientists to be true – that the mind and body are inextricably bound up one with the other.

FLEXIBILITY AND STRENGTH

In addition to oxygenating ourselves, we need to include exercises for suppleness and strength to ensure all-round fitness.

Flexibility exercises involve putting the major muscle groups and joints through a wide range of movement. They are carried out in a relaxed fashion, without any strain. To strengthen muscles, they have to work against resistance at above normal daily requirements. I find there is no better way of getting the system going first thing in the morning than to have a short workout that involves these two types of exercise. As an added bonus, the chance of accidental injury is greatly lessened because the body is more ready to cope with unexpected demands. I start with my head and neck, then move down the body. The following is my workout before breakfast. If I am unable to fit all the exercises in I make a selection.

Early morning workout
1 Stand tall, but relaxed, feet a little apart, shoulders down. Turn the whole head as far as it will go to look to the right, keeping it straight. Move no other part of the body. Turn the head to the left similarly. Avoid jerking. Repeat both movements three times.

2 Drop the head directly backwards, releasing the jaw; then drop it forwards. Stay very relaxed throughout. Repeat three times.

3 Circle the head slowly, dropping it forwards, then rolling it to the right, the ear moving towards the shoulder, then dropping it back and round to the left. Repeat three times, then reverse.

4 Shrug the shoulders, lifting and dropping them several times.

5 Make big circles with the arms, first swinging them backwards, then forwards, stretching out as far as possible. Repeat five times each way.

6 Bend the arms at the elbows, so that the fists almost touch at chest level, palms down. Keeping the legs and hips still, twist the upper half of the body from the waist, first to the right, with the elbow leading the way. When you have reached your limit do a gentle 'bounce'. Repeat to the left. Do five times.

7 While keeping the whole body facing front, bend sideways to the left from the waist by sliding your fingers down your leg. Do not twist or move your hips. You will feel a good stretch up your right side. Now bend to the right. Repeat five times.

8 Place your hands on the back of your hips for support, then bend your knees, pushing your hips forward. Meanwhile drop your head back, making a smooth arch with your spine. Hold for a few seconds. You will find this easier if you release your jaw. Remember to keep your feet apart.

9 Place your hands on your hips and loosen them by making big circles with them, to left and to right.

10 Bring your feet together and, keeping the back straight, bend your knees and put your hands on them. Make gentle circles with your knees to left and to right.

11 (See drawing A.) Hold on to the back of a chair with one hand and stand at right-angles to it in first position; that is, place the heels together with the toes pointing out at about ten to two. Make sure you don't roll over on to your insteps, but stand on the outer edges of your feet. Now rise up gently on to the balls of your toes, keeping the knees straight. Tighten the muscles all the way up the legs and in the buttocks as you do this. Hold. Lower. Now, keeping the heels on the floor, bend the knees out so that they are directly over the feet. Keep your bottom tucked in. Straighten. Repeat the whole exercise five times.

12 (See drawing B.) Slide your outer foot along the floor directly in front of you and point it, feeling the stretch. Slide it back to first

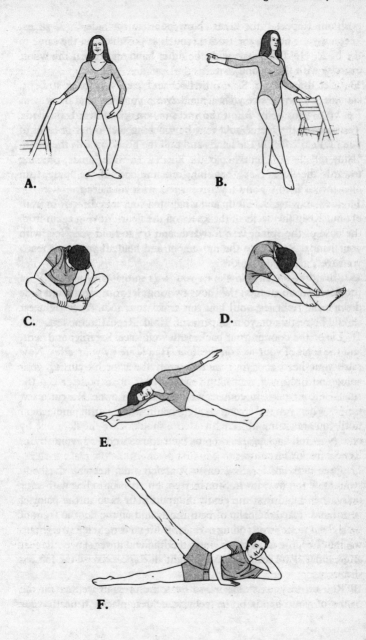

A.

B.

C.

D.

E.

F.

position. Repeat three times. Now point to the side three times, keeping your heel to the front as much as possible. Do the same to the back. Hold the chair with the other hand and repeat the whole exercise with the second foot.

13 (See drawing **C**.) Sit on the floor and keep your back straight, shoulders down. Place your arms between your legs and draw your feet up to your body. Allow the knees to flop open towards the floor. The soles of the feet should now be touching each other in front of you. Take the feet in the hands and pull the heels towards the groin. Using the elbows, gently coax the knees even wider apart, pressing towards the floor. Now, bending from the base of the spine, lean over forwards to try and touch your feet with your head.

14 (See drawing **D**.) Sit up and straighten your legs directly in front of you. Keep the backs of the knees on the floor. Moving again from the base of the spine, lean forwards and try to hold your feet with your hands. Relax into the movement and hold. If you can't reach your feet, grasp your ankles.

15 (See drawing **E**.) Now open your legs so that they make a V on the floor. Sit up straight. Without twisting, let your right hand slide down your right leg until you can grasp your foot. Your right ear should be resting on your upper arm. Hold. Repeat to the left.

16 Lie on the floor on your back, with your knees together and bent, and the soles of your feet on the floor. Hands are by your sides. Now raise your head and your shoulders off the floor by curling your spine and dropping your chin towards your breastbone. Keep the small of your back in contact with the floor. Lower. Repeat a few times. When you feel strong enough, continue the curling movement until you are sitting up. Each vertebra should leave the floor one by one. Now roll back again, keeping your spine curved to avoid strain. Repeat five or seven times.

17 (See drawing **F**.) Roll on to your left side, keeping the body straight all the way down. Stretch your left arm out in line with your body, then bend it at the elbow. Support your head in the palm of your hand. Place the palm of your right hand on the floor in front of your chest to stop you rolling over. Now lift your right leg straight up without bending it, as far as you can. Hold and lower slowly. Repeat a few times. Roll over on to your right side and exercise the left leg similarly.

18 Roll on to your stomach and do some press-ups either on the palms of your hands or on your knuckles, placed beneath your shoulders. Keep the body completely straight as you raise and lower it. If you have never done these before, practise against a wall first.

Now you should feel supple and strong and ready to face the day.

AEROBIC EXERCISE

When carefully and regularly practised, this type of exercise will increase the efficiency of the heart and lungs and improve the circulation. You can tell how hard the heart muscle is working by taking your pulse. Do this by placing the tips of the first three fingers of your right hand on to the inside of your left wrist (beyond the base of the thumb) and feel for the pulse. Count the beats for 30 seconds and multiply by 2. It is best to take your resting rate first thing in the morning. If it is under 70 you are reckoned to be fit; 70–80 is average; over 90 is unfit. As you exercise, your pulse rate will go up, because the heart beats faster to satisfy the increased demand for oxygen: the muscles need large amounts to work properly. As you become more fit the efficiency of your heart and lungs will improve, and your resting pulse rate will drop. Thus the heart is no longer forced to work with so much effort and is likely to last longer. The aim is to keep your pulse raised without exceeding your personal training rate. Calculate this by subtracting your age from 200. Then, if you are unfit, take off a further 40 points. For example, if your age is 45 you work out your personal training rate as follows:

	200	
less age	-45	
	155	
less unfitness handicap	-40	
	= 115	personal training pulse rate

As you become more accustomed to aerobic exercise, your handicap can be lessened.

Do not exercise after eating. Allow two hours after a snack, and four after a full meal. Always start with a gentle warm-up (see below).

To begin with, if you are very unfit, test your pulse every minute (or as often as practicable) and make sure you are not going above your personal rate. Stop, also, if you experience any chest pains or excessive fatigue. Your rest periods may exceed your amount of exercise at first. But this is fine. Gradually you will improve as your lungs become more elastic and your heart muscle stronger, until you can sustain minutes on end of your selected activity, without raising your pulse above your threshold.

The following types of exertion give the best aerobic effect: aerobic dance, cycling (hard), jogging, continuous skipping, swimming (hard), squash, badminton, rowing, cross-country skiing, team sports such as hockey and soccer. Moderate aerobic effect is derived from these: rounders, netball, tennis, judo, disco dancing, brisk hill walking, downhill skiing, climbing stairs. A small amount of benefit will be gained from: cricket, ballroom dancing, golf, sailing, yoga, walking, digging garden, moderate housework, mowing lawn (hand mower).

It really is best to choose something that you enjoy. Consider your needs. If you genuinely have very little time, take to doing housework without some of those electrical gadgets. Walking upstairs is marvellous for you, so give up lifts and escalators. Skipping you can do in any spare minutes and all you need is a rope and comfortable shoes that support your feet well. Another easy way of exercising is to put some music on and just allow it to move you. Invent your own spontaneous dance.

If you are lacking in self-discipline join a regular class. Other people will help give you that extra bit of energy and motivation. If you enjoy socialising you might choose badminton or ballroom dancing. Perhaps you are the competitive type, in which case a sport such as hockey or squash might appeal; or if you are an individualist you will probably prefer swimming or yoga.

What sort of person are you? Maybe you can select a form of movement that not only tones you up physically, but also balances out your personality in some way. Just as your body language subtly reveals who you are, so, conversely, body shapes that you make impress themselves on your unconscious mind. An obvious example is that of a shy, withdrawn person signing up for a martial arts class. Not only will the student learn the techniques of self-defence, combined with a superb form of exercise, but s/he will also acquire alertness, confidence and determination. The big, powerful movements of karate quickly dispel feelings of inadequacy and inferiority – another guaranteed way of moving out of the victim position (a poor place to be if we wish to stay well).

Whatever exercise you decide on, make sure you include a combination of movement for flexibility and strength as well as for stamina (aerobics). All it takes to stay fit is three twenty-minute sessions of aerobics per week, plus three ten-minute bouts of flexibility and strength exercises. Every so often, maintain your selected aerobic activity for about an hour and a half, or until you have arrived at your 'second wind'. You will return home feeling glowing and marvellous. Strenuous exercise of this type releases endorphins in the brain, nature's happiness hormones, that give you a glorious feeling of well-being, while enhancing immunity. Just imagine those natural killer cells racing around and firing their poisons at unwanted foreigners!

Warm-ups
Just a few minutes spent warming up before strenuous exercise will keep strains and sprains at bay.

a) Select a few exercises from the early-morning workout described earlier. For example, the circling movements for head (3), arms (5) and hips (9) will help to loosen you and get the circulation going. Number 11 will exercise the leg muscles.

b) Now, with your feet a little apart and keeping your legs more or less straight, but not rigid, bend down slowly until you can touch the floor between your feet. Let your head hang loosely. Slowly straighten up and stretch your arms high above your head. Push your hips forward, arch your back and bend your head back for a bigger stretch up your body. Repeat four times.

c) Give your calves and Achilles' tendons a gentle stretch. Stand facing the wall and put your hands flat on to it, arms straight. Place your left foot about 18 inches/45 cm behind the right. Keeping the left leg straight and the heel on the floor, bend the right knee until you feel a pull in your left calf. Hold a few seconds. Repeat with the right leg.

d) Stretch your thigh muscles next. Hold on to a chair with your left hand. Stand erect and, keeping the thighs parallel, bend your right leg straight up behind you from the knee and hold your foot with your right hand. Gently pull backwards on the foot until you feel the stretch in the thigh. Hold for several seconds. Repeat with the other leg.

e) Jog gently on the spot for a few minutes.

Now you are ready for your chosen activity. Afterwards, do some gentle walking, then repeat some of these exercises while you cool off. This way you will be less likely to suffer from muscle aches. It is also essential to have the correct footwear, to cushion any shock to the legs and give adequate support to the arches. A good sports shop will advise you. Gym shoes are useless.

WEIGHT LOSS

According to research carried out in 1983–4 in conjunction with Britain's Health Education Council, about two-thirds of healthy adults lose weight if they follow a regular exercise programme (three brisk aerobic sessions per week of twenty minutes each) for one year and continue to eat whatever they like. Sometimes increased muscle bulk makes up for loss of fat, which accounts for the retention of weight in some cases. One-third sees a marked improvement in body shape, with loss of flab especially from the waist and buttocks.

In its wisdom, the body stores surplus energy in the form of fat, in case of unexpected demand. A sedentary lifestyle will inevitably lead to an accumulation of this unused energy. Only by changing your diet or by regular physical exercise – preferably both – can you begin to improve your body shape and overall condition. Statistics show that many cancers, diabetes and other degenerative diseases are more common among overweight people, so anything that helps to reduce excess fat is well worth doing.

A NOTE FOR THE ELDERLY OR UNWELL

If you are elderly or ill or disabled please do not skip this chapter, because there is plenty you can do, even from a wheelchair. Deep breathing will keep you well oxygenated, so practise this every day near an open window. Massage and skin brushing are also very beneficial, both of which stimulate the circulation and encourage the flow of the lymph.

Multiple sclerosis sufferers who have included regular physiotherapy in their régime from an early stage do better than those who do no exercise at all, according to a study carried out at the Middlesex Hospital in London. Although deterioration in voluntary movements could not be altogether halted, it was significantly slowed down as compared with the control group, and patients were well able to continue with normal everyday activities. So make sure your doctor refers you to a physiotherapist.

The same principle applies to arthritis sufferers. Experience shows that it really is best to keep the body moving as much as possible, otherwise muscles atrophy and range of movement will be quickly lost.

If your illness makes you feel weak or nauseous, then try exercising lying on your back on the floor, with your head on a cushion. Most patients at the Bristol Cancer Help Centre can manage a simple routine similar to this one. It can also be performed from a chair with some modifications. First, put on some dreamy music and keep your movements gentle.

1) Relax, then waggle your jaw from side to side. Open your mouth wide. Close it and grin.

2) Roll your head from side to side. Now raise it to look at your toes. If you can, raise your shoulders too.

3) Keep your elbows on the floor beside you, but raise and lower your forearms. Then circle your wrists in both directions. Now shake your hands.

4) Fan your arms out in an arc along the floor until they reach above your head. Enjoy the stretch. Return them to your sides.

5) Bend your knees up, placing your feet flat on the floor slightly apart. Now try raising your hips towards the ceiling.

6) Stretch out your legs, first pushing with the heels, then pointing the toes. Relax. Bend one leg up and hug it to you, then let it straighten up at right angles in the air. Lower it to the floor (keeping it straight if possible). Repeat with the other leg.

7) Bend one knee and rest the other leg on it, so the ankle is free. Rotate the ankle in one direction, then in the other. Repeat with the other leg.

8) Bend both knees, keeping the feet together on the floor. Stretch your arms out on the floor at shoulder level. Now rock your knees from side to side as far as you wish, to give your spine a twist.

9) Relax completely, roll on to your side and get up very slowly to avoid any dizziness.

DEEP BREATHING

However unwell or disabled you are, you can still oxygenate yourself by regular deep breathing. The first rule is to breathe through the nose. Take advantage of the immune system's number one line of defence: the tiny hairs along the nasal passage that trap dust particles, and the mucous membranes that guard against infection. Dust and bacilli can be actively expelled by exhaling very vigorously through the nose. Do this before starting. Then breathe in slowly through your nose from the bottom of your lungs as you raise your arms in a big arc out to the sides and up above your head. Hold your breath for as long as comfortable. As you breathe out, slowly let your arms float down to your sides again. This exercise is effective either sitting or standing, but keep your spine straight throughout. Make sure you have a supply of fresh air.

Yoga breathing
This is particularly beneficial if you are suffering from chest tension, palpitations, or any other stress-related problems, as the extended, regulated breathing slows the heart rate and induces a feeling of calm. As with any deep breathing, it increases the oxygen supply to the blood.

Expel the stale air from your lungs, and then take your pulse and use its beat for your counting. The first two exercises can be carried out either standing, sitting or lying on your back. Keep the spine straight.

1 Complete yoga breathing
In this, the trunk is animated by a wavelike motion. Breathe in slowly to a count of 8: first expand your abdomen, then your ribs and finally the upper chest. Retain the breath for as long as comfortable. Breathe out, also to a count of 8, by first drawing in the abdominal wall, then contracting the ribs, and finally compressing the chest. Repeat 7 times, starting the motion always with the abdomen and working up the trunk. Practise three times a day.

2 Healing breathing
The basis of this is complete yoga breathing, described above. As you draw in the air, imagine that you are storing up healing energy in your body. On your outward breath, direct this healing energy to whichever part of your body most needs it. See this part becoming well again.

3 Cleansing breathing
The expulsion of stale air from the bottom of the lungs helps to eliminate toxins that can accumulate in the blood. It is also reputed to fortify the immune system.

Choose a place where the air is really fresh. Stand straight with your legs apart, but not stiff. Inhale slowly through the nose to a count of 8, as in complete yoga breathing. Press the lips close to the teeth, until only a narrow slit is left. Force the air out in a number of detached bursts. It should take a great effort on the part of the abdominal, diaphragm and rib muscles to eject the air.

Hatha yoga

The word 'hatha' is derived from 'ha' meaning 'sun' and 'tha' meaning 'moon', symbolising the positive and negative currents in the body. The aim is to have these energies in complete equilibrium and at the same time to bring body and mind into unison. It sets out to perfect the body, to compensate for physical defects and to release the natural healing forces. Even the workings of the autonomic nervous system can be brought under conscious control by an expert yogi. We already know this is true from the experience of meditation. After a few months' practice, I myself could suppress the rush of adrenalin when startled by something unexpected, as for instance when a low-flying military jet comes squealing across the peaceful Suffolk sky. It is so much better for my health not to have those damaging hormones racing uselessly around in my bloodstream. Thus, the postures of yoga offer more than physical flexibility; they offer protection from illness through mental and physical control. Equally, practice of the discipline helps those who are already ill, and symptoms, such as those suffered by MS patients, can be lessened or kept at bay.

Some of the postures help to stimulate internal organs, such as the thymus, liver and spleen, and can thereby have a therapeutic effect on the body's defence systems. Other postures accelerate healing of wounds, offer protection against colds, strengthen various parts of the body, such as the back, influence the pancreas (of great benefit to diabetics) and so on. Whatever your physical weakness, you will find something in hatha yoga to help you.

If this form of meditative movement appeals, then do sign up with a well-qualified teacher, preferably someone who understands the mental and spiritual aspects as well as the physical.

MASSAGE AND BODYWORK

Touch is of vital importance to humans. Babies will pine if they are rarely picked up and cuddled; they may even fail to develop properly, despite being fed adequately. It is through touch that they first experience warmth and care. For adults, any sort of massage can be both soothing and relaxing; it can also be deliciously sensual, and it is delightful for us to be able to enjoy our bodies in this way, especially if we are ill. It seems a shame that this ancient form of therapy has become associated in people's minds with sex parlours. There are various types which have been specifically developed as a means of healing, the best known being shiatsu, or acupressure. When skilfully applied, massage can alleviate stress, headaches, muscular tension and a variety of other conditions. It is sensible, however, to find a well-qualified practitioner who has experience of treating your particular disorder. The first hour or so should consist of a detailed account of your medical history and present state of health. From this, the masseur will decide upon the approach which is best for you.

Shiatsu has been evolved over the centuries by first the Chinese and then the Japanese to provide a very caring form of healing based on touch. Although rubbing and kneading movements are sometimes used on specific areas to relax the muscles and increase circulation, the principal mode of treatment is a firm pressure on the acupuncture points. Additionally, gentle shaking, pulling and stretching increase flexibility, and loose clothing needs to be worn for sessions. The overall aim is to create a balance within the body and to encourage the energy to flow so that the natural healing processes are maximised.

The practitioner may work along the meridians, if your condition calls for it. These are lines of acupoints connected with various organs. For example the meridian running up the inside of the shin bone is connected to the spleen, an integral part of the immune system. A well-trained practitioner will know how to apply pressure to the lymph nodes and other key points, to stimulate various aspects of the immune defences. Any tender spots can be treated with gentle palm healing, which involves very little pressure. Moxibustion, or application of heat to the acupoints, is also practised for particular conditions.

Having experienced shiatsu myself, I can wholeheartedly recommend it. For a whole hour I was pressed, kneaded, shaken, pulled, stood on and knelt on, and at the end of it I felt as light as air and floated out of the room feeling truly wonderful.

Biodynamic massage is another form of healing through touch. Here again, the aim is harmonisation through energy distribution. Practitioners are trained to listen to the inner language of the body by using a stethoscope, and massage will be adjusted according to the information received from this form of biofeedback. Some of them may also work with the aura. It is best to choose a masseur who is trained in biodynamic therapy as well, since the two go together. Founded by the Norwegian psychologist and physiotherapist Gerda Boyesen, the theory is that every unresolved emotional conflict is quite literally embodied. For example, a child who is frequently punished for expressing anger, may end up 'holding down' his anger with muscular effort, causing permanent tension. Wilhelm Reich, a psychoanalyst, referred to this many years ago as 'body armouring'. As we have seen, powerful emotions that are locked into the body in this way can eventually lead to serious illness. A biodynamic therapist can treat the tense areas directly and as these are freed up, so the long-held emotions are released. To do this kind of work, you will need to feel comfortable and safe with the therapist.

A rather different relationship is encouraged by an Alexander teacher: you will be treated more as a pupil rather than a client. Although you will be gently held and stretched, the idea is to learn how to use your body in a more natural, relaxed way. The technique was developed by an Australian actor who suffered from recurring hoarseness, which became a real threat to his career. He eventually cured himself by devising a new 'manner of doing', which involved releasing all extraneous tension. Actors and musicians have benefited greatly from this technique, and many people now use it to improve their health. Here again, anyone suffering from tension, back pain, or any other disorders affecting posture will find it helpful. After about twenty lessons you will be living your life in a totally different, effortless way. For a while, I was taught the cello by a devotee of the Alexander Technique, and was astonished how my playing improved. By allowing the relaxed weight of my arm to rest on the bow, rather than pressing down or forcing it with my fingers, a vibrant new richness of tone emerged. I learnt something very important from this: the harder I tried to do anything, the more tense I became and the more difficult it seemed, but once I gave up trying, everything was a lot easier! There were many areas of my life in which I could usefully apply this principle.

SKIN BRUSHING

You will remember from the earlier part of the book how important the lymphatic system is to our immune defences. Not only is it home to our patrolling lymphocytes, but it also helps to clear unwanted debris, toxins, metabolic wastes and bacteria from the tissues. Yet this system has no pump to move it around; it relies on gravity or the action of muscles. It is important that it should be kept on the go, so that the unwanted matter can be filtered and cleaned up in the lymph nodes. If the fluid becomes trapped in the tissue spaces, it can build up and cause uncomfortable and unsightly swelling.

One pleasurable way to stimulate the flow of this drainage system is to do skin brushing. It also assists the elimination of toxins through the pores. All you need is a long-handled brush with real bristles, firm but soft enough not to scratch. A rough hemp glove is an alternative. Using one or the other, dry-brush your skin with long, firm strokes, starting with your feet and working upwards, always brushing towards the heart. Thus, you will brush your arms from your fingertips to your shoulders. Ask someone to do your back for you if you are unable to reach. Treat your front more gently, with soft, circular movements.

The tingly sensation that results from skin brushing is truly delightful. Finish off with a warm shower, and then, if you can stand it, a cold one.

6 Feeding your defences

Since switching to my immunity-boosting régime, the contents of my store cupboard and fridge have changed dramatically. Gone are those standard ingredients of milk, cheese, bacon and mince, the tins of plum tomatoes, tuna, and ham and pea soup, and the packets of Earl Grey tea and Kenya coffee. Instead, there are tofu and tempeh and large glass jars full of brightly coloured beans and many sorts of nuts and dried fruits. Pumpkin seeds, raisins and almonds provide an instant snack and many varieties of herb and fruit tea offer refreshment when needed. The fruit bowl tends to contain the odd treat, such as a pineapple or mango, while my allotment provides carrots and other vegetables, rich in minerals and vitamins, straight from the earth.

If you think this sounds a little stringent, please don't be deceived. The Peak Immunity Diet, which relies mainly on vegan cooking, with the addition of a little fish and a few eggs, can be very creative and really tempting. Above all, you know that every mouthful is not just filling you up; it is truly nourishing you and doing you good. I wouldn't go back to grease and stodge for anything.

IMMUNITY-DEPLETING FACTORS

If you wish to attain peak immunity and your present diet is 'normal', then you are going to have to change it. The fact is that the average Western diet is seriously deficient in vital nutrients, as a result of processing, refinement and depleted soil. A recent estimate showed that as many as 35 per cent of cancers are clearly linked with dietary factors. Happily, wholefoods have had plenty of publicity in the last few years and people are becoming much more aware of the value of eating food in its natural, unrefined state. Yet much of what we eat is still poisoned by preservatives, insecticides or artificial ferti-lisers, and organic fruit and vegetables can be very hard to obtain.

Here are a few facts, which I hope will help to convince you that organic wholefoods really are best:

1 Plants are only as healthy as the soil in which they grow. Artificial fertilisers lock up certain minerals in the soil, notably zinc and magnesium, by forming insoluble compounds with them; vegetables therefore cannot take them up. This results in mineral deficiencies in our diet. Zinc is important for many functions, such as growth of bones, appetite, vision and sexual functioning. Magnesium assists in the relaxation of muscles. If you are under stress, your requirements will be increased. Both minerals are essential for proper immune functioning.

2 The important trace element selenium also helps the immune system to function and deficiencies are associated with cancer and heart disease. Cereals grown in soil-eroded areas will not contain sufficient selenium to maintain health, and food processing destroys it entirely.

3 Iron deficiencies can be caused by the food preservative EDTA and the phosphates used as additives in such foods as ice cream, pies and cakes and soft drinks. These can prevent the body from absorbing the iron by as much as half, and can result in anaemia.

4 The refining of food destroys both natural sodium chloride and potassium, minerals that are closely related. The salt alone is returned to the food, but in excessive amounts, causing an imbal-ance. Potassium deficiency can result in weakness of the heart and other muscles, while excessive sodium leads to swelling of the cells, reduced kidney function and raised blood pressure.

5 Food processing destroys almost half the natural content of vitamin A. This vitamin is essential for growth, vision and reproduction. It also helps to heal wounds, and a nineteen-year study in Chicago con-cludes that it reduces the rate of lung cancer in men. Some chemicals, including the nitrates in artificial fertilisers, attack this vitamin.

6 Refining of carbohydrates to create white flour and sugar, robs them of their nutrients. In turn, they leach the body of vitamins during their metabolic process, particularly the B complex. Of the twenty-two natural nutrients in wholemeal flour, only a few are returned after refining, with none at all to sugar, which provides only empty calories. These foods cause over-production of insulin to correct high levels of blood sugar. They are instrumental in

causing diabetes, which can produce blindness and early death. It is therefore not an exaggeration to say that refined carbohydrates are dangerous.

7 Fibre does not provide nutrients as such, but a mixture of soft and hard fibres is essential for the easy passage of food through the intestine. Ingestion of cereals that have their fibre removed not only causes constipation, but can result in diverticulosis (inflamed intestine) and cancer of the colon, through fermentation of food in the gut which produces unhealthy bacteria.

8 Western diets rely heavily on meat for protein. This means that fat consumption is very high. Steak, for example, contains 17.4 per cent complete protein by weight, but 25.3 per cent fat; by contrast, soya beans are 34 per cent complete protein by weight and only 18 per cent fat, of which 11 per cent is polyunsaturated. The damage to the arteries and the resultant heart disease caused by an excess of fat is well known. Less publicised is the way in which fat interferes with the metabolism and leaches vitamins and minerals needed by other parts of the body. The connection with other degenerative diseases, including cancer, is well established.

Do you still believe that the average Western diet is good for you?

ASSESSING YOUR DIET

The following questionnaire will help you to evaluate your own diet. Select which type of food you normally eat, or which alternative you would prefer, and mark the appropriate letters.

1 For breakfast do you generally have:
a   Slice of white toast with butter and marmalade; coffee or tea?
b   Cornflakes with milk and sugar; fried egg, bacon or sausage; slice of white toast; coffee or tea?
c   Sugar-free organic muesli or wholegrain porridge with soya milk; slice or two of wholemeal bread with tahini or sun-flower seed spread?

2 At mid-morning do you have:
a   Cup of coffee or tea?
b   Sweet biscuits and coffee?

c   Herb tea or fruit juice and a handful of nuts and raisins?

3 At lunchtime do you have:
a   Ham or beef sandwich made with white bread and butter; cup of coffee or tea?

b   Steak and kidney pie or fried fish, peas and chips; pint of beer?

c   Slice of nut roast with mixed salad?

4 At teatime do you have:
a   Cup of tea?

b   Cup of tea and cake?

c   Herb or fruit tea and banana?

5 For dinner do you have:
a   Tinned soup; frozen ready-made meal, such as shepherd's pie, with frozen spinach or tinned carrots; ice cream; coca-cola?

b   Onion soup; boeuf bourgignon with white rice and courgettes; fruit pie and cream; half bottle of wine?

c   Salad; lentils and brown rice with lightly steamed broccoli; fresh fruit?

6 Before bed do you have:
a   Tea and biscuit?

b   Mug of hot chocolate?

c   Small cup of chamomile tea or slippery elm?

Scoring
1a   Far too little protein. The carbohydrate will provide some instant energy, but you will be hit by a drop in blood-sugar level at around mid-morning. This may be characterised by a loss of concentration, fatigue or headache setting in. Constipation can result from the low fibre content. Score 10 points. Add 1 if you take sugar in your drink. Take off 1 if your toast was made with wholemeal bread.

1b   This solid breakfast will keep you going all morning, as you are giving yourself good protein. However, unless you are doing physical work, the fat in the meat, frying oil and butter could be storing up trouble for the future. Score 7 points. Add 1 for sugar in your drink.

1c   The whole grains provide a rich variety of nutrients, with additional protein available in the spreads. The low fat and high fibre content are healthy. Score 4 points.

2a   The caffeine will give you a temporary boost, but it is a slow poison and can do you harm in the long term (see 'Drinking and eating' later in this chapter). Score 3. Add 1 if you take sugar.

2b   The sugar and fat in the biscuits will raise your blood-sugar level temporarily, but will grab nutrients from your body. Score 2. Add 1 for sugar in your coffee.

2c   Natural fructose in the raisins will give you energy, and the nuts will provide protein and other nutrients to see you through the morning. Score 1.

3a   Lunch unbalanced. While protein is provided by the meat, the sodium content is very high – not good for your tissues unless you are going to be sweating it out. Vitamin content very low, and fat content high: bad for your arteries. Score 10. Add 1 for sugar in your drink.

3b   It is preferable not to wash your food down with liquid, because the nutrients have insufficient time to be absorbed. The fat content of the pastry, fried food and chips is too high. The peas will provide some vitamins, including A and C, but only if they are not over-cooked. Score 7.

3c   A fresh salad will give you plenty of vitamins and minerals. If the nut roast contains some cereal, then the combined ingredients offer good-quality protein. Otherwise include a slice of wholemeal bread. Score 4.

4a   Poor nutritional value. Score 3. Add 1 for sugar.

4b   The refined flour and sugar will steal nutrients from your body. Score 2. Add 1 for sugar in your tea.

4c   Vitamins and minerals available in some herb and fruit teas, also in the banana. Score 1.

5a   Canned and prepared frozen meals are low in nutrients and high in sodium. The additives that they often contain are poisons and will make your liver work unnecessarily hard. Score 10. Add 1 for salt on the table.

5b   A good, filling dinner with a balance of nutrients. However, beware of the high fat content of the meat, pastry and cream. Score 7. Add 1 for salt on the table.

5c The salad activates the correct enzymes for easy digestion of the rest of the meal. Lentils and rice together form complementary amino-acids. Plenty of nutrients in this meal. Also, it is low in fat. Score 4.

6a Tea won't help you to sleep; sweet biscuits at night are likely to end up on your thighs. Score 3. Add 1 for sugar in your tea.

6b Good calcium from the milk, but you would be better off without the fat. Score 2.

6c Will aid sound sleep. Score 1.

Immunity rating

35-45 You are poorly nourished and rely too heavily on convenience foods. You need to take much better care of yourself and eat more fresh fruit and vegetables. Low immunity.

27-33 Your diet is too high in saturated fats and sugar and rather low in fibre. Although you will feel well fed and probably enjoy your food, you are storing up trouble for the future. Eating grilled fish and roast chicken rather than red meat would be an immediate improvement, as would the use of whole grains rather than refined ones. Moderate to low immunity.

19-26 You eat sensibly and are aware of the value of whole, fresh foods, but there is still room for improvement. Moderate immunity.

15-18 You have a low-fat, high-fibre diet, with a wide variety of nutrients. High immunity.

HEALTHY EATING

The latest scientific evidence coming from archaeologists, anthropologists and primatologists suggests that our prehistoric ancestors were not predominantly meat-eaters, but hunted mostly for wild cereals, plants, roots and berries. In other words, they were mainly herbivores. Animal life was taken only when absolutely essential and consumed in quite small amounts. The slow pace at which evolution progresses leads to the supposition that humans are not well adapted to heavy meat-eating and that people in affluent societies are exceeding their biological capacity to tolerate such a rich, fatty diet. The result is a host of health problems, ranging from obesity and diabetes to coronary heart disease and several types of cancer.

If we look at other cultures around the world today, it is noticeable that the people who live the longest and suffer the least from degenerative diseases have a mainly vegetarian diet, combined with plenty of outdoor exercise. During the years 1904–11, a British surgeon named Robert McCarrison travelled around a remote Himalayan kingdom known as the Hunza. He was astonished to discover that many degenerative and infectious diseases, common in the West, were completely unheard of in this area. 'I never saw a case of asthenic dyspepsia, of gastric or duodenal ulcer, of appendicitis, of mucous colitis, or of cancer,' he wrote. The diet of the Hunza people consisted mainly of wholemeal chapatis, maize and barley, with green vegetables, beans and legumes and both fresh and dried apricots. Dairy products including goat's milk were occasionally allowed on feast days. Some years later, McCarrison ran a series of experiments in which he fed the Hunza diet to rats over a period of four years. The same number of rats were fed with the standard Indian diet for the same length of time, which included such items as white rice, sugar, black tea and spices. The result was that the rats on the Hunza diet remained free of disease, while those on the refined Indian diet contracted cysts, abscesses, heart disease and cancer of the stomach.

An article published by the *National Geographic* magazine a few years ago included an analysis of the Hunza diet. The average daily caloric intake was 1,923 calories, with 50 grams of protein (principally from vegetable sources), 35 grams of fat, and 354 grams of carbohydrate. The average American consumes 3,300 calories per day, with 100 grams of protein (mainly from animal sources), 157 grams of fat and 380 grams of carbohydrate. Not only do the Hunza people remain disease-free, the concept of retirement is unknown to them. They stay vigorous into their eighties and nineties and often live well past one hundred years.

The people of Vilcabamba in Ecuador have a comparable diet and are also noted for their vitality and longevity. The elders continue to walk long distances, to farm and to teach until the end of their days. By contrast, many people from affluent societies decline during their sixties, having lost the use of their bodies after a sedentary way of life and too much rich food.

As long ago as the 1820s, there was positive evidence in America that a low-fat, high-fibre diet was directly linked with enhanced immunity. The vegetarian religious sect, known as the Bible Christians, had settled in Philadelphia, where the local citizens ate hearty meals rich in red meat, fried food and sweet puddings. An outbreak of cholera swept over the town and many people succumbed to the disease, yet the Bible Christians remained healthy, even though they were nursing many of the victims. Their diet was simple, consisting of vegetables, cereals, nuts and plain spring water. Despite true stories such as this, the abstemious eating habits of many religious sects have continued to be derided.

The Yogis have studied the effects of different foods on the body. Meat they consider to be too heavy, with the result that the body becomes lethargic and the consciousness blurred. All vegetables must be eaten fresh and preferably raw, with maximum 'life force'. Scientific analysis proves that when eaten this way, vegetables retain their maximum goodness in terms of vitamins and minerals. Cooking and processing destroys many important nutrients.

Also using Eastern ideas is the macrobiotic diet, well known for its curative qualities. This balances 'yin' and 'yang' energies in food, so that the body chemistry is harmonious. The word is derived from *macro*, Greek for long, and *bios* meaning life, and indeed, research from the Harvard Medical School demonstrates that it does contribute to a long life by lowering cholesterol levels and high blood pressure. With its low fat and sugar content, the diet helps to prevent cancer also. It was brought to Paris from Japan in the 1920s by George Ohsawa and is adaptable to individual requirements, taking account of climatic conditions, age, amount of activity and general state of health. Basically, it consists of 50-60 per cent cooked whole cereals, 5-10 per cent soups, 25-30 per cent fresh vegetables, 5-10 per cent beans and seaweeds, and some locally grown fruit. All dairy foods and sugar are banned, but a little mineral-rich sea salt is allowed, as is white deep-sea fish. Macrobiotics is not just about food, but involves a whole way of life based on living in harmony with nature.

It is wise to take heed of these traditional ways of eating, and, indeed, the Peak Immunity Diet includes many ancient precepts, combined with modern scientific understanding of the chemistry of food. For decades, healthy eaters have been dismissed as 'cranks'. Even the National Cancer Institute in the USA refused to admit that diet might be associated with cancer, until finally in 1982 it published a report that clearly endorses the approach taken by advocates of natural health. Reduce fat consumption, it said, avoid alcohol, eat more whole cereals, cut down on salty and smoked foods, and emphasise fresh fruit and vegetables.

THE PEAK IMMUNITY DIET

There is no better way to take vitamins and minerals than in their natural state, as constituents of food. The Peak Immunity Diet is carefully worked out so that your body will obtain maximum nourishment. Only in this way can the digestion, metabolism and immune system work to peak efficiency, unencumbered by refined carbohydrates, too many saturated fats or poisonous additives. The emphasis, therefore, is on fresh, organically grown wholefoods, with fruit and vegetables eaten 70 per cent raw, low in fat, high in fibre, salt- and sugar-free. This means no more 'dead' or processed foods from packages or tins, no more high-fat red meat, no dairy products except goat's milk yoghurt and 'ghee', no more stimulants such as coffee or tea, no junk food or drink, no more white bread or sugar, no more sickly cakes, sweet biscuits or jams, no added salt. You may well be exclaiming, 'But what is there left to eat?' Plenty. You will be trying all sorts of new dishes with whole grains, beans, tofu and nuts that you have probably never considered using in cooking before now. Instead of red meat you can switch to occasional deep-sea fish. This is a real opportunity to be creative!

The chart on the following page summarises which foods are best avoided and which should be included.

Who is it for?

Prevention, of course, is always better than cure and the Peak Immunity Diet is ideal for anyone who wishes to remain disease-free and retain their vitality for many, many years to come. It is especially suitable for patients suffering from all kinds of degenerative diseases. Cancer patients and those infected by the HIV will benefit greatly if they follow it strictly for at least six months, preferably longer (initially excluding the white meat and eggs), to give the body a good clean-up. It will encourage you to know that some patients at the Bristol Cancer Help Centre who also had symptoms of arthritis or diabetes, and who followed a similar diet to this one, discovered that

Foods to avoid	Foods to include
White bread	Stoneground, wholemeal bread
Shop-bought cakes and biscuits	Home-made, low-fat, sugar-free cakes
Marmalade and jam	Sugar-free jams and fruit spreads
Sugar	Malt extract, honey, black molasses
Salt	Herbs, mild spices, seeds
Malt vinegar	Cider or wine vinegar
Salted butter, margarine, lard, cooking oils	Ghee, cold-pressed sunflower oil, olive oil
White rice, refined cereals and packaged breakfast foods	Whole grains and cereals, including brown rice, barley, rye, maize, millet, oats, buckwheat
Red meat	Occasional white deep-sea fish
	Beans, peas, lentils; nuts and seeds; tofu and tempeh
Battery poultry and eggs	Free-range chicken or turkey (not more than once a week); up to 4 free-range eggs per week
Cow's milk and cheese	Soya milk
Frozen or tinned vegetables and fruit; commercial desserts and ice cream	Fresh, organic vegetables and fruit, sun-dried fruit; home-made, sugar-free desserts
Coffee, tea, cocoa, coca-cola, soft drinks	Herb and fruit teas, bancha tea; fresh vegetable and fruit juices
Tap water	Filtered tap water, spring water

not only did their tumours regress, but that their other conditions began to clear up too. It will be a tremendous help to those who persistently fall prey to respiratory infections, and the problems of allergy sufferers will almost certainly be reduced, if not cured, on this fresh, wholefood diet. ME is a strange, little-understood disease, but patients have discovered that plenty of raw food definitely keeps the symptoms at bay. Needless to say, the low-fat, low-sodium content of the Peak Immunity Diet makes it ideal for heart-disease patients. Certain adjustments may be necessary for those with delicate stomachs and yeast infections, as well as for arthritics and allergy sufferers, and these readers should refer to 'The PI Diet and special conditions' later in the chapter.

Patients with a wide variety of disorders have been helped with a diet such as this. Early this century Dr Max Gerson cured himself and many patients of severe migraines by means of this natural remedy. One of these patients happened to be suffering from lupus, too, and Gerson was amazed when this condition cleared up at the same time. Other chronic diseases responded similarly, including ulcerative colitis and multiple sclerosis. Albert Schweitzer was cured by Gerson of his diabetes, and the doctor later became famous for his success at treating cancer patients. Always the emphasis was on organically grown raw vegetables and fruit. He believed that 'the entire organism must be attacked in its totality, especially in degenerative diseases'. Referring to the adulterated, refined diet of the time, he maintained that a body fed on such unnatural stuff 'loses the harmony and cooperation of the cells, finally its natural defences, immunity and healing power'.

It is, of course, difficult to change your eating habits, however highly motivated you may be. Some readers may prefer to make modest improvements for general maintenance of their health, by cutting down gradually on their fat, salt, and sugar intake, while placing more emphasis on fresh vegetables and salads and whole cereals. By using the main principles as guidelines, they will give their immune defences a greater chance of operating more effectively.

Today, there are many witnesses to the beneficial effects of a wholefood, mainly raw, low-fat, low-sugar, salt-free diet, not least among the patients at the Bristol Cancer Help Centre. Stories of unexpected remissions do occur, and some patients who had been given only a few months to live are now enjoying a greatly improved quality of life many years later. The following comment is typical:

> X-rays had shown a regression of the tumour in my lungs
> and my friends had all commented on how much better
> I was looking. The first thing that people noticed was
> how much clearer my skin and eyes were, and this really
> proved to me that the diet was working. It also helped my
> diabetes. . . . Now I found I could give myself less insulin,
> eat more carbohydrates, and suffer fewer hypoglycaemic
> attacks.

One thing is certain, the PI Diet will change your body chemistry for the better. It is important, however, to approach the diet scientifically and, since you will be giving up red meat, to ensure that your protein requirements are met, which brings us to the next topic.

IMMUNITY-ENHANCING NUTRIENTS

Amino-acids

Proteins are the basic building-materials of our bodies, and they form approximately one-fifth of our weight. Their complex fibrous structures provide a framework, not only for our internal organs, but also for our bones, hair and nails, cartilages, tendons and muscles. They are essential for growth and for the repair and replacement of tissues. Some proteins are hormones that regulate the metabolism; others are enzymes that act as catalysts for chemical reactions, essential for the functioning of the digestive system. Vital for proper immune functioning is the synthesis of new protein for the formation of antibodies to fight bacterial and viral infections.

Proteins are made up of twenty-two amino-acids in different combinations, most of which can be synthesized in the body according to demand. Eight of these, however, known as the essential amino-acids, must be obtained from external sources and are needed every day from our food. They are also needed simultaneously for synthesis to occur, otherwise their value to the body is very low or even non-existent. To make matters more complicated, they are needed in the right proportions.

Eggs, fish and chicken are high in complete usable protein, as are soya beans, but other sources of plant protein contain only some of the essential amino-acids and not others. It is important, therefore, when planning a vegan menu, to select foods that complement each other and combine to produce the eight essential amino-acids needed by the body.

There are three main sources of plant protein: beans, peas and lentils; grains; nuts and seeds. Grains, nuts and seeds are low in the same amino-acids, but are particularly well complemented by legumes which have an opposite pattern. A meal which incorporates, say, rice and beans will therefore provide high-quality usable protein. Remember that you can include protein in your desserts, so sprinkle on seeds or add nuts. Tofu, blended with fruit, makes delicious high-protein creams. If your main course consisted of, say, nut risotto, tofu in your dessert would greatly increase the total value of usable protein in the meal. Most Western people eat more protein than they actually need, especially in the form of meat, and the excess is converted into carbohydrates and used up as energy. This is not an efficient process, however; it is rather like your car burning up oil, and some strain is put on the system. It makes sense, therefore, to keep protein levels to the desired amount. Although individual requirements vary, it is estimated that an average of 0.28 grams of usable protein per pound of body weight is needed each day. In other words, a 9-stone woman will need 35.3 grams (1¹/₅ oz) of usable protein per day, whereas an 11-stone man will need 43.1 grams (1¹/₂ oz). These amounts may seem extremely small to you, but remember that we are talking about usable protein only, pure protein that contains all eight essential amino-acids. There are many other substances in what you eat apart from protein, in particular fat and carbohydrates. When converted into a food table, the daily allowance is as follows:

Body weight	Daily allowance of usable protein	Equivalents in terms of food Fish or	Eggs or	Nuts or	Beans (dry)
9 stone (126 lb)	35.3 g (1¹/₅ oz)	8¹/₄ oz	6	12 oz	12³/₄ oz
11 stone (154 lb)	43.1 g (1¹/₂ oz)	10 oz	7	14¹/₃ oz	15¹/₃ oz

I am not suggesting that you eat six eggs in one day – please don't! The table is simply to give you an idea of the amount of protein your body needs. You may already have an instinctive feel for this. I am a high-protein person. If I don't have a good dollop for breakfast, my concentration deteriorates by mid-morning and I may even feel faint.

The food chain
Apart from the high fat content of meat, there are other reasons why the Peak Immunity Diet excludes it. Animals are at the top of a long food chain. In the 1960s it was discovered that chlorinated pesticides such as DDT, previously thought to be safe, were causing damage to the nervous systems of large fish such as salmon, and impairing the reproductive process of predatory birds like falcons. How had the DDT collected in the bodies of these species? It happens like this: if grubs eat contaminated vegetables, small animals such as moles may consume many such grubs and the contaminant is stored in the mammals' fat. Then a predatory bird such as an owl may eat

poisoned moles, so that the pesticide becomes even more concentrated in the owl until serious damage to the organism is caused. This process is known as 'biological magnification'. As carnivores, humans are at the top of many food chains and are therefore likely to be eating concentrated stores of pesticides from the animals and fish. If, however, we decide to eat plants, which are low on the food chain, chemicals can mostly be removed by washing. We do not yet know what long-term damage is being caused to humans by the continual use of pesticides. Cancerous tumours occur in laboratory mice if they are fed with seriously contaminated foods over a long period. It makes sense, therefore, to steer clear of these poisonous chemicals if we wish to retain our health.

Vitamins, minerals and trace elements
The word vitamin is derived from the Latin *vita* meaning life. Thus, vitamins are regarded as nutrients essential for the maintenance of life. Without them, we die. Minerals are even more essential because they can only reach our bodies via food, whereas some vitamins can be manufactured inside our bodies. The two groups work together, facilitating reactions with one another. For example, vitamin B_6 and zinc work together, as do calcium and vitamin D. Thus, vitamin D aids the absorption of calcium from the intestine and regulates the interchange of this mineral between the blood and bones.

In order to counter the onslaught of disease and infection the immune system has to produce millions of new cells. This is only possible if the diet is rich in vital nutrients. Eating raw vegetables and fruit is the very best way of obtaining these nutrients – the reason why this is such an important part of the PI Diet.

VITAMIN A   This vitamin is essential for the production of the white T- and B-cells, the main fighting troops of your immune system, whose job it is to protect your body against disease. Vitamin A is also important for the health of membranes, where immunoglobulins (which are specialised antibodies) are secreted. If you are even slightly deficient in vitamin A, your body will be unable to produce the full complement of these antibodies, and unwanted invaders will become established more easily. Very serious deficiency will actually cause your spleen and thymus to shrink in size, resulting in severely restricted output of white cells. Clearly, with your body in such a deprived state, you will be highly vulnerable to infection.

Apart from helping to keep the immune system fully operational, vitamin A has several other functions. It is essential for healthy vision, and it is involved in the healing of cuts together with vitamins C and E.

If you take this vitamin as a supplement, then buy it in the form of beta-carotene, from which your body will make the vitamin A that it requires. Even better is to drink a glass of fresh carrot juice. The old saying that carrots help you to see in the dark really is true! A word of warning: if vitamin A is taken in its oily form, your liver will store it up, and doses exceeding 50,000 IU per day will cause toxicity; 5,000 IU per day is thought to be adequate for the average male and 4,000 for a female, although your needs will rise during cold weather. Diabetics and cancer patients have particularly high requirements for vitamin A and supplements are recommended of up to 25,000 IU per day. Recent research in Cambridge confirms that carotinoids protect against cancer by preventing any pre-malignant disease from progressing to full malignancy. Don't worry if your skin turns slightly yellow; this is likely to happen on a high dosage. I constantly had to reassure my friends that I wasn't suffering from jaundice.

Apart from animal liver, fish-liver oils (especially halibut) are very rich in retinol (the chemical name for vitamin A). Carrots, sweet potatoes, apricots, spinach, pumpkin, broccoli, watercress and cantaloupe melon are prime sources of beta-carotene.

B VITAMINS Of this group of vitamins, the most important for successful immune functioning is B_6, or pyridoxine. Along with B_2 (riboflavin) and, to a lesser extent, some of the other B vitamins including folic acid and pantothenic acid, pyridoxine is vital for the health of your mucous membranes; you will remember from the first chapter how these provide the first line of defence against the onslaught of viruses and other organisms that cause disease. It also works in cooperation with B_2 in the formation of antibodies. As with vitamin A, if you are deficient in pyridoxine your immune response will be seriously lowered; once again, your thymus will shrink and there will be far fewer white T- and B- cells circulating in your bloodstream. Your spleen will become equally less effective.

Vitamin B_6 has other important functions. Animal studies have shown that it protects against hardening of the arteries (atheroma). Also, you need it to metabolise the amino-acids in your food, so your requirements are related to the protein content of your diet. The average recommended daily allowance (RDA) is 1.75 to 2.2 mg, but if you are on the Pill, or in later life, you will need more. This vitamin needs the assistance of the mineral zinc in order to be fully effective. So, if you take supplements, balance these two together. (The RDA of zinc is 15 mg.) Pyridoxine is found in many foods, including brewer's yeast, wheat germ, brown rice, molasses, avocado pears, soya beans, sunflower seeds, walnuts, bananas, cauliflower, spinach, Brussels sprouts, kale, eggs, chicken and fish. If vegetables are frozen, a 20 per cent loss will occur.

Vitamin B_2 taken as a supplement is also advisable for those suffering from immune deficiency diseases, or for anyone under excessive stress. The RDA is 1.2 – 1.7 mg for an adult. Apart from milk and cheese, foods that contain riboflavin are watercress, turnip greens, mushrooms, broccoli, asparagus, dandelion leaves, Brussels sprouts, kale, spinach, parsnips, avocado pears, dates, prunes, beans, cauliflower, almonds and sunflower seeds, as well as molasses, brewer's yeast, wheat germ, whole grains, soya flour and eggs.

In order to become active, folic acid needs certain enzymes and vitamin B_{12}. This can be a problem for vegans, since B_{12} is found mainly in meat and dairy products and deficiency can cause pernicious anaemia. The solution is to take B-complex tablets. The PI Diet, however, does offer two sources in the form of fish and eggs. All the B vitamins work together and too much of one can result in too little of others. Folic acid is an indispensable component of your body tissues, being involved in the formation of DNA (deoxyribonucleic acid) and RNA (ribonucleic acid), which are essential for cell division and transmission of inherited characteristics. It assists in the formation of red and white blood cells in the bone marrow and in their maturation. Thus it is a vital ingredient for the building of your defence forces. It is known that people who are low in this vitamin are more likely to succumb to carcinogenic substances and develop cancer. Conversely, folic-acid therapy has proved valuable in treating women with a pre-cancerous condition of the cervix. Arthritics are often deficient in this vitamin, although this may be a result of taking large quantities of aspirin. People with Hodgkin's disease or leukaemia have particularly high requirements. Folic acid is widely available in foods, especially wheat, beans and dark-green leafy vegetables. It is sensitive to ultra-violet light and is spoilt by boiling – more good reasons for eating your greens fresh and raw. The RDA is 400 mcg.

Pantothenic acid (vitamin B_5), also called calcium pantothenate, helps wounds to heal up quickly and fights infection by promoting the building of antibodies. It is a well-tested antidote to many allergies and can alleviate arthritis. Apart from offal, it is found in eggs, whole grains (especially wheat germ and bran), brewer's yeast, mushrooms, peas, nuts and royal jelly, but heat and food processing are its enemies.

VITAMIN C Despite the fact that vitamin C (ascorbic acid) is a popular supplement with the general public, this vitamin is still somewhat surrounded by mystery and has been the cause of heated controversy. We still do not know exactly how it helps to protect us against viruses, but experience shows that it prevents, or lessens the severity of, colds and 'flu if taken in large doses. (NB: aspirin negates its effect, so do not take this along with vitamin C.) Nobel prize-winner Dr Linus Pauling, together with a Scottish surgeon, Ewan Cameron, noted distinct improvements in cancer patients when given doses of 10 grams a day or more. Indeed, it has now been shown that vitamin C stimulates the activity of macrophages, the large white blood cells that gobble up invaders and help to fight tumours. A recent study also suggests that it encourages antibodies to respond to tumours and that it aids the production of T killer cells, which also devour cancer cells.

If you suffer from allergic reactions you will be interested to read that ascorbic acid reduces the effects of many allergy-producing substances. So do give it a try.

Together with A and E, vitamin C is important as an anti-oxidant – i.e. it neutralises carcinogens, those cancer-causing substances that are taken into the body in the form of, for example, burnt or smoked food.

Vitamin C is vital in countering the effects of corticosteroids, the immuno-suppressive hormones that are produced when the body is under stress. If you are going through strenuous times, therefore, make sure you protect yourself by taking at least 2 grams of vitamin C per day as a supplement. You will also need more ascorbic acid if you live in a city, since carbon monoxide destroys this vitamin, as do cigarettes. Women on the Pill need extra too.

Cancer or Aids patients may wish to discover their own maximum tolerance level. This is done by taking the supplement until it causes diarrhoea, then cutting back the amount by 10 per cent. Ascorbic acid is not toxic and will pass through the body if not needed. Very high doses can be taken intravenously. Need for the vitamin is increased while you are undergoing radiotherapy or chemotherapy, but be careful, since side-effects can be occasionally exacerbated.

Ascorbic acid can be found in green peppers, broccoli, kohlrabi, Brussels sprouts, kale, turnip greens, watercress, cauliflower, cabbage, tomatoes, spinach, cantaloupe, strawberries and citrus fruits. It is easily destroyed by cooking, so do eat these vegetables raw in salads as often as you can. The RDA is 60 mg for adults.

VITAMIN E   A recent study showed that if vitamin E supplements were included in the diet of laboratory animals their ability to produce antibodies to ward off viruses was considerably enhanced. If the trace element selenium was also included, antibody production was increased even more significantly.

Its anti-oxidant properties are well established. Animal experiments proved that it could reduce tumours caused by carcinogens. It can also help to prevent damage to the lungs from air pollution – worth knowing if you live in an industrial area. Macrophages, those large white blood cells, are easily harmed while doing their work of killing bacteria, but their health is maintained by the presence of vitamin E.

Apart from these vital immune-response functions, vitamin E is thought to improve fertility; at any rate, it does so in rats. It certainly helps to prevent thromboses, and contributes to the health of the muscles and nerves. Additionally, it may act in a similar way to vitamin C, by reducing the harmful effects of corticosteroids released into the bloodstream when a person is under stress.

A rich source of vitamin E is wheat germ, which can be sprinkled on to your muesli. On its own, it has rather a weird, slightly bitter taste, but this is easily disguised by the sweetness of raisins or a little honey. Other good sources are cold-pressed vegetable oils and unrefined cereals, with small amounts available in almonds, pecans, walnuts (if fresh), soya beans, green vegetables and eggs. Refining of flour gets rid of 90 per cent of vitamin E, while freezing destroys nearly all of it. It is estimated that modern Western diets contain less than one-tenth the amount of this vitamin than they did a century ago. Some experts have linked the increase of degenerative diseases with the decrease of this vitamin. So the inclusion of stoneground, wholemeal flour in your diet really will help to protect you from serious illness.

A supplement of around 200 IU is recommended for people suffering from lowered immunity, together with 25 mcg of selenium, while the daily requirement for the average adult is put at around 30 IU – more if the intake of polyunsaturated fatty acids is high. Some experts suggest that very large doses could cause increased blood pressure, so if you suffer from heart disease or diabetes, take the supplement under medical supervision only. Since vitamin E can enhance the production of oestrogen, supplements may not be a good idea for breast cancer patients, especially if there is evidence that the tumour is hormone receptive.

VITAMIN D AND CALCIUM   These two cooperate with each other, since the absorption of calcium is dependent upon the availability of vitamin D. Your own body makes and stores this vitamin, provided your skin receives sufficient ultraviolet light from the sun. If you live in a country that experiences inclement weather, therefore, do spend as much time out of doors as possible. Vitamin D is also available in egg yolks, butter and fish liver oils. Supplementation is not necessary. Indeed, there is a possibility that this vitamin in excess actually lowers immune function; a Californian study demonstrated that the vitamin suppressed the activity of white cells in humans. If you already have lowered immunity, it would therefore not be wise to take supplements of this vitamin.

When people give up dairy products they sometimes worry that they are not obtaining sufficient calcium, the main constituent of our bones and teeth and important for nerve conduction, muscular contraction and regulation of the heart. Dark tahini, made from whole, crushed sesame seeds, is an excellent source. Spread it on rice cakes, or use it to make vegetarian pâtés. Other good sources are wholemeal bread, muesli, sunflower seeds, almonds, sprouting seeds and grains, soya beans, molasses and sardines. The mineral also occurs in an odd assortment of other foods: rhubarb, dates and figs, broccoli, kale, watercress, dandelion leaves and turnip greens. Supplementation can be linked with vitamin C intake in the form of calcium ascorbate – a gentle way to take ascorbic acid.

COPPER   There is a possibility that copper may protect humans against cancer of the liver. Experiments with animals show this to be true. This apart, it is important for the healing of tissue, for the formation of bones and blood, and for the development of the central nervous system. Deficiencies will certainly leave your body more vulnerable to infection. On the other hand, too much of this trace element can lead to less effective antibody response, so keep within the standard supplement range of 2-5 mg per day, unless you are taking large amounts of zinc, which interferes with copper absorption. Apart from liver and seafood, legumes (especially soya beans), green vegetables, whole grains, nuts, raisins, prunes and molasses all contain this mineral, as will your water supply if it runs through copper pipes.

IRON Many people take iron as a supplement, particularly women who are anaemic, and it is often prescribed by doctors. It is very important for health because it is necessary for the production of haemoglobin, the main constituent of red blood cells and an efficient transporter of oxygen. White T- and B-cells have a high requirement for oxygen and this is the main reason why the immune system needs a healthy level of haemoglobin in the blood. Although malignant cells have a hard time thriving in well-oxygenated blood, they do like iron, and the body has a natural mechanism for withholding this mineral from tumours.

It is important to note that an excess of iron as well as a deficiency can cause problems within the immune system. You will need to know, therefore, that the recommended daily intake is 10 mg for adult males and 18 mg for women of childbearing age. Because many invading microbes need iron in order to reproduce, it makes sense not to take iron supplements if you are suffering from an illness caused by a virus.

Some experts reckon that excess iron may be involved in the damage to joints evident in rheumatoid arthritis, since this disease is rare among iron-deficient populations.

Clearly, a balanced intake of iron from natural sources is best. Apart from meat, it is available in many foods, including apricots, dates, prunes, dandelion leaves, spinach, Brussels sprouts, turnip and beet greens, watercress, artichokes, broccoli, asparagus, cauliflower, strawberries, soya beans, bean sprouts, peas, molasses, eggs, whole cereals and wheat germ, nuts and sesame and sunflower seeds.

MAGNESIUM Because heavy use of artificial fertilisers is now prevalent, magnesium deficiency is common among people on Western diets, for the reason mentioned earlier: this, and other minerals, become locked up in the soil and unavailable to plants. Moreover, a high intake of phosphorus from preserved foods, soft drinks and meat can bind up magnesium, zinc and copper, so that they cannot be digested. If you avoid all such junk foods and eat plenty of raw green vegetables, organically grown, then any deficiency will be naturally corrected, but bear in mind that stress will increase your need for it. Other sources of magnesium are figs, lemons, grapefruit, corn, honey, nuts and kelp.

Magnesium has to be balanced with calcium in the body: for instance, it helps muscles relax, while calcium aids contraction. So if you are taking a calcium supplement, it is best to take the same amount of magnesium also.

There is an established link between magnesium-deficient diets and cancer, especially cancer of the oesophagus. The exact reason is not understood, since magnesium deficiency alone does not seriously affect immune functioning, but it could be linked with the collective effects of mineral imbalance.

Diabetics and people with kidney abnormalities, as well as those suffering from stress, and pregnant and lactating women, all have extra requirements for magnesium. A daily intake of about 350 mg is standard for adults.

POTASSIUM AND SODIUM CHLORIDE (COMMON SALT) Some of the dangers of an imbalance between potassium and sodium have already been described, yet the average Westerner eats between ten and twenty times more salt than the body needs. Because excessive intake of sodium leads to a deficiency in potassium, many people in affluent countries have a potassium level which is too low and can produce not just fatigue and constipation but weakness in the muscles, particularly the heart. The excess salt raises the blood pressure and weakens the heart still more. Potassium assists immunity because it acts as an ascorbate transporter. In other words, it aids the passage of vitamin C through the cell membrane.

If you follow the Peak Immunity Diet, with an emphasis on green vegetables without added salt, your potassium-sodium levels will return to normal. Other rich sources of potassium are haddock, potatoes, raisins, whole grains, mint leaves and bananas.

SELENIUM This trace element is vital to health on account of its anti-oxidant properties; in other words, it prevents oxygen from combining with other compounds and thereby damaging cells. It promotes immune functioning in a number of ways, especially by protecting the large white cells called macrophages and reinforcing their ability to reduce tumours, and also by enabling phagocytes to kill and dispose of invading microbes. It cooperates with vitamin E in encouraging antibodies to deal with offending organisms. Selenium has yet another useful function: like zinc it assists the

Immunity–enhancing Nutrients and their Best Sources
(excluding red meat and dairy products)

	Vitamin A (retinol)	Vitamin B$_2$ (riboflavin)	Vitamin B$_5$ (pantothenic acid)	Vitamin B$_6$ (pyridoxine)
	Vegetables sweet potatoes carrots spinach pumpkin turnip greens broccoli asparagus lettuce (romaine, iceberg) tomatoes chicory dandelion greens kale watercress *Fruit* watermelon cantaloupe apricots peaches nectarines prunes *Other* eggs	*Vegetables* spinach broccoli asparagus Brussels sprouts mushrooms turnip greens watercress dandelion leaves kale parsnips cauliflower soya beans *Fruit* avocados peaches dates prunes *Nuts & seeds* almonds cashew nuts sunflower seeds *Cereals* wheat germ barley *Fish* most *Other* brewer's yeast molasses eggs	*Vegetables* broccoli cabbage cauliflower mushrooms peas legumes *Fruit* elderberries *Nuts & seeds* peanuts sesame seeds *Cereals* wheat germ & bran most whole grains *Fish* salmon *Other* brewer's yeast molasses royal jelly eggs chicken	*Vegetables* soya beans black-eye beans lentils broccoli potatoes tomatoes corn spinach kale asparagus cabbage *Fruit* cantaloupe bananas raisins avocados *Nuts* walnuts *Cereals* brown rice wheat germ & bran malt extract *Fish* salmon halibut tuna *Other* chicken brewer's yeast molasses eggs
Enemies	heat, air; food processing; metals; artificial fertilisers	light, water (by leaching), refining; alkalis; alcohol; stress; the Pill	heat, refining; caffeine, alcohol; sleeping pills, oestrogen; stress	storage; heat, freezing; food processing, refining; alcohol; the Pill
RDA (average adult)	4,000–5,000 IU	1.2–1.7mg	10mg	1.75–2.2mg

Folic acid	Vitamin C (ascorbic acid)	Vitamin E	Calcium	Copper
Vegetables asparagus spinach turnip greens broccoli Brussels sprouts cauliflower pumpkin carrots beans lentils *Fruit* melon apricots avocados *Nuts* walnuts hazelnuts almonds *Cereals* whole wheat dark rye flour *Other* egg yolks	*Vegetables* green peppers broccoli Brussels sprouts spinach cabbage, kale watercress tomatoes cauliflower potatoes sweet potatoes parsley kohlrabi turnip greens *Fruit* oranges strawberries lemons grapefruit rosehips kumquats kiwi fruits pineapple guava	*Vegetables* soya beans cold-pressed oils broccoli Brussels sprouts spinach *Nuts & seeds* pecans walnuts most seeds *Cereals* wheat germ & bran whole grains *Other* eggs	*Vegetables* turnip greens spinach broccoli kale beans carrots garlic kelp watercress dandelion leaves *Fruit* prunes oranges rhubarb dates figs *Nuts & seeds* peanuts walnuts almonds sesame seeds (dark tahini) sunflower seeds *Fish* sardines salmon	*Vegetables* beans peas lentils *Fruit* prunes raisins cherries *Cereals* whole wheat *Other* seafood molasses
heat, light, air, water; refining; alkalis; alcohol; aspirin; stress	heat, air, light, water; bruising and cutting of food; alkalis; metals/ heavy metals; aspirin, the Pill; carbon monoxide (from fumes); stress	heat, air, freezing; food processing; chlorine	water (by leaching); saturated fats	water (by leaching)
400mcg	60mg	30 IU	800–1,200mg	2–5 mg

Iron	Magnesium	Potassium	Selenium	Zinc
Vegetables spinach beans, beansprouts asparagus lettuce (iceberg) peas dandelion leaves Brussels sprouts turnip & beet greens watercress artichokes broccoli *Fruit* watermelon prunes apricots peaches dates raisins strawberries *Nuts & seeds* most nuts sesame seeds sunflower seeds *Cereals* wheat germ whole grains oatmeal *Other* molasses egg yolks	*Vegetables* spinach kale Brussels sprouts broccoli corn kelp legumes *Fruit* figs lemons grapefruit apples *Nuts & seeds* almonds sesame seeds sunflower seeds *Cereals* whole grains *Other* honey	*Vegetables* cabbage kale spinach mint potatoes watercress legumes *Fruit* oranges lemons grapefruit bananas raisins *Seeds* sunflower *Cereals* whole grains *Fish* haddock	*Vegetables* (depending on soil) onions garlic tomatoes broccoli asparagus legumes cold-pressed oils *Cereals* (depending on soil) wheat germ & bran whole grains *Nuts* most *Fish* tuna *Other* brewer's yeast	*Vegetables* corn beetroot peas carrots spinach mushrooms soya beans *Fruit* cherries pears *Nuts & seeds* most nuts pumpkin seeds sunflower seeds *Cereals* wheat germ *Fish* herring *Other* brewer's yeast eggs
water (by leaching), preservatives, additives	water (by leaching); artificial fertilisers; alcohol; stress	water (by leaching); refining; sugar, coffee, alcohol	soil erosion; food processing; heavy metals	sweating; food processing; artificial fertilisers; heavy metals; alcohol
10–18mg	300–400mg	900mg	25–50mcg	15mg

excretion of heavy metals from the body, such as cadmium, lead and mercury, all of which have immuno-suppressive effects.

Studies carried out in the 1970s and '80s provide conclusive evidence that selenium protects against cancer, heart disease and arthritis. For example, Dr Larry C. Clark at Cornell discovered that people in the lowest tenth of blood selenium levels have six times the incidence of skin cancer as those in the highest tenth. W.C. Willett found that American men in the lowest fifth of all blood selenium levels have twice the incidence of any cancer as those in the highest fifth. When considered together with blood levels of vitamin E, those people in the lowest third, who are also low in selenium, are more than eleven times likely to die of cancer as those in the upper two-thirds of blood vitamin E and selenium levels; this last study was conducted in Finland by Dr J.T. Salonen.

Since people who suffer from cancer, arthritis, multiple sclerosis or heart disease are likely to be deficient in selenium, a supplement of around 200 mcg per day is recommended. This mineral is toxic in high doses (over 2,000 mcg per day), so do be careful not to take too much. If you live in a glaciated or soil-eroded area and eat local produce, it is highly likely that your selenium level is too low and that you will need a supplement. Take the natural sort that is organically bound in yeast cells. Remember that food processing destroys it entirely. Hair analysis will show if you are deficient.

Should you be unlucky enough to suffer from arthritis, you will be fascinated to read that veterinary surgeons have been using selenium combined with vitamin E to treat arthritic horses for many years. In humans, selenium supplementation combined with the anti-oxidant vitamins A, C and E has successfully relieved pain in inflamed joints. In fact the British Arthritic Association now recommends this treatment to its members.

Whole cereals and wheat germ, brewer's yeast, green vegetables (especially asparagus and broccoli), nuts, legumes, unrefined oil, butter, onions and garlic contain selenium in varying amounts according to soil quality. Fish is another source.

ZINC This mineral works in balance with copper. If too much copper is ingested, then less zinc can be absorbed and vice versa. It also cooperates with vitamin B_6. Zinc is probably the most important mineral for effective immunity, and significantly assists in the production of the white T-cells. It is also involved in healing and many other functions, such as appetite and digestion, sense of smell, vision and growth. The average Western diet is almost certainly deficient in this mineral as chemical fertilisers bind it up in the soil. It is further removed in food refinement and by boiling vegetables – unless the water is also kept and used for soups and sauces. So don't throw that precious juice away. If your lifestyle is physically very vigorous, it is possible that you are losing up to 3 mg of zinc per day through perspiration. Eating too much bran can equally reduce amounts in the body.

The recommended daily allowance is 15 mg. Supplements of up to 100 mg in the form of zinc orotate will certainly assist patients suffering from degenerative diseases. Incidentally, it helps to form insulin, so diabetics will especially benefit. However, do not take this if you have a bacterial infection or candida, since recent reports state that zinc in excess inhibits phagocytic activity – in other words, although T-cell growth is promoted, some of the other cells are less able to gobble up invaders.

Apart from meat and cheese, very good natural sources of zinc are fish, brewer's yeast, wheat germ, soya beans, spinach, mushrooms, sunflower and pumpkin seeds, nuts and eggs.

Essential fatty acids

These have nothing to do with cream cakes or greasy sausages. On the contrary, fatty foods of this kind can inhibit the metabolism of EFAs. In fact, they are rather like a vitamin in action and are sometimes referred to as vitamin F. Only very small amounts can be stored in the body, yet we have an enormous demand for EFAs, which are fundamental to the health of the skin, the blood and kidneys. More than half of your daily intake will be used for the formation of cell membranes. Presence of EFAs ensures that the membranes are flexible; in their absence they go stiff. This in turn can affect the health and activity of the lymphocytes, the white blood cells produced by the thymus gland that play such an important part in fighting off unwanted invaders. Approximately one-third of your brain consists of EFAs – so you see how important these are!

A further function of EFAs is for the formation of prostaglandins. These are similar to hormones, but they tend to stay within certain areas of the body rather than travelling around, and regulate cells, enzymes and organs. They are very short-lived and need to be constantly re-created. Of the thirty or more prostaglandins, E1 has the most amazing qualities: it prevents thrombosis, lowers high blood pressure, and lowers cholesterol levels; and it is thought to suppress arthritic inflammation. Additionally, E1 directly affects the immune system by stimulating T-suppressor lymphocytes, that is it prevents other white cells from attacking the body's own tissue; failure of this function results in auto-immune diseases. It also inhibits the multiplication of abnormal cells.

Essential fatty acids are freely available in our foods, yet deficiencies of prostaglandins can occur because the process of conversion can be interrupted by certain factors. For instance, the linoleic acid family (contained in foods such as sunflower seed oil, corn oil and legumes) is no use just as it is; it becomes biologically active only when metabolised, and it has to go through three more stages before being converted to prostaglandin E1. The second stage is the most hazardous, the transformation into gammalinolenic acid, because many foods which are commonly eaten in our Western diet can act as blockers here. These are foods rich in saturated fats (fatty meats, dairy products, cooking fat, cakes and so on) and cholesterol; also, too much alcohol (more than two glasses of wine per day) has a similar effect. There is another hazard to watch out for: when linoleic acid is processed and hydrogenated (in other words, when oil is turned into margarine), what was originally an EFA is transformed into a trans-fatty acid which behaves just like a saturated fat. So, do not be seduced by those margarine advertisements that declare their health-giving properties! They are no good for you at all. In fact they produce EFA deficiencies by competing with the EFAs in your body. If you have to eat margarine, make sure it is soft and that it is unhydrogenated – available from health-food shops.

Some scientists suspect that the switch from butter to margarine has simply resulted in a switch from heart disease to cancer. An excess of polyunsaturated fats can depress immune functioning. Additionally, these sorts of fats, when processed by the body, can release free radicals which are positively dangerous: they damage cells and are carcinogenic. Remember that most shop-bought pastries, cakes and biscuits are made with margarine – another good reason to avoid this kind of food.

It is best to consume your EFAs in a pure form, for instance in a salad dressing made from cold-pressed sunflower or soya oil, and in raw leafy vegetables, especially cabbage, Brussels sprouts and spinach, and sprouting shoots (which contain both linoleic and linolenic acids). Oily fish and seaweeds are also prime sources. If you are immune deficient, or suffer from the auto-immune disease of multiple sclerosis, a supplement of evening primrose oil of 3 grams per day can be very helpful – especially if you are a woman. This oil contains the precious gammalinolenic acid, and therefore is already at the second stage of the conversion to prostaglandins, so is unlikely to be blocked. I personally can testify to the soothing effect that evening primrose oil has during the last half of the menstrual cycle. Most of my adult life was afflicted by recurring dysmenorrhoea, accompanied by excruciating pain, until I took 3 grams of the oil per day. Now, having also altered my lifestyle with the assistance of counselling, I am totally free of this trouble. It has also been successful in alleviating benign breast disease. When I went for my last hospital check-up, my consultant was amazed that my lumpiness had completely subsided, but, afraid of scepticism, I kept my remedy a secret. Most capsules contain a small amount of vitamin E; make sure that they do, because this vitamin is an anti-oxidant and prevents those dangerous free radicals from forming in the body. You will notice from the chart below how many other vitamins are required

---

Conversion of essential fatty acids

Stage 1   **EFA: Linoleic acid**
(available in sunflower seed oil, corn oil and legumes)
↓
helped by zinc, magnesium, vitamin B₆, biotin (vitamin H)
↓
blocked by saturated fats, cholesterol, trans fatty acids, or too much alcohol

Stage 2   **Gammalinolenic acid**
(evening primrose oil, borage oil, blackcurrant seed oil)
↓
with vitamin E prevents oxidation

Stage 3   **Dihomo-gammalinolenic acid**
↓
helped by vitamin C and vitamin B₃

Stage 4   **Prostaglandin E1**
(important for immune functioning)

---

for the conversion of EFAs. This collective, or synergistic, action is crucial to our health.

Fibre
High-fibre diets have been fashionable recently among slimmers. However, shovelling bran on to your food is not recommended here. Wheat bran contains phytates, compounds of phosphorus, which can combine with important minerals such as zinc, magnesium and iron and prevent their absorption by the body, thus lowering your immunity. The Peak Immunity Diet is naturally high in fibre and will provide you with all the roughage you need to speed up elimination of toxic waste. The combination of soft and hard fibres from fruit and vegetables also appears to promote the formation of healthy bacteria in the intestine, another way of lessening the risk of colorectal cancer.

It is the fibre in food that gives you that satisfied, 'full' feeling. If you squeeze an orange and drink it, you won't feel as if you have eaten anything. But if you eat the orange whole, your stomach will notice the difference.

CHANGING TO THE PEAK IMMUNITY DIET

Frankly, changing one's diet is not easy. It is quite natural to crave foods that we found satisfying as children. Foods not only sustained our bodies, but very often they were an expression of mother's attention and love. By continuing to eat those same foods, we feel psychologically as well as physically nourished. However, the fact is that mother may have had little or no knowledge concerning nutrition and she may well have fed you on a high-fat, high-sugar, highly refined diet. What about all those soggy chips dripping with grease, or those stodgy puddings and pies that we remember with such affection? One of my favourite treats as a child was a 'sugar butty', a large slice of white bread spread thickly with butter with white sugar sprinkled on top, then folded over so that there was a sweet, sticky centre to the sandwich. No doubt this supplied plenty of instant energy for more ballet dancing or tree-climbing, but what else did it do to my growing young body? Were treats such as this storing up trouble for the future?

During my late teens I began to develop my own ideas about food.

As an animal-lover, I wanted to be a vegetarian, but utter scorn was poured on to me. I was told I wasn't 'eating properly', that I would become ill through lack of protein, and my mother clearly thought I was just 'being difficult'. In those days, vegetarians were considered to be very cranky and health-food shops were unheard-of. I persevered for a number of years, but was finally worn down by the repetitive taunts and social disapproval. Modern scientific research into nutrition has since proved that my instincts were right. If only I had listened to my own inner wisdom and ignored the criticism of others! How difficult it is to be different from the crowd.

During the years before my illness, I had always assumed that I was being fairly sensible about food. I ate wholemeal bread, plenty of fruit and vegetables and fish rather than meat. However, my diet was high in dairy fats: I loved milk and cheese. Endless Cheddar sandwiches satisfied those hunger pangs in the office and sleep at night was impossible unless I had my half pint of all-milk hot chocolate. The truth is, however, that cows' milk is meant for calves rather than humans. Since reading that dairy products cause women to create the enzyme lactase in their bodies, thought to be involved in the formation of breast cancer, I have cut them completely from my diet – hard to do, but well worth while. To compensate, I occasionally indulge myself in live yoghurt and cheese made from goat's milk (the hard sort avoids any slight risk of listeria), which doesn't adversely affect the body in the same way.

Nowadays, people are far more tolerant of unusual diets. When asked why I don't eat meat, the replies 'Doctor's orders', or 'I have to keep to a low-fat diet for my health' often stimulate interested questions and friendly conversation. However, when people hear that I eat 'peculiar' things like millet and tofu, the going gets a bit rougher. In the end, my present high energy levels and glowing state of health convince them that I must be doing something right!

Eating out can be a bit tricky – especially with business colleagues. On these occasions I ignore the white rolls and butter, steak and sickly desserts and stick to fish and vegetables, followed by fresh fruit salad. If invited to a dinner party, I simply point out that I'm on a low-fat régime and don't eat red meat, but that fish and chicken are acceptable. Most hosts and hostesses cope with these limitations very well. If they produce an elaborate Pavlova for the dessert which has obviously taken hours to concoct, I exclaim how wonderful it looks, but that I am very full and can only manage a tiny spoonful. This way, no offence is caused. To be honest, having been on the PI Diet for more than five years, my body is so unused to sugar that the very sight of a sweet dessert makes me feel quite ill. As far as wine is concerned, if I drink it slowly not only do I enjoy each sip, but manage not to exceed the limit of two glasses per day (see 'Drinking and eating' later in the chapter).

Try and aim to balance psychological health with physical. It is far better to enjoy a real binge and go back to your diet having satisfied your cravings than to beat yourself up and make the whole thing into a miserable penance. It really is important to enjoy your food.

Motivation

The speed at which you are able to make the switch from your present food to the PI Diet will depend on your motivation and on whether you have to cook for other people, or, indeed, on whether you generally rely on someone else to cook for you. If others are involved, this can be either a tremendous blessing or a terrible hindrance, depending on their attitude. However, enthusiasm on your part will surely convert the sceptical. As you and your family try out the new vegan recipes, you will soon discover what you like best and meat will become less and less important.

I was highly motivated. That mysterious 'hot spot' that had appeared on my bone scan so terrified me that the only way I could manage to crawl through those endless three months of waiting was to dedicate myself wholeheartedly to my new régime. Caring for myself in practical ways helped to focus my mind on staying alive, rather than brooding over the possibility of dying. I didn't want to die; I wanted to live! As a cancer patient I decided to follow a cleansing vegan diet for six months, reintroducing fish and eggs gradually (see 'The PI Diet and special conditions', later in this chapter). So I cleared out my food cupboard, fed all the tinned fish, meats and soups to my dog (who was delighted at these unexpected treats!) and gave the white flour, sugar and other sweet things to my neighbours. In return I acquired from them spare glass storage jars and purchased more from the local sweet shop. Then followed a trip to the health-food shop. Where possible, I chose organic produce, even though it was more expensive. This is what I bought:

Shopping list

Grains and cereals
Brown rice
Millet
Jumbo oats
Pot barley
Cornmeal
Wholemeal and rye flours
Muesli base (no sugar or
milk powder)
Rice cakes (salt-free)

Nuts and seeds
Almonds
Hazelnuts
Cashew nuts
Dried chestnuts
Sunflower, sesame, pumpkin,
fenugreek and alfalfa seeds

Dried pulses and legumes
Haricot beans
Soya beans
Mung beans
Butter beans
Aduki beans
Chick peas
Lentils, red and brown
Split green peas

Pasta
Wholewheat spaghetti
Wholewheat macaroni

Soya products
Tofu
Tempeh
Soya milk (salt- and sugar-free)

Dairy products
Unsalted butter
Live goat's milk yoghurt

Seaweeds
Kelp Powder
Nori flakes
Hijiki
Arame
Agar-agar flakes

Sun-dried fruits
Dates
Figs
Sultanas
Raisins
Hunza apricots

Spreads and sweeteners
Brown tahini
Honey
Molasses
Malt extract
Sugar-free jam

Herbs, spices, flavourings
Basil
Oregano
Tarragon
Thyme
Marjoram
Sage
Dill and caraway seeds
Coriander
Cumin
Cinnamon
Miso

Drinks
Herb teas: limeflower and
mint, mixed fruit, chamomile
etc.
Bancha tea
Apple juice, fresh pressed

Oil and vinegar
   Cold-pressed sunflower oil
   Olive oil
   Cider vinegar

My protein intake was now assured for several weeks. Luckily, the same health-food shop also sold organically grown fruit and vegetables. It looked as if food shopping was going to be easier than previously. No more waiting in long supermarket queues! Another bonus was that beans were a great deal cheaper than meat.

Utensils

Aluminium and Teflon pans were clearly not a good idea, since they can cause poisoning over a period of time, so all of mine were dispatched to the next jumble sale. Little tugs of regret at losing such faithful old items made this job more difficult. One ancient stewpan had belonged to my mother and its battered lid and pock-marked interior brought back vivid memories of childhood, most especially the glorious cooking smells that had filled the kitchen. Oh well, it was all in a good cause. After shopping around I managed to find stainless-steel pans and a vegetable steamer that weren't too appallingly expensive. Luckily, my casseroles were Pyrex and Le Creuset, both of which were fine. I also bought a water filter. A very kind friend gave me a juicer, which had been sitting unused in her parents' attic, so now it was possible to make highly nutritious drinks from fresh vegetables and fruits. My blender with nut-grinding attachment was soon in use nearly every day – an indispensable piece of equipment.

Early experiments

Having the incentive to try out totally new recipes was actually quite fun and I was proud of my successes. But there were a few problems. Although salads had always been part of my diet, so had those convenient slices of cheese and cold ham and tins of tuna fish. The protein part now had to be replaced with something else and this needed some imagination. In the end I learnt how to make bean pâtés, which were delicious. My old stand-by, the cheese sandwich, was replaced by a tahini and banana filling, rich in calcium and potassium. Quick meals could be made out of lightly fried cubes of tempeh (cultured beancurd), with, say, mushrooms, brown rice and green vegetables. Tofu was also new to me, but I soon discovered that I could make glorious creamy desserts with it, as well as high-protein savoury dishes. Millet became a useful ingredient, and when boiled, mixed with ground almonds and herbs and baked in the oven, provided another easy meat substitute. Cooking, which used to be a real chore, was suddenly interesting and creative. Every so often a yearning for a sweet snack, such as chocolate biscuits, would overwhelm me, but dates and sultanas soon satisfied those sugar cravings.

Food preparation and cooking methods
Some bad old habits had to be abandoned – no more boiling or deep-fat frying – just light steaming for vegetables and quick stir-frying when the recipes required it. This way, most of the vitamins and minerals could be retained. The water from the steamer was religiously preserved and used in soups and bean stews. Vegetables contain natural sodium, so there is no need to add extra salt. After a short time on the Peak Immunity Diet my taste buds seemed to become more sensitive and I began to appreciate the many subtle flavours of food that hadn't been smothered with condiments.

If you find it impossible to buy fresh, organic produce, you can successfully eliminate traces of most pesticides by washing vegetables in a malt vinegar solution: add two tablespoons to the water. Root vegetables are frequently sprayed with fungicides, and hormones to prevent them from sprouting, so careful scrubbing is essential.

It is very important to avoid burning food, since this produces carcinogens (substances capable of causing cancer), so when frying keep the heat very low and use ghee or olive oil, both of which tolerate fairly high temperatures. Do not, for instance, allow onions to go brown, but just cook gently until transparent. (You will find instructions for making ghee in the 'Peak immunity dairy' section in chapter 7.) Be careful of oven temperatures; if you accidentally burn something, throw it away. The same applies to toast.

Until your body adjusts to the unaccustomed foods, flatulence can be an embarrassing problem, but, since beans are the main culprits, there is an easy remedy. After soaking them overnight, boil rapidly in water for ten minutes to remove the toxins from the skins. Discard this juice and cover with fresh, filtered water. Simmer gently until tender.

Ingredients

Tofu is readily available at most health-food shops. However, in case you are unable to buy it locally, recipes are given in this book for making both soya milk and tofu. Being high in protein, soya-bean products will become an important part of your new diet. Natto, fermented soya beans, has a slightly bitter taste, rather like coffee, and provides an instant, high-protein snack. Seitan, which is made from the gluten of wheat, has a meaty texture and is also a good source of protein, so do try this if you can find it.

Miso, another soya-bean product from Japan, may also be new to you. It is a brown paste made with a cultured grain base and fermented, and is valuable as a flavouring especially in soups and stews. Although it contains salt, its nutritional benefits outweigh this disadvantage. In 1945, a Japanese doctor and his staff in a Nagasaki hospital survived atomic radiation, while everyone around them was dying. He attributed their continuing vitality to their daily intake of miso soup, brown rice and wakame seaweed. Patients undergoing radiotherapy may well find that a regular intake of miso helps to reduce side-effects.

I have to confess that it has taken me a long time to get used to seaweeds, but since they are a prime source of trace elements it is worth persevering. Try arame first; it has quite a mild flavour and blends nicely with vegetables in casseroles. It can also be used cold in salads. Hijiki goes well with rice dishes. Cooking instructions generally appear on the packets. As for nori flakes, these are excellent sprinkled on soups and have a subtle flavour.

Eggs are restricted to four per week on account of their high cholesterol content. Choose species of fish from the deep seas, as these are less likely to be polluted than flat fish or river fish, and eat them no more than once a week. On the other days you will be enjoying mainly vegan food.

The Peak Immunity Diet places considerable emphasis on whole grains, which are highly nutritious. They can be incorporated into any meal in one form or another, greatly increasing the repertoire of recipes. Limit your intake of potatoes; brown rice or pot barley are much better for you, containing protein, minerals and B vitamins. You may not be familiar with millet, but this has a pleasant flavour and can be used in either savoury dishes or desserts. The protein content is almost as high as wheat. People in Africa, Asia and northern China have depended on this crop for a very long time, but it is unjustifiably neglected in Europe and America.

Storage

Freshness really is vitally important, especially where oils are concerned, as rancidity causes harmful free radicals to form in the body. Remember that nuts are oily, so if they are shelled it is best to store them in the refrigerator, especially if they are ground. Brazil nuts and walnuts are particularly prone to rancidity, so buy them in their shells.

Foods containing vitamin C should also be eaten as soon as possible since this vitamin is quickly lost when exposed to the air. Refrigeration aids its retention. Anything containing B_2 and B_6 needs to be kept in the dark, as these vitamins are unstable to light.

Freezing should be used selectively. Vitamin C in foods can be preserved if frozen quickly, whereas vitamin E is almost completely destroyed and B_6 is significantly reduced. Do not therefore freeze bread, any other grain dishes, nor nuts, green plants or anything containing vegetable oils.

If your salad oil leaves a white deposit when stored in the fridge it has gone off, so throw it away.

Stainless-steel containers are useful for left-overs. Avoid wrapping food in cling film unless it says 'non-PVC' or 'plasticiser free'. One plasticiser, DEHA, is a known carcinogen and it is possible for such substances to migrate into foods.

The bottom of the refrigerator is a good place for salads and vegetables. Of course, there is nothing better than growing your own and eating them fresh from the earth. I now rent a large allotment for the princely sum of £5 per annum. Yes, the digging is hard work, but a satisfying way of obtaining healthy outdoor exercise. And the flavour and crispness of my fresh organic produce is unbeatable. Everyone can at least grow a few herbs on their windowsills. Another important part of your diet will be sprouting seeds and beans, which are very easy to grow. You will find details in the 'Salads' section in chapter 7.

At least, if you eat seasonally, the fruit that you buy is more likely to be ripened on the tree rather than in transit. Your vegetables will also be fresher. The longer it was since they were growing, the poorer their nutritional content. If possible, buy only small quantities at once, so that you don't have to keep them for too long.

Drinking and eating

Avoid drowning your food with liquid. This way, maximum nutrients can be absorbed. It is best to have a drink half an hour or more before your meal. Then wait at least an hour after the meal before drinking again.

The Yogis have a saying that the faster you eat, the younger you will die. Modern research reinforces this ancient wisdom: hastily swallowed food predisposes people towards stomach and digestive disorders, because the stomach has to produce more acid to make up for their ineffective chewing. Michio Kushi in his *Cancer Prevention Diet* recommends that you chew each mouthful fifty times! At all events, make sure you use your teeth to grind your food to a mush before swallowing it. Good chewing is also a first line of defence in our immune system, since unwanted bacteria can be destroyed in the mouth by the naturally antiseptic saliva before penetrating further into the body.

Adapting to the Peak Immunity Diet also means changing the order in which you eat courses. You will notice from the sample menus that salad comes before soup; this may seem somewhat eccentric, but there is a good reason for it. If cooked food enters the stomach first, it is regarded as foreign by the immune defences, which respond by mustering white blood cells, a process known as leucocytosis. If this happens repeatedly, immunity can become depleted. When raw food starts the meal, however, this process does not occur. The salad stimulates the correct enzymes and the digestive system works efficiently. Always start your main meal with a helping of salad, therefore.

You will find the PI Diet very filling, but always aim to eat to only 80 per cent of your capacity in order not to overburden your digestive system. Thus, after a meal, you should feel satisfied but definitely not 'FFTB', as my grandmother used to say, that is 'full fit to bustin'!

Filter your tap water to remove the heavy metals, such as lead and cadmium, which depress the immune system. A few filters will also remove at least some of the nitrates – important if you live in an agricultural area; their consumption has been linked with stomach cancer. Keep the jug clean (vinegar removes the limescale) and change the cartridge regularly, to avoid build-up of unwanted bacteria. Otherwise, if you can afford it, buy pure spring water in bottles.

Alcohol in small quantities is reputed to stimulate the production of prostaglandin E1, an important part of immune functioning. So enjoy up to two glasses of wine per day. More than this has the reverse effect and in large amounts will cause damage to the organs, particularly the liver, which is vital to our health. Contrary to popular belief, regular consumption of too much alcohol actually raises anxiety levels.

When possible, always make your own fruit juices. Shop-bought ones made from concentrates have been heat-treated and have lost much of their goodness.

It really is best to avoid tea and coffee. Coffee inhibits the absorption of zinc, so vital for immunity. An international study, reported in the *British Journal of Cancer* in 1970, concluded that prostate cancer mortality was directly linked with *per capita* coffee consumption. The following year the *Lancet* said that women who drink coffee regularly have a two and a half times higher risk of developing cancer of the urinary tract. A more recent report (1981) from the Harvard School of Public Health stated that people who drink a cup of coffee a day are nearly twice as likely to develop cancer of the pancreas as those who do not drink it. Another article appeared in the *Lancet* (1988) confirming that caffeine causes increased infertility in women by up to 50 per cent. Are these facts sufficient to convert you to herb teas? I hope so. It may be a little while before you grow accustomed to their tastes, but allow yourself to experiment and you will quickly find some that you like. My favourite is a fruit tea consisting of whole dried chunks of strawberries, orange peel, apple and hibiscus flowers – truly delicious! Others that I like are limeflower and mint – very refreshing first thing in the morning – nettle and elderflower blend during the day and chamomile to send me to sleep.

My herbalist recommended three teas to boost my immune system: red clover, sweet violet and mistletoe. You can purchase these dried, by the ounce, from a herbal apothecary (see address list at the end of the book). Alternatively, the red clover is very easy to grow. Allow them to infuse for about ten minutes and drink three cups a day of one kind. The mistletoe has a slightly odd taste, but you will become used to it. Iscador, an extract of mistletoe, has long been used by homoeopathic doctors as a booster of the immune system and is regularly prescribed for cancer patients. Sage tea, which should be boiled for three minutes to release the enzymes, is also considered beneficial.

Bancha tea is made either from the leaves or twigs of the bush and has health-giving properties. The stem tea is best as it contains calcium and other minerals.

A word of warning: if you wish to take any of the less usual herb teas on a regular basis, do consult a professionally qualified herbalist first. Some of these are quite potent and can occasionally be harmful to certain people, for example pregnant women, or those with weak hearts. The herbalist will take a full medical history and will prescribe only those teas and medicines that will do you good.

Always allow drinks and food to cool a little before consuming them. Equally, refrain from eating or drinking anything very cold, which can upset the stomach. Both extremes harm the delicate mucous membranes of the mouth and throat, and can pave the way for cancers. Have you noticed how your pets will wait until their food is the right temperature? My golden labrador would never touch her dinner if it was too hot, no matter how hungry she was.

A delightful way to improve the quality of your life is to eat in calm, relaxing surroundings. In the evening, I often light a candle, even if I am eating on my own, and put on some soothing music. I really allow myself to appreciate my food. By avoiding irritating external stimuli, your system will operate smoothly and your blood supply will be where it is needed – around the stomach and digestive tract. Occasionally I watch television while eating, but have discovered that exciting programmes definitely cause upheavals in my stomach, and are not a good accompaniment to a meal. During the day, I can gaze through the window and contemplate the graceful silver birches at the bottom of my garden.

Sit quietly for a while after eating and avoid vigorous exercise for several hours.

Your weight
One immediate advantage of the Peak Immunity Diet is that, because it is low in fat and salt, you will lose weight! Most people lose approximately seven pounds. Even though I ate like a horse, I lost nearly twice that amount, but later put a few pounds back on again after my body had become adjusted to the different types of food. A shopping spree definitely confirmed that I was back to size ten clothes. It's good to feel so lean and fit.

The dangers of obesity have been well publicised, yet half of the retired population is overweight, and almost 40 per cent of men and around 32 per cent of women are heavier than they should be. Surplus fat increases the body's need for all nutrients, and large people often suffer from vitamin and mineral deficiencies. The immune system is put under a strain in a fat body and all sorts of miscellaneous problems can occur, from fluid retention, shortage of breath or wearing-out of the joints, to heart failure, thrombosis and diabetes. There is a higher incidence of cancer and of arthritis in overweight people. Dr Robert Good, former head of the Memorial Sloan-Kettering Cancer Center in America, has estimated that obese women are ten times more likely to develop a malignancy than their slim sisters. If you have a tendency to produce excess rolls of fat, therefore, the Peak Immunity Diet will certainly help you. Not only will it trim your figure down, but it will provide you with high-quality nutrients, correctly balanced, so that your body chemistry can operate to maximum efficiency.

Detoxification
The more our food is treated with artificial additives and other chemicals, the harder our livers have to work to deal with them. If confronted with an 'unrecognisable' toxic element, the liver will refuse to process it, and instead make fat to store it in. Thus, toxins can build up in the body to unhealthy levels.

At the start of the Peak Immunity Diet, therefore, it is a good idea to give your system a thorough clean-out. Set aside two days in which you are able to have a reasonable amount of rest and on the first day eat nothing but grapes. You will need approximately 1 1/2 lbs/700 g. Eat every two hours and include the skins and pips, which are full of goodness. Take up to six glasses of water within the twenty-four hours. On the second day, eat only salads or raw vegetables and sprouting seeds, and fruit. There are several suggestions in the 'Lunch' section in chapter 7. Add a few nuts. Instead of dinner, have a large bowl of uncooked vegetable soup. Liquidise small pieces of carrot, broccoli, spinach, onion and so on in some vegetable stock and eat cold or just tepid; do not allow it to become too warm. Drink no more than 2 pints/1.1 l of liquid within the twenty-four hours.

Repeat the fruit and salad day each week for a month or longer, depending on your general state of health. Patients with degenerative diseases will especially benefit from such a clean-out.

An excellent tea for stimulating the kidneys to excrete toxins and waste products from the body is nettle tea. Wearing rubber gloves, pick the tender tops, free of flowers, wash them, place in a jug and pour boiling water on to them. You will need about 12 tops to ³/4 pint/425 ml of water. Allow to cool. Drink about half a cup three times a day.

Remember that it takes some time for the body to become free of toxins, and that a 'healing crisis' can occur – in other words you may get worse before improving. Persevere through this difficult patch and the diet will help to alleviate your condition.

Planning the menus
To give you an idea of how to balance menus, the following is a typical day from the Peak Immunity Diet:

> *On waking*
> Cup of limeflower and mint herb tea.
> *Breakfast*
> Muesli served with stewed apricots and a little goat's milk yoghurt.
> Tempeh toast.
> *Mid-morning*
> Rosehip tea or dandelion coffee.
> Banana.
> *Lunch*
> Waldorf salad.
> Leek broth with slice of wholemeal bread.
> Tofu cream.
> *Tea*
> Strawberry fruit tea.
> Slice of sticky bread.
> *Dinner*
> Carrot juice half an hour before eating.
> Chicory salad.
> Nut loaf, jacket potatoes and lightly steamed spinach.
> Poires belle Hélène.
> *Before bed*
> Cup of chamomile tea.

If you work in an office or factory, take your homemade soup with you in a thermos flask. The salad you can pack in a lunch box. Yes, this is more effort than hastily gobbling a sandwich, but a very great deal better for you.

THE PI DIET AND SPECIAL CONDITIONS

Readers suffering from particular conditions may need to exclude certain items from the Peak Immunity Diet, to help themselves still further, or, alternatively, emphasise various elements. These are discussed below.

Allergies and food intolerance

Strictly speaking, a true food allergy occurs when a protein or carbohydrate in the substance eaten triggers off a specific immune response and antibodies are formed. The subsequent release of histamine and other chemicals results in severe local inflammation. If these enter the circulation in large amounts there can be a sudden drop in blood pressure that puts the person into anaphylactic shock, which can be fatal. More usual is an intolerance to certain foodstuffs that produces a feeling of tiredness or general malaise. The reason for this reaction is not yet proven, although modern research indicates that it could be due to enzyme deficiencies or disturbances in the gut flora. Live yoghurt made from goat's milk or soya milk will help to provide the correct balance of bacteria.

At present, the main solution is avoidance of the offending substances. Many foods that most commonly cause reactions, such as preserved meats, smoked fish, cow's milk, tea, coffee and chocolate and artificial additives are already excluded from the PI Diet, so the chances are that you will notice an improvement in your condition after about two weeks of following this. However, if you find that symptoms still persist, your food intolerance may be caused by another substance. In this case, try excluding eggs altogether, also wheat, oats, barley, rye, corn and yeast, potatoes, onions and sweetcorn, citrus fruits and drinks, alcohol and tap water, all of which are well-recognised sources of allergies. Eat rice cakes instead of bread and include millet and buckwheat in your diet. Stick to bottled spring water. Admittedly, it will be difficult to begin with, but you only have to keep it up for a fortnight! If the symptoms disappear, one of these foods is the culprit, so add each back gradually into your diet until you discover which it is.

If you are still suffering, your condition may be a result of some other cause entirely, so do consult your doctor.

A more direct way to spot a food intolerance is to ask yourself which items you most crave. A three-stage process seems to be involved, very similar to the General Adaptation Syndrome described in chapter 3. Initially, the intolerance is experienced as a symptom, such as a rash, feeling faint, or a headache. In the second stage, the body adapts to it. In fact, the person may feel pleasantly stimulated for a short time, as with that early morning cup of coffee. Then a craving develops for that item, to the point where withdrawal symptoms occur if the need is not satisfied. Thus, the hangover will be fixed with yet another drink to ease the pain of the headache. In the final stage, exhaustion sets in and the 'boost' experienced by the food or drink is no longer a pleasure, but an addiction. At this stage the body becomes really ill with repetitive headaches, fatigue, depression and so on. It is, of course, hard for the sufferer to accept the cause for the malaise, because the 'addiction' was once experienced as pleasurable.

Arthritis and rheumatism

Detoxification is especially important if you suffer from inflammatory arthritis, gout or rheumatism, because your condition has probably been exacerbated by a build-up of uric acid in your body. This substance, because it has an affinity with the organic lime within the bones, is particularly attracted to joints and it is here that it is very often deposited. The result is swelling and pain within these areas. The same acid can become deposited in the muscles, and the effect of this is the discomfort of rheumatism.

There is no medical cure for these conditions, although symptoms may be relieved by powerful anti-inflammatory drugs, many of which have undesirable side-effects. Surgery is useful in some cases, but again this will not cure the disease, which will reassert itself in another area of the body.

Switching to the PI Diet will help with detoxification and will supply the nutrients essential for the neutralization of the acid. Formation of uric acid will be reduced, since the main culprits, such as meat, have already been eliminated. However, acidic fruits must be avoided as well, and these include the following: oranges, lemons and grapefruit, also pineapples, plums, damsons, gooseberries, rhubarb, strawberries, blackcurrants, redcurrants, blackberries and tomatoes. Instead, eat peaches and apricots, pears, apples, melons and bananas, and take a supplement of vitamin C with bioflavonoids. Drink plenty of apple and carrot juice, but avoid all alcohol, which is high in acid. If this is too hard to bear, an occasional glass of Guinness is acceptable.

Paradoxically, cider vinegar has proved very useful in the treatment of arthritis, because the malic acid which it contains is able to dissolve the hard deposits of uric acid in the joints. Use this in salad dressings and cooking. A drink can be made by dissolving 1 tsp honey in a mug of warm water and adding a dsp of cider vinegar. Take three times a day.

Molasses is also thought to be beneficial, being rich in minerals, especially potassium, and B vitamins. Stir this into your cereal. Alfalfa contains similar properties, so grow plenty of this and use it in your salads. It is also reputed to reduce the pain and swelling that accompany toxic accumulation. However, if your condition is rheumatoid arthritis, watch your iron intake, since it has been noticed that iron-deficient populations are rarely troubled by this disease.

Thousands of people suffer from the crippling arthritic condition of ankylosing spondylitis, which initially affects the spine and most often attacks young males. New evidence from the Middlesex Hospital and King's College Hospital in London suggests that it may have auto-immune connections and that a bacterium in the bowel called Klebsiella triggers this disease. Since the bacterium thrives on starch, cut out potatoes altogether and reduce your intake of rice and foods such as bread and pasta made from flour. This will help to control the illness. Both AS and RA patients will benefit from regular doses of live yoghurt to keep the gut flora healthy.

Patients given calcium pantothenate have shown improvement in arthritic conditions and a supplement of at least 25 mg daily is recommended. Keep up your intake of wheat germ, an anti-stress food that is a good source of B vitamins and vitamin E, and take around 200 mcg of selenium. Also, make sure your calcium supply is adequate, since this will decrease your sensitivity to pain. (See also under 'Rheumatoid arthritis' below.)

Cancer and Aids
As has already been mentioned, the PI Diet is ideal for anyone suffering from immune-deficiency diseases, including cancer patients and those diagnosed as being HIV positive. Eat as much raw vegan food as you can manage and (unless you have digestive problems) avoid returning to fish and eggs until you are feeling stronger.

Vitamins and mineral supplements are also highly recommended. This is what I take each day, based on the suggestions given to me by the Bristol Cancer Help Centre: beta carotene 10,000 IU (now reduced from an initial 27,000 IU), vitamin B complex 500 mg, vitamin C as calcium ascorbate 2 g (if you are seriously ill, take at least 6 g per day), evening primrose oil 3 g, selenium 200 mcg, zinc orotate 100 mg.

A supplement of folic acid can be helpful to patients with leukaemia and Hodgkin's disease, since these conditions increase the need for the nutrient.

Candida albicans (thrush)

This uncomfortable disease is best corrected by including plenty of goat's milk yoghurt along with your PI Diet. This must be the live sort, containing the bacterium *Lactobacillus acidophilus*; make sure this is stated on the carton. Severe cases may need around 3/4 pint/ 425 ml daily, so use it on your cereal and make drinks out of it by blending with a banana or other fruit and soya milk. It can also be used in desserts along with a little honey. In a short time the flora in your gut will be restored to a healthy balance, and unwanted bacteria, including yeast infections, will be kept at bay.

Biotin deficiency is common among candida patients. This allows the mild, yeasty form of thrush to develop into a more severe case of fungal infection which can be difficult to eradicate. By keeping up your intake of biotin, therefore, this conversion is prevented. Well-cooked free-range eggs provide a rich source of biotin, so use plenty of these until your condition is corrected. Then revert to four per week. Oleic acid is equally effective and this is found in cold-pressed olive oil. Use this generously every day in your salad dressing.

The PI Diet will provide essential nutrients for healing the damaged mucous membranes as the disease clears up, but it may be wise to take extra zinc, vitamin E and calcium pantothenate for a while.

Should you reduce your yeast intake? Doctors cannot agree on this. Some say yes; others that the yeast used in food and drink is completely different from candida and that it makes no odds. Perhaps it is sensible to reduce your yeast intake while recovering from the disease.

Colds and 'flu

You will be much less susceptible to respiratory infections once your body has adjusted to the PI Diet. It was two years before I even caught a mild cold, despite my husband's coughs and sneezes. If you do succumb, increase your intake of citrus fruits and eat plenty of fresh beansprouts all of which are rich in vitamin C. The traditional hot lemon-and-honey drink really is good for you. In fact, make sure you take plenty of liquids to counteract any sweating caused by the feverishness associated with 'flu.

Diabetes and hypoglycaemia

If you are a diabetic, it is important that you consult with your doctor before considering any change in the food that you eat. However, diets commonly prescribed for diabetics have strong similarities with the one described in this book, being high in fibre and low in sugar, fat and salt, with an emphasis on fresh vegetables and whole cereals. At the University of Kentucky, Dr Anderson developed the HCF (high-carbohydrate, high-fibre) diet especially for diabetics, after discovering that it lowered the body's need for insulin and the fat levels in the blood, and this is similar to the PI Diet. Of the patients with adult-onset diabetes who were on daily insulin of less than 25 units, eighteen out of twenty were able to discontinue their injections altogether after adapting to the diet. Among juvenile-onset cases, insulin needs were lowered by 25 per cent.

Glucose tolerance can be improved by a supplement of 4 g per day of brewer's yeast, which is rich in chromium. But be patient. Results will not be obvious for at least three months. Zinc has a similar effect.

Hypoglycaemia is very rare in countries where sugar consumption is low and fibre intake is high, but it is common in the West. A refined, low-fibre meal, such as a breakfast consisting of cornflakes, milk and sugar, followed by a slice of white bread, butter and marmalade, will cause the blood sugar to soar rapidly and then to drop below the level that it was before the meal. At this point, you will feel utterly wretched. The PI Diet will correct this problem, but, for maximum well-being, make sure you keep your protein intake high, especially early in the day.

Multiple sclerosis

MS sufferers can be particularly sensitive to pollutants, so detoxi-fication is really important. Follow the guidelines given earlier. Additionally, supplements of zinc and selenium are helpful. There is a theory that poisoning from lead and mercury can exacerbate the condition of MS. However, these heavy metals will bind with trace elements such as zinc and selenium and can thus be expelled naturally from the body. Otherwise, they may accumulate and cause further damage. Certainly, they depress the immune defences. Unfortunately, mercury can gradually leach from the amalgam fillings in your teeth. One study by a dentist in 1984 indicated that removal of fillings results in an increase of T-cells, which then drop again when the fillings are replaced. It is possible to have tests carried out to determine whether you are hypersensitive to mercury. Some MS sufferers have noticed a reduction in symptoms after the removal of amalgam fillings, but this is not recommended unless hypersensitivity has been established.

Symptoms of the disease can appear to be worse because of food intolerances, so do test yourself for reactions to different substances. Changing to the Peak Immunity Diet will automatically remove many of these. The diet will also drastically reduce your intake of saturated fats, of great significance to MS patients, since they have difficulty in metabolising them. One theory suggests that a build-up of fats in the blood damages the vessels and thereby contributes to the onset of multiple sclerosis. A twenty-year study was carried out by R.L. Swank, from which he produced convincing evidence that a low-fat diet, if maintained over a long period, slows down the disease process and reduces the frequency of new attacks. Of equal importance is the inclusion of essential fatty acids in the diet. It has been noticed that MS is unheard of among Eskimos, who have a diet rich in fish oils. In 1973 Dr J.H.D. Millar of Belfast and Dr K.J. Zilkha of the National Hospital, London, carried out carefully controlled trials on the therapeutic effects of polyunsaturated oils; the conclusions were that they shortened relapses and reduced their severity. Read especially, therefore, the section on 'Essential fatty acids' in this chapter, and do take the evening primrose oil recommended. Also, make sure that you include fish in your diet and don't forget the salad dressing.

Rheumatoid arthritis
The good news is that more than 50 per cent of sufferers overcome the disease spontaneously with the assistance of natural therapies. Wholesome food is vital, because the inflammatory process can result in both malabsorption of nutrients and in increased nutritional

requirements. Zinc levels are often particularly low, so supplements of this mineral are recommended, especially as it can help reduce inflammation, as can vitamin E and selenium. Patients treated with zinc sulphate for more than three months showed improvement over those who took none. If you are using aspirin, your need for ascorbic acid will be greatly increased, so ensure that your intake of vitamin C is high. RA patients are often low in B_6, too. In addition to a B-complex supplement, good natural sources of vitamin B_6 are soya beans, brown rice, lentils, raw broccoli, bananas and chicken.

Those on steroids will probably need potassium supplements, balanced by a restricted salt intake.

Freshly pressed raw fruit and vegetable juices are highly recommended for all RA patients – the best way to absorb those essential vitamins and minerals – and wheat germ for the vitamin E.

Poor digestion

Patients with serious disorders affecting any part of the digestive system, such as cancer of the intestine, are likely to find the high-fibre content of, for instance, beans too much for them. Instead, eat free-range chicken and turkey and deep-sea white fish and well-cooked eggs. High protein drinks made of tofu and soya milk (see 'Drinks' in chapter 7) are very nutritious and easily digested by anyone. These will help to keep your energy up when solid foods cause problems. Important also are fresh vegetable juices, which will provide you with the vitamins and minerals that you need in an easily digestible form.

A note for the faint-hearted

If life without red meat is truly unbearable, have a little lean lamb every so often. Avoid pork, which is high in fat, and beef, which is heavily contaminated with hormones and antibiotics, and make sure any chicken or turkey you eat is organically produced.

If you are well, small amounts of skimmed milk are acceptable – but this is definitely not for anyone who has ever suffered from breast cancer or has a history of it in the family. Occasional goat's milk cheeses are fine (choose the hard ones), and a little cottage cheese now and then – but note that this can prevent absorption of zinc in your body, a mineral that is vital to healthy immunity.

Take a step at a time. For example, include a raw vegetable such as broccoli in your salads or learn to grow alfalfa sprouts. Every so often introduce a nut roast or bean casserole instead of the usual meat dish. Old favourites can be adapted: make your rice pudding from brown rather than white rice and with soya milk instead of cow's. This gradual familiarisation with the new ideas will make them seem more manageable and accessible. Remember that each modest improvement that you make to your diet is yet another step towards immune efficiency.

7 Recipes for peak immunity

The emphasis in this chapter is on recipes that you may not easily find in other books. None includes salt, sugar, baking powder or saturated fats (except ghee) and all are egg-free. Fish and chicken recipes you will find in abundance elsewhere and you can simply adapt them to suit the diet. There are plenty of high-protein vegan meals to choose from here, which incorporate the ingredients already discussed, and each has been put together with maximum nutritional value in mind. You will even find some really tempting treats!

BREAKFAST

Have you noticed how many recipe books omit breakfast altogether? This is symptomatic, unfortunately, of the general apathy regarding this important meal. If you eat your dinner early enough in the evening you will feel hungry for your breakfast the following morning. High immunity needs the right sort of fuel first thing. In addition to energy-giving carbohydrates, vitamins and minerals are essential, plus a good source of protein; aim for one-third of your day's supply, that is 12 grams (1/3 oz) of usable protein for a 9-stone (126-lb) woman and 14.5 grams (1/2 oz) for an 11-stone (154-lb) man.

Meagre breakfasts can result not only in general fatigue, but in dizziness, headaches, poor concentration, constipation and a host of other complaints. Start your day well and treat yourself to two courses. I find that if I follow my cereal or fruit with a cooked dish I can work at peak efficiency all morning without needing to stop for a snack. In fact, the good effect lasts all day, even with a light lunch, because my blood-sugar level never sinks too low.

If you have to resort to a packaged cereal choose a natural one that is additive free, such as Shredded Wheat or Weetabix. There is no need to add bran. The Peak Immunity Diet is already high in fibre, and too much bran can leach minerals from the body.

Muesli

This Swiss breakfast dish is full of goodness, and, although packets of muesli can be purchased, it really is best to make your own. This way, you will avoid unwanted additives, milk powder or sugar, and freshness will be guaranteed. It will also taste a lot better!

Dr Bircher came across this health-giving food while on a walking tour in the Swiss mountains earlier this century. After a tiring day, he found a shepherd's hut and was asked in to supper. The meal was muesli. The shepherd was now seventy, had never had an illness in his life, and was still climbing mountains with ease. Thereafter, this peasant dish was offered to patients at the Bircher-Benner clinic in Zurich. In those days vitamins were still unidentified, but the mountain folk had discovered through experience what was best for them.

Grain flakes are the basis of muesli, generally either oats, wheat, barley, rye or millet, and it is best to soak these overnight. Apart from carbohydrates, the grains provide us with dietary essentials: protein, iron, phosphorus, thiamine, riboflavin, niacin, vitamin E and some calcium. They also contain valuable trace elements and enzymes. Of the grains mentioned, wheat, oats and millet have the highest protein content and inclusion of seeds and nuts will enrich the usable protein still further, as will goat's milk yoghurt, soya milk or a nut milk (see 'The peak immunity dairy' for recipes). Fruits, either dried or fresh, will increase the number of vitamins. As for kelp powder, this takes a little getting used to, but it has several important minerals and trace elements. Its strong seaweed flavour will be well disguised by the raisins and other fruits.

FOR SOAKING OVERNIGHT

6 tbsp jumbo oats or other grain flakes such as millet
1 tbsp sunflower seeds
2 tsp sesame seeds
1 tbsp wheat germ
1/4 pint / 150 ml spring water
1 dsp raisins
1/2 tsp kelp powder

NEXT MORNING ADD

    1 dsp chopped almonds
    1 dsp hazelnuts
    a few pumpkin seeds
    1 apple, sliced
    1/2 tsp lemon juice
    1/4 pint / 150 ml soya milk or nut milk (see 'The peak
    immunity dairy')

After soaking, mix in the nuts and the pumpkin seeds and spoon
into serving bowls. Place the apple slices on top and sprinkle with
the lemon juice. Add the soya or nut milk.
Serves 2

Muesli with yoghurt

Instead of the milk, add 2 tbsp goat's milk yoghurt, sweetened with
1 tsp honey.

Fruit Muesli

Replace the apple with a few Hunza apricots soaked overnight, or
some stewed prunes. Alternatively, use any fresh fruit in season.

Crunchy granola

Better by far than anything bought in a packet, is this delicious
breakfast cereal. Dried okara will boost the protein content still
further (see 'The peak immunity dairy').

    1 lb / 450 g jumbo oats
    3 oz / 75 g millet flakes
    2 oz / 50 g wheat germ
    2 oz / 50 g desiccated coconut
    3 oz / 75 g almonds, chopped
    3 oz / 75 g hazelnuts, chopped
    2 tbsp sesame seeds
    2 tbsp sunflower seeds
    2 tbsp pumpkin seeds
    3 tbsp honey

3 tbsp olive oil
6 oz / 175 g raisins

Combine the oats, millet flakes, wheat germ, coconut, nuts and seeds in a large mixing bowl. In a small pan, warm the honey and oil over a low heat, stirring. Pour this over the oat mixture and stir thoroughly so that all the ingredients are coated.

Spread the cereal on a large, shallow baking dish and toast lightly in the oven at 325°F / 170°C (gas mark 3) for about 15 minutes. Stir two or three times to prevent sticking or burning. When cool, add the raisins.

Store in a tightly covered jar and use as a cereal, adding soya milk, stewed fruit, or goat's milk yoghurt.
Makes about 2¹/₂ lb / 1.25 kg cereal

Nutty wheat germ

For speed and personal choice, members of the family can mix their own cereal at the table. Place the following ingredients in separate bowls:

wheat germ
walnuts (fresh ones)
cashews
desiccated coconut
sunflower seeds
pine nuts
raisins or sultanas
fresh fruit in season
jug of soya milk or nut milk (see 'The peak immunity dairy')

Simply mix the dry ingredients with the milk, according to individual taste.

Scottish porridge

Made from nutritious jumbo oats, this is best started the night before and allowed to soak. The prepared 'quick' oats have been heat treated and have lost some of their goodness, so avoid using them.

1 pint / 570 ml soya milk

1 pint / 570ml filtered water
4 oz / 110 g jumbo oats
2 tsp malt extract

Bring to the boil the milk and water in a large saucepan. Remove from the heat and stir in the oats. Leave to soak overnight.

Return the pan to the heat and boil again. Reduce the heat and simmer gently, stirring all the time, until the oats are tender. This will take about 15 minutes.

Stir in the malt extract and serve immediately.
Serves 4 to 6

Quick millet porridge

In my view, the taste of millet is far superior to oats. This is my favourite porridge.

4 oz / 110 g millet flakes
3/4 pint / 425 ml soya milk
3/4 pint / 425 ml filtered water
2 tbsp raisins

Put the millet flakes, the milk and water into a large pan and cook gently for about 10 minutes until the porridge is formed, stirring meanwhile. Add the raisins and serve hot.
Serves 4 to 6

Polenta

Unfortunately, badly prepared, lumpy porridge has put many people off hot cereals. Forget your prejudices and try this traditional Italian dish, with its delicious delicate flavour. Cornmeal is lower in protein than other grains, so include the ground almonds which also add calcium. It is very quick to prepare.

1/2 pint / 275 ml filtered water
1/2 pint / 275 ml soya milk
2 1/2 oz / 60 g cornmeal
2 tbsp sultanas

2 tbsp ground almonds
1 tbsp desiccated coconut
pinch of ground nutmeg

Pour the water and soya milk into a medium saucepan. Sprinkle the cornmeal into the cold liquid, stirring meanwhile, then cook over a gentle heat until it thickens (about 5 minutes).

Stir in the sultanas and ground almonds and put into individual bowls. Sprinkle each with a little nutmeg.
Serves 3

Scrambled tofu on toast

As easy as scrambled eggs and better for you.

3 oz / 75 g mushrooms
knob of ghee, for frying (see 'The peak immunity dairy')
6 oz / 175 g firm tofu
2 tsp tarragon
2 large slices of wholemeal or rye bread, lightly toasted

Wash the mushrooms and cut into pieces. Using a small saucepan, fry them gently in the ghee with the tarragon, until they start to give up their juices. Meanwhile mash the tofu in a bowl until crumbly. Stir this into the mushrooms and heat through thoroughly.

Pile on to the toast to serve.
Serves 2

Variations:
Substitute 1 courgette for the mushrooms, chopped finely. Tomatoes and onions are equally good.

Tempeh toast
Tempeh is a really first-class breakfast food. It is high in protein, with one small portion of $3^{1}/_{2}$ oz / 100 g providing about one-third of your daily requirements, depending on your weight. It is also a rich source of iron, with the same portion contributing almost half of your daily needs. In addition, it contains phosphorus and calcium, and vitamins B_1, B_2 and B_3 (niacin).

Keep several packets in the freezer and slice or grate one as necessary.

2 or 3 slices of tempeh
2 field mushrooms, peeled
1 tomato, quartered
2 slices of wholemeal bread
sunflower oil for frying

In a large pan, gently fry the tempeh, mushrooms and tomatoes in a little oil until cooked. Turn the tempeh once, when golden on the first side. Meanwhile, toast the bread, being careful not to burn it.

Pile the tempeh and vegetables on to the toast when ready.

Serves 1

Herb sausages

3 oz / 75 g hazelnuts, ground
3 oz / 75 g almonds, ground
1 large piece wholemeal bread, in crumbs
1 tbsp soya flour
1 tbsp arrowroot
2 tsp mixed dried herbs
1 1/2 tbsp millet flakes
1/3 pint / 190 ml soya milk
2 tbsp oat flakes
2 tbsp sunflower oil

Mix all the ingredients together, with the exception of the oat flakes and oil, making sure that the consistency is stiff. Divide into 8 portions and roll each into a sausage shape. Coat with oat flakes and fry gently in the oil.

Makes 8 small sausages

Boston baked beans

Originally cooked long and slow in the oven by Pilgrim women on Sundays, this version of the traditional Boston recipe makes a really nourishing breakfast meal. You will never want to open a tin of baked beans again after tasting this!

Cook a large batch and store in the freezer in separate portions. Then warm these up quickly as required and serve on lightly toasted wholemeal bread.

1 lb / 450 g haricot beans, soaked overnight
2 onions, chopped
1 lb / 450 g tomatoes, skinned and chopped
3 tbsp molasses
1¹/2 tbsp cider vinegar
1¹/2 tsp mustard powder
2 tbsp olive oil
2 tsp basil
2 tsp oregano

Drain the beans, place in a large saucepan, and boil rapidly in fresh water for 10 minutes. Drain again and cover with filtered water. This time simmer gently until almost done (about 50 minutes). Drain and reserve the cooking water.

Mix in all the other ingredients except the oil and add ¹/2 pint / 275 ml of the bean water. Stir well. Tip into a large casserole. Pour oil evenly over the surface.

Bake in a moderate oven at 350°F / 180°C (gas mark 4) for one hour or until the beans are soft. Check for dryness after 30 minutes and, if necessary, stir in a little more bean water or vegetable stock.
Serves 8

MID-MORNING SNACK

If you have been used to a quick energy boost from the sugar and fat in biscuits, you will notice a difference as you replace them with protein ingredients such as nuts; these will sustain you for longer.

Crunchy squares

It is possible to buy fruit and nut bars without sugar, if you shop around. Generally these are sweetened with apple juice. Alternatively, you can make your own.

5¹/2 oz / 160 g jumbo oats
4¹/2 oz / 120 g mixed seeds and nuts (e.g. sunflower and
sesame seeds, cashew pieces, chopped almonds and hazelnuts)

2 tbsp wheat germ
4 tbsp sunflower oil
3 tbsp malt extract
2 tbsp molasses

Stir all ingredients together thoroughly. Cover a baking sheet with foil or grease-proof paper or wipe with oil. Using moistened hands, press the mixture on to this until about 1/2 in / 12mm thick and 9 in / 22.5 cm square.

Bake for 15 minutes at 350°F / 180°C (gas mark 4). Allow to cool for a few minutes, then score the squares with a fork. Turn over on to a cooling rack and peel off the paper. Break into squares when cool.
Makes 9

Indian nuts

1 tbsp sunflower oil
1 tsp coriander
1 tsp cumin
6 oz / 175 g mixed nuts and seeds (e.g. slivered almonds, cashew and walnut pieces, and sunflower and pumpkin seeds)

Heat the oil in a heavy frying pan on a low heat and sprinkle in the spices to blend for a few minutes. Stir in the nuts and cook lightly for 3 to 5 minutes. Eat when cool.

Store in an airtight container.
Makes 6 oz / 175 g

Trail mix

Invent your own mixture. Dried fruits give it a sweeter flavour.

4 oz / 110 g pumpkin seeds
4 oz / 110 g almonds
2 oz / 50 g sunflower seeds
2 oz / 50 g chopped dates
2 oz / 50 g shredded coconut

Mix together and store in an airtight container.
Makes 14 oz / 400 g

BREADS

During the second half of the nineteenth century, Dr T.R. Allinson was the foremost advocate of wholemeal bread in Britain: 'If a law could be passed forbidding the separation of the bran from the fine flour, it would add very greatly to the health and wealth of the nation and lessen considerably the receipts of the publican, tobacconist, chemist, dentist, doctor and undertaker,' he wisely said. We now know that wholemeal flour, which includes the bran and germ of the wheat, is rich in B vitamins, vitamin E and essential fatty acids, nearly all of which are removed by refining.

Quick sunflower bread

The texture of this bread is quite dense. However, eaten very fresh, it is both acceptable and healthy. You may find salt-free loaves a little strange at first, but the sunflower seeds add flavour. If you really must, add a little Biosalt, which is correctly balanced with potassium.

1 dsp honey
1$\frac{1}{2}$ oz / 40 g fresh yeast
1$\frac{1}{4}$ pints / 750 ml filtered tepid water
2$\frac{1}{2}$ lb / 1.25 kg stoneground wholemeal flour
3 tbsp sunflower seeds
2 tbsp sunflower oil

Cream together the honey and yeast with a fork. Mix well with $\frac{1}{2}$ pint / 275 ml of warm water, cover with a clean cloth and leave in a warm place for a few minutes until it starts to bubble.

Put the flour into a large mixing bowl and stir in the sunflower seeds. Make a hollow in the centre.

Beat the oil into the frothing yeast with a fork, then pour this into the flour gradually, stirring meanwhile. Also stir in the remaining warm water to form a stiff dough.

Turn the dough on to a floured board and knead thoroughly for at least 5 minutes. Add extra flour if necessary.

Divide the dough into two and put one piece in each of two well-oiled large loaf tins. Cover with a cloth and leave in a warm place to rise (about 45 minutes).

When the dough has doubled, place the loaves in a hot oven at 400°F / 200°C (gas mark 6) for 10 minutes. Reduce the heat to 350°F / 180°C (gas mark 4) and bake for a further 30 to 40 minutes.

Makes 2 large loaves

Pumpernickel

A surprising number of people are allergic to the gluten in wheat, often without realising it. Being made of rye flour, which is very low in gluten, German Pumpernickel provides a useful alternative. It will not, however, rise in the same way as wheat flour.

1½ lb / 675 g rye flour
2 oz / 50 g ghee
2 tbsp black molasses
½ pint / 275 ml soya milk
¾ oz / 20 g fresh yeast
¼ pint / 150 ml filtered tepid water
2 tsp caraway seeds

Put the flour into a large mixing bowl. Cut the ghee into small pieces with a knife and rub it into the flour.

Stir the molasses into the soya milk, using a small saucepan over a very low heat. When the molasses has dissolved, the milk should still be only lukewarm.

Blend the yeast in the tepid water. Make a well in the centre of the flour mixture and pour in the yeast liquid and milk and molasses. Do this gradually, mixing meanwhile, until a sticky dough has formed. Add more tepid water if necessary.

Turn the dough on to a floured board and knead for 10 minutes, until the dough is firm. Add more flour if needed. Return the dough to the mixing bowl, cover and leave in a warm spot to rise. This will take about one hour, by which time the dough should have doubled in bulk.

Knead again for 3 minutes on the floured board, then divide the dough into two, forming each into a smooth oval. Put them on a greased baking sheet. Sprinkle the caraway seeds over the loaves, pressing them lightly into the dough. Cover with a cloth and allow to double in size again in a warm place.

Bake for 45 to 50 minutes at 400°F / 200°C (gas mark 6). Test with a skewer, which should come out clean.

Makes 2 small loaves

Mixed-grain herb bread

2 oz / 50g fresh yeast
1 dsp honey
1/2 pint / 275 ml filtered tepid water
6 oz / 175 g oatmeal
2 oz / 50 g buckwheat flour
3/4 lb / 350 g stoneground wholemeal flour
2 tbsp mixed dried herbs

Dissolve the yeast and honey in the water and leave the mixture in a warm spot until it starts to bubble.

Mix together the flours and herbs in a large bowl, then add the frothy yeast. Stir well to form a stiff dough. Knead this for at least 10 minutes on a floured board, then return the dough to the bowl. Cover with a clean cloth and leave to rise in a warm place (about 45 minutes). It should double in bulk.

Knead again for a few minutes on the floured board. Oil a large loaf tin and form the dough into a regular oval. Place this in the tin and allow to rise in the warmth until it reaches the rim.

Bake at 400°C / 200°F (gas mark 6) for 10 minutes. Turn the oven down to 350°F / 180°C (gas mark 4) and bake for a further 35 minutes.

Makes 1 large loaf

Almond rolls

1 oz / 25 g fresh yeast
1 tsp honey
1/3 pint / 190 ml filtered tepid water
3/4 lb / 350g stoneground wholemeal flour
3 oz / 75 g cornmeal (polenta)
1/3 pint / 190 ml soya milk, warmed
a little extra soya milk

4 oz / 110 g ground almonds
12 whole almonds

In a small bowl, cream together the yeast and honey and warm water. Leave in the warmth for 10 minutes until it bubbles.

Put the flour, cornmeal and ground almonds in a large bowl, mix together and make a well in the centre. Pour in the yeast liquid, stirring all the time. Then add the warm soya milk gradually until a firm dough is formed.

Sprinkle flour on a board and knead the dough for 10 minutes. Return the dough to the mixing bowl, cover with a cloth and allow to rise in a warm place. It should have doubled in bulk in about 45 minutes.

Knock back the dough for a further three minutes, then divide it into 12 equal portions. Roll each into a round ball and press a whole almond well into the centre. Place the rolls on a well-oiled baking tray in a warm spot, allowing gaps between them of about 1½ in / 3.5 cm. Let them rise again for 30 minutes.

Using the extra soya milk, brush the rolls over their tops, then put them in the oven at 400°F / 200°C (gas mark 6) for 10 minutes. Reduce the heat to 350°F / 180°C (gas mark 4) and bake for a further 15 minutes.
Makes 12 rolls

Pitta bread

¾ oz / 20 g fresh yeast
½ pint / 275 ml filtered tepid water
2 tsp malt extract
1 tbsp olive oil
12 oz / 350 g stoneground wholemeal flour

Put 2 tbsp warm water into a large mixing bowl and stir in the yeast and 1 tsp malt extract. Keep warm. In about 15 minutes, when bubbly, add remaining water, malt extract, oil, and work in about two-thirds of the flour.

Knead the dough for about 5 minutes on a floured board, using up the remaining flour as necessary. Return the dough to the bowl, cover with a clean cloth, put in a warm place and leave to rise for 2 to 10 hours, as convenient.

About 45 minutes before baking, knock back the dough and divide into 8 balls. Roll out each until 1/8 in / 3 mm thick and 5 or 6 in / 12.5 or 15 cm round. Place on a floured baking sheet, cover with the cloth and leave to rise again for 30 minutes in a warm place.

Bake at 425°F / 220°C (gas mark 7) for 10 or 12 minutes until puffed up. Remove and wrap each in a napkin to retain softness. Eat within 24 hours.

Makes 8

LUNCH

Salads

I had always been brought up to believe that salads were rather boring dishes, consisting of a piece of limp lettuce, half a tomato and a dollop of salad cream. It has taken me a long time to appreciate that, with imaginative use of ingredients, they can really excite the taste buds. Vegetables have a much more pronounced flavour when uncooked, and, if finely chopped or grated and combined in a variety of ways, they provide unusual dishes. Try in particular carrots, beetroots, turnips, Jerusalem artichokes, fennel, kohlrabi, Brussels sprouts, red and white cabbage, cauliflower, broccoli and courgettes. I also discovered that it was well worth increasing my repertoire of salad dressings to enhance the flavours still further.

If you find it impossible to buy fresh organic vegetables, then add 2 tbsp malt vinegar to the washing water. This will help to remove unwanted chemicals. Don't peel root vegetables; just scrub them. Most of the vitamins are immediately under the skin.

The importance of raw salads cannot be overemphasised. They are a prime source of vitamins and minerals, vital for the efficient functioning of your immune system. Make sure you eat two salads a day: one good big one for lunch and another smaller one as the first course of your dinner. The recipes here are especially high in nutrients. Doubtless you will soon be creating your own.

Sprouts

Seeds, beans and grains which are actively growing and sprouting are especially important, because their vitamin content multiplies by up to ten times. They are also high in essential amino-acids. They can be sprouted successfully at home, although some are easier than others. Alfalfa never goes wrong, whereas sunflower seeds only grow in spring or summer and need nurturing in compost, and sesame seeds often produce nothing at all. Experiment, and discover which you like best. Bags of sprouts are now available in some health-food shops, but it's very much cheaper to grow your own. They are delicious in salads or as a snack in wholemeal rolls.

Method:
You will need several large glass jars. Remember that beans and seeds increase between eight and ten times in size when sprouted, so scatter only a thin layer at the bottom of each jar. Add filtered water and soak for several hours; chick peas and soya beans need eighteen hours, with changes of water.

Place a sieve over the neck of each jar, invert and drain well. Lay each jar on its side in the light, close to the sink. Rinse and drain them three times a day until the sprouts appear. This will take three to five days.

The following are my favourite sprouts:

Aduki beans	3-5 days	1½ in/3.5 cm	Beneficial to kidneys.
Alfalfa	5-6 days	1½ in/3.5 cm	Easy to grow. Rich in vitamin A and essential amino-acids (EAAs). Good source of vitamin B6.
Chick peas	3-4 days	1 in/2.5 cm	Valuable source of protein.
Fenugreek	3-4 days	½ in/1.25 cm	Very cleansing. Contains iron and vitamin A.
Lentils (whole)	3-5 days	1 in/2.5 cm	Good protein content.
Millet (whole)	3-4 days	½ in/1.25 cm	Rich in EAAs.
Mung beans	3-5 days	½-2½ in/1-5 cm	Easy to grow. Good source of B vitamins.
Radish	4-5 days	1 in/2.5 cm	Needs no soaking. Hot flavour; good for mucous membranes.
Rye grains	2-3 days	½ in/1.25 cm	Beneficial to glands.
Wheat grains	2-3 days	½ in/1.25 cm	Contains B vitamins. Use the soaking water in cooking.

Crisp beansprout salad
  4 oz / 110 g mixed beansprouts
  3 oz / 75 g alfalfa sprouts
  6 oz / 175 g tender Bobby beans, sliced

1 large courgette, sliced thinly
1/2 Webbs lettuce, shredded
2 oz / 50 g pumpkin seeds

Dressing:

4 tbsp olive oil
2 tbsp cider vinegar
a little grated fresh ginger

Mix together the salad ingredients in a large bowl. Whisk up the dressing, pour over the salad and toss.
Serves 4

Arab Salad

8 oz / 225 g wheat sprouts
1 onion, finely chopped
sprig parsley, finely chopped
several mint leaves, chopped
2 tomatoes, sliced
black olives, to decorate

Dressing:

4 tbsp olive oil
1 tbsp cider vinegar
squeeze garlic

Mix in with the wheatsprouts the onion, parsley and mint leaves. Whisk together the dressing ingredients, pour over the salad and toss. Put in the serving bowl, topped with the sliced tomatoes and black olives.
Serves 4

Italian salad

4 oz / 50 g red kidney beans, soaked overnight
6 oz / 175 g wholewheat pasta shells

a few drops olive oil
12 oz / 350 g tomatoes, sliced
1 green pepper, sliced
2 oz / 50 g green olives

Dressing:

4 tbsp olive oil
1 tbsp wine vinegar
1 tsp oregano
a squeeze of garlic

Boil the kidney beans rapidly in water for 10 minutes, then drain. Replenish water from filter jug so that the beans are just covered. Bring to the boil, then simmer gently until tender (about 1¼ hours). Allow to cool.

Cook the pasta in a generous amount of boiling water, together with a few drops of olive oil; this will take about 10 minutes. When cool, mix the pasta with the beans in a large bowl and add the tomatoes, pepper and olives.

Whisk together the dressing ingredients, pour over the salad. Stir thoroughly and serve.
Serves 4

Waldorf salad

This salad goes very well with a serving of soya cheese (see 'The peak immunity dairy').

2 dessert apples
1½ tbsp lemon juice
2 satsumas
1 bulb fennel, chopped
3 sticks celery, sliced
4 oz / 110 g fresh walnut pieces

Dressing:

3½ oz / 85 g firm tofu
2 tbsp sunflower oil

1 tbsp lemon juice
3 tsp cider vinegar
2 tsp tarragon

Wash the apples and dice, leaving the skin on and including the pips. Toss in the lemon juice and place in a large bowl. Peel the satsumas and add the segments, followed by the fennel, celery and walnut pieces.

To make the mayonnaise, whisk the ingredients in the blender, then stir it into the salad.
Serves 4

Root salad

6 oz / 175 g carrots, scrubbed and grated
6 oz / 175 g raw beetroot, scrubbed and grated
4 oz / 110 g turnip, scrubbed and grated
3 slices fresh pineapple, cubed

Dressing:

6 tbsp sunflower oil
1 tbsp wine vinegar
3 tbsp pineapple juice
1 level tbsp chopped chives

Stir together the root vegetables and pineapple in a serving bowl. Whisk up the dressing ingredients and combine with the salad.
Serves 3

Rice and spinach salad

8 oz / 225 g cooked brown rice
3/4 pint / 425 ml filtered water
8 oz / 225 g fresh spinach
4 oz / 110 g button mushrooms

Dressing:

6 tbsp olive oil
2 tbsp cider vinegar

2 tsp caraway seeds

Put the rice into a bowl. Shred the spinach, slice the mushrooms, then mix them with the rice.

Put the dressing ingredients into a screw-topped jar and shake vigorously. Pour over the salad and toss.

Serves 4

Chicory salad

    1/4 cauliflower
    1 head chicory, shredded
    6 radishes, sliced
    1/2 cucumber, diced
    1 grapefruit

Dressing:

    1 small carton goat's milk yoghurt
    1 tbsp chopped fresh mint

Take the outer leaves off the cauliflower and cut the florets into small pieces. Place in the salad bowl, together with the chicory, radishes and cucumber. Peel the grapefruit and add the segments to the bowl.

Stir the mint into the yoghurt and pour over the salad.

Serves 4

Red and green salad

    1/2 lb / 225 g broccoli or calabrese
    6 oz / 175 g mung bean sprouts
    2 oz / 50 g sunflower seeds
    small bunch watercress
    4 tomatoes, sliced

Dressing:

    1 avocado pear
    1 tbsp lemon juice
    3 oz / 75 g firm tofu
    1 small carton goat's milk yoghurt

2 tsp finely chopped parsley
1 tsp tarragon
1/2 clove garlic

Cut off the broccoli florets and slice into small pieces. Mix with the mung bean sprouts in the serving bowl and add the sunflower seeds, watercress leaves and tomatoes.

To make the dressing, scoop the flesh of the avocado into the blender and add the lemon juice, tofu, goat's milk yoghurt and herbs. Squeeze in the garlic. Blend briefly until smooth, then pour over the salad.
Serves 4

Soups

Always keep the water from the steamer after cooking vegetables; this absorbs many nutrients and can be used in soup. Alternatively, make a stock by boiling up cast-off leaves and peelings. Strain off the juice when done.

Bortsch

This famous soup from Russia can be served hot or cold.

1 medium onion, chopped
1 oz / 25 g ghee
1 small potato, diced
1 lb / 450 g beetroot, scrubbed and diced
2 pints / 1.1 l vegetable stock or filtered water
3 tbsp cider vinegar
1 tsp nutmeg
2 tsp caraway seeds
1 small carton goat's milk yoghurt

Using a large saucepan, sauté the onion gently in the ghee until transparent. Add the other vegetables and stock and bring to the boil, then lower the heat and simmer for 1/2 hour. Remove from heat and stir in the cider vinegar, nutmeg and caraway seeds. Blend in a liquidizer until smooth.

Cool or reheat gently as desired, and stir in the yoghurt just before serving.
Serves 6

Cream of pea

> 8 oz / 225 g green split peas
> 1³/4 pints / 1 l vegetable stock or filtered water
> 1 large onion, chopped
> 1 carrot, scrubbed and diced
> 2 tsp tarragon
> ¹/4 pint / 150 ml soya milk

Bring the peas to the boil in the stock, stirring occasionally. Add the onion and carrot and tarragon, then lower the heat and simmer until the peas are soft (about ³/4 hour).

Remove from the heat, stir in the soya milk and liquidize until smooth. Adjust the amount of milk to suit preferred consistency.
Serves 4 to 6

Carrot and cashew

> 2 pints / 1.1 l vegetable stock or filtered water
> 1 lb/ 450 g carrots, scrubbed and chopped
> 1 large onion, chopped
> 1 small potato, diced
> 1 orange
> juice ¹/2 lemon
> 2 oz / 50 g ground cashew nuts

Boil up the stock and put the vegetables into it. Simmer until tender (about 20 minutes). Take off the heat, add the orange segments and lemon juice, then stir in the cashews. Blend in a liquidizer and serve.
Serves 4 to 6

Leek broth

> 4 oz / 110 g butter beans, soaked overnight
> 2 pints / 1.1 l vegetable stock or filtered water
> 2 oz / 50 g ghee
> 3 large leeks, sliced
> 2 tbsp chopped parsley

1 tbsp cider vinegar

Boil the beans rapidly in tap water for 10 minutes. Drain and reboil in the stock or filtered water, then simmer until soft (about 40 minutes).

Melt the ghee in a large saucepan and cook the leeks gently for 4 or 5 minutes. Add the beans together with their water. Stir and simmer for 15 minutes. Remove from heat, stir in the parsley and cider vinegar, then purée in the blender.
Serves 4 to 6

Melon and almond

Cold 'raw' soups are highly recommended as part of the PI Diet. Here is one idea.

1 large melon
1/4 pint / 150 ml soya milk
3 oz / 75 g ground almonds
1/2 tsp ground ginger

Remove the flesh from the melon, chop roughly and place in a bowl. Add the soya milk, almonds and ginger. Blend until smooth.
Serves 4

Miso soup

1 large onion, finely chopped
2 large carrots, scrubbed and diced
1 oz / 25 g ghee
1 tsp thyme
2 pints / 1.1 l vegetable stock
1 dsp miso
1 tbsp cress, to decorate

Sauté the vegetables in the ghee for a few minutes over a low heat, using a large saucepan. Add the thyme and stock, bring to the boil, then reduce the heat and simmer, covered, for 20 minutes. Take off the heat and stir in the miso until dissolved. Pour into individual serving bowls and sprinkle a little cress on each.
Serves 4

Pâtés and savoury spreads

These are designed to boost the protein content of your lunches and go well with salads or wholemeal bread. Alternatively, they can be used as dips, with crisp raw vegetables to complement them. Some are also suitable as breakfast foods.

Oriental lentil pâté

    8 oz / 225 g red lentils
    1 red pepper, chopped finely
    knob ghee
    1 tsp coriander
    1 tsp cumin
    a little grated root ginger
    1 pint / 570 ml filtered water
    2 oz / 50 g creamed coconut, grated
    2 tbsp tahini
    1 tbsp lemon juice
    1/4 pint / 150 ml goat's milk yoghurt

Remove any grit from the lentils and rinse. Using a large saucepan, gently sauté the red pepper with the spices in the ghee for a few minutes, then stir in the lentils and water. Bring to the boil, turn down the heat and simmer until soft, about 20 minutes.

Sprinkle the grated coconut into the simmering lentils and stir until dissolved. Remove from the heat.

Beat in the tahini and lemon juice until smooth. Turn into a pâté dish and allow to cool. Pour on the yoghurt and serve.
Serves 6 to 8

Butterbean pâté

    4 oz / 110 g butterbeans, soaked overnight
    juice 1/2 lemon
    2 sprigs parsley, chopped
    1 clove garlic, chopped
    1 tsp coriander
    2 oz / 50 g ground cashew nuts

Boil the butterbeans quickly for 10 minutes. Discard the water and bring to the boil again in filtered water to cover. Lower the heat and simmer gently until soft. Allow to cool.

Put the lemon juice and butterbeans with their liquid into the blender. Add the parsley, garlic and coriander and liquidize. Add the ground cashews gradually until you achieve the desired consistency.
Serves 4

Chestnut terrine

> 4 oz / 110 g dried chestnuts, soaked overnight
> 2 bay leaves
> 1 medium onion, chopped small
> 3 oz / 75 g mushrooms, chopped small
> 1 dsp ghee
> 1/4 pint / 150 ml soya milk
> 1 tbsp arrowroot
> 4 bay leaves to decorate

Simmer the chestnuts with the two bay leaves in filtered water to cover, until soft (about 50 minutes). Top up the water if necessary. Meanwhile, gently fry the onions and mushrooms in the ghee until the onion is transparent.

Roughly mash the chestnuts in their juice, then transfer to the liquidizer goblet together with the onion and mushrooms. Add the soya milk and arrowroot. Run the machine until a fairly stiff paste is formed. Pour into an oiled ovenproof dish.

Bake at 325°F / 170°C (gas mark 3) or until set (about half an hour). Allow to cool, then ease the edges and turn out on to a serving plate. Decorate with the four bay leaves.
Serves 4

Carrot pâté

> 7 oz / 200 g tofu
> 3 tbsp carrot juice
> 1 tbsp sunflower oil
> 2 tomatoes
> 1 tbsp wheat germ
> 1 large carrot, grated
> 1/2 tsp basil
> 1/2 tsp paprika

Put the tofu, carrot juice and oil, followed by the other ingredients with the exception of the wheat germ, into the blender. Liquidize until smooth. Gradually sprinkle in the wheatgerm until a fairly stiff pâté is formed.
Serves 4

Guacamole

> 2 ripe avocado pears
> juice of 1 lemon
> 1 small onion, chopped finely
> 2 tsp chopped fresh sage
> 1 tomato, skinned and chopped

Scoop out the flesh of the avocados, then put this with the lemon juice, onion, coriander, cumin and tomato into the blender. Whir until smooth.
Serves 4

Hummus

Very good with wholemeal pitta bread. It also makes a tasty dip, using slices of carrot and celery.

> 8 oz / 225 g chick peas, soaked overnight
> 3 tbsp olive oil
> juice of 1^1/2 lemons
> 4 tbsp goat's milk yoghurt
> 2 cloves garlic, chopped
> sprig of parsley, chopped

Boil the chick peas rapidly for 10 minutes and discard the water. Bring to the boil again in filtered water, just covering the beans, then lower the heat, cover and allow to simmer for about 30 minutes until done. Check from time to time if more water needs to be added. Allow to cool.

Put oil, lemon, yoghurt and garlic into the blender, then add half the chick peas and their liquid. Whir briefly and add more chick peas and liquid gradually until they are all included. Adjust consistency as necessary.

Pile into a serving dish and garnish with parsley.
Serves 6

Japanese spread

Served with warm, wholemeal rolls, this provides a quick, high-protein snack, rich in calcium, with an intriguing flavour.

    4 tbsp brown tahini
    1¹/₂ tbsp miso
    ³/₄ pint / 425 ml spring water
    3 or 4 wholemeal rolls, warmed in the oven (see 'Breads')

Beat the tahini, miso and water to a smooth paste. Turn into a small saucepan and heat through very gently until just warm.

Cut the rolls in half, spread the paste thickly in the centre, and enjoy the unique flavour.

Serves 3 to 4

Almond paste

    2 tbsp ground almonds
    1 tbsp soya flour
    1 tsp sunflower oil
    a little warm water

Mix together to form a spreading consistency.

Serves 2

THE PEAK IMMUNITY DAIRY

Long-lasting health means avoiding full-fat cow's milk, cream and cheese; if you wish to attain peak immunity, these really are out. Take heart, however! There are plenty of nutritious substitutes that are low in fat and can only do you good.

Soya milk

This can be bought in cartons in some supermarkets and most health-food shops. Make sure it is organic and salt- and sugar-free and without any other flavourings. Some varieties taste better than others, so do shop around. Of course, none will taste better than your own. The milk will keep for four or five days in the fridge, or it can be frozen and stored for up to three months. Keep the pulp (okara) for use in other recipes (see below).

7^1/$_2$ oz / 210 g soya beans
filtered water

Wash the beans and soak them for 1 to 2 days, changing the water to prevent fermentation. To test if they are ready, split one open; it should be flat and of uniform colour in the centre. If it is concave and darker yellow in the centre, they need longer. Soaking times can be reduced to 8 hours by putting the beans into hot water. Rinse and drain the beans and divide into two equal portions.

Line a colander or sieve with a dampened clean cloth or muslin and sit it in a large bowl or pan so that it is suspended.

Boil up some water in a kettle and pour ^{3}/$_4$ pint / 425 ml into your blender, taking care that the goblet will sustain the heat. (It may be best to warm it first with a little hot water.) Add one portion of the beans and purée for 1 minute. Pour the hot purée into the lined colander. Repeat the process with the second portion of beans.

Twist together the corners of the straining cloth to form a bag and press the soya milk from the pulp (okara) with the bottom of a clean glass jar, collecting it in the bowl or pan beneath.

Rinse the blender with ^{1}/$_4$ pint / 150 ml hot water and add this to the contents of the straining cloth. Press once more. Retain the okara.

Pour the soya milk into a large, heavy pan and cook gently for 20 minutes, stirring frequently to avoid burning.

Cool the milk quickly by sitting the pan in cold water.
Makes 1^1/$_2$ pints / 900 ml

Okara
This is the pulp that remains after making soya milk or tofu. It is high in fibre and contains about 3.5 per cent protein, which is about the same as cow's milk or cooked brown rice, so don't throw it away! If you haven't time to use it in baking feed it to your pets, who will love it. Alternatively, store it in the freezer.

It is excellent in cakes in the place of eggs, giving a lighter texture. If included in pancake batters, bread and biscuit recipes, it will add a pleasant nutty flavour; substitute okara for about one-fifth of the flour. As a crumble topping it is really special; use equal amounts of okara and wholemeal flour.

You can also include it in savoury roasts, burgers and patties. Just substitute it for the nuts, beans, lentils, or some of the flour.

To enrich your Granola recipe, dry out some okara by spreading it on baking sheets and putting it in the oven at a low temperature. This will take about an hour. Use it instead of some of the grain.

Tofu
Tofu is a white bean curd which is available in many health-food stores and some supermarkets. It has a higher protein content than any other food of equivalent weight, including meat, and is therefore an indispensable part of a vegetarian diet. Another bonus is that it costs only a fraction of any meat, especially steak. Because the taste is so bland, it can be used in innumerable ways, as an ingredient in either savoury or sweet foods. As with the soya milk, you will be left with the delicious okara pulp. The whey can also be saved for use in soups.

Traditionally, the Japanese have always used nigari to curdle the milk and this makes the firmest tofu. Ask your health-food shop to order it for you. Lemons or cider vinegar are suitable alternatives.

7 oz / 200 g soya beans
juice of 2 lemons (or 3/4-1 tsp nigari dissolved in a cup
of water)
filtered water

Soak the beans in plenty of filtered water overnight, putting the bowl in a cool place. Drain and rinse.

Using one cup of water for each cup of beans, liquidize them until creamy. Meanwhile, boil up 6 cups of water in a large pan and add the slurry. Bring to the boil again and keep at boiling point for 20 minutes, stirring from time to time to prevent burning. If the mixture foams, a little cold water can be sprinkled on it to stop it from boiling over the sides of the pan.

Place a colander over a clean bowl and line the inside with dampened muslin. Pour the slurry into the muslin and allow the soya milk to drip through into the bowl. Gather up the corners of the muslin and press as much soya milk as possible from the bag with a wooden spoon. Okara is left in the muslin; keep this for use in other recipes.

Pour the soya milk into a clean pan. Bring to the boil, then pour it into another bowl. Very gently, stir in the lemon juice (or nigari solution), then leave the milk to curdle. Should this fail to happen, return the liquid to the pan, boil once again and add more lemon juice. The curds should float on a clear yellow liquid, the whey. Scoop out the curds with a perforated spoon into the colander lined with dampened muslin. Allow any surplus whey to drip into the bowl beneath. You now have a soft or silken tofu.

If you need a firm beancurd, wrap up the corners of the muslin over the soft tofu, leaving it in the colander, and place an inverted saucer or plate over it. Stand a weight on top of this, such as a jar full of water. Drain for at least 15 minutes for a firm tofu.

To store, leave it in a bowl of water in the refrigerator. It will keep for about three or four days. Change the water each day.

Makes 10 oz / 275 g tofu and 10 oz / 275 g okara

Tofu cream

Particularly good on breakfast cereals, this cream can also be used for desserts. Vary the flavouring by adding banana, orange juice or coconut. The consistency can also be altered by adjusting the amount of soya milk, or by adding milled nuts. Eat as much as you like! You won't get fat on this.

1/2 pint / 275 ml soya milk
3 1/2 oz / 85 g firm tofu, crumbled
3 drops real vanilla essence

Put ingredients into the blender and whir until smooth.

Makes 2/3 pint / 380 ml

Cashew and sesame milk

Nut milks provide a nutritious alternative to soya milk and are very easy to prepare. The pulp can be reserved for further use.

3 1/2 oz / 85 g broken cashews
1 oz / 25 g sesame seeds
2/3 pint / 380 ml spring water

Grind together the nuts and seeds. Pour the water into the blender and add the ground cashews and sesame seeds. Liquidize thoroughly, then leave to stand for 1 hour. Pour through a fine sieve, reserve the pulp and store the milk in the refrigerator.

Makes 3/4 pint / 425 ml

Almond milk

    3 oz / 75 g fine oatmeal
    3 oz / 75 g ground almonds
    3/4 pint / 425 ml spring water

Blend ingredients in a liquidizer. Allow the milk to stand for 1 hour, then pour through a sieve. Retain the pulp for inclusion in baking and store the milk in the refrigerator.

Soya cheese

This can be used in place of cottage cheese, in rolls or with salads. Do try it. It is easy to make and surprisingly tasty. If you wish to use it as a dip, straining may not be necessary.

    4 oz / 110 g soya flour
    1 pint / 570 ml filtered water
    juice of 2 lemons
    1 clove garlic
    a few fresh herbs, chopped finely

Put the soya flour in a large mixing bowl and add about half of the water. Stir to form a paste.

Boil up the remaining water, stir into the soya paste, then return the mixture to the saucepan. While stirring, bring it to the boil, then simmer gently for 5 minutes. Remove from the heat, stir in the lemon juice and allow to cool.

Line a large sieve or colander with damp muslin and suspend over a basin. Pour the soya mixture on to the muslin and let the liquid drain through. Put the curds in a bowl and stir in the crushed garlic and herbs.
Serves 4

Ghee

This is the only cow's milk product recommended as part of the diet, but even so, be frugal with it. The skimming removes the impurities, leaving the clarified butter. Keep in the fridge and then use in cooking when more suitable than oil.

    1/4 lb / 110 g unsalted butter

Cut the butter into pieces and place in a small pan. Heat very gently until it begins to bubble. A white froth will form on the surface; scoop this off carefully with a spoon until the butter is completely clear. Pour into a bowl and allow to cool.

Makes 3 oz / 75 g

TEATIME TREATS

Shop-bought cakes and biscuits really are not at all good for you. In addition to their high sugar and fat content, and the tendency to use refined flour, the bicarbonate of soda destroys vitamin B in the stomach. How, then, is it possible to produce any treats at all for tea, you may wonder, if the sugar, fat, eggs and raising agent are banned? Well, it is, and here are some recipes to prove that it really can be done.

Banana and pear cake

2 bananas, mashed
1 pear, finely chopped
2 oz / 50 g ground almonds
6 tbsp sunflower oil
4 oz / 110 g sultanas
3 oz / 75 g jumbo oats
5 oz / 150 g stoneground, wholemeal flour

Turn the oven to 375°F / 190°C (gas mark 5). While it is heating up, mix all the ingredients together until evenly moist. Grease a 71/2-in / 19-cm cake tin and spoon the mixture into it.

Bake for about 1 hour. Insert a skewer into the cake to test it; it should come out clean. Cool for a few minutes, then turn on to a rack.

Makes one 71/2-in / 19-cm cake

Sticky bread

1 oz / 25 g fresh yeast
1/2 pint / 275 ml tepid filtered water
1 tsp clear honey
1 oz / 25 g ghee
3 tbsp malt extract

2 tbsp molasses
1¼ lb / 550 g stoneground, wholemeal flour
4 oz / 110 g sultanas
2 oz / 50 g dates, chopped small
3 oz / 75 g apricots, chopped small

Dissolve the yeast in the tepid water with the honey and leave for a few minutes in a warm place until frothy. Put the ghee in a small pan and melt it with the malt extract and molasses, stirring until well combined.

Put the flour in a large mixing bowl, make a well in the centre and pour in the bubbling yeast. Stir in the melted ingredients and the fruit until all are well blended. Add a little more flour if necessary to give a firm dough.

Divide the dough into two, form each into an oblong shape and put into two well-greased medium loaf tins. Cover with a clean cloth and allow to rise in a warm place until double in size (about 1/2 hour). Bake for 3/4 hour at 400°F / 200°C (gas mark 6).
Makes two 1¼-lb / 550-g loaves

Carob cake

Don't expect this cake to rise. It is delicious none the less.

3 oz / 75 g ghee
5 oz / 150 g carob powder
3 oz / 75 g desiccated coconut
3 oz / 75 g soya flour
2 oz / 50 g millet flakes
2 oz / 50 g stoneground, wholemeal flour
8 oz / 225 g sultanas
2 tsp cinnamon
1 tsp nutmeg
4 tbsp sunflower oil
1/2 pint / 275 ml apple juice

Filling:

2 tbsp tahini
2 tbsp carob powder
a little soya milk
1 tbsp clear honey

Cut the ghee into small pieces and put into a large bowl with the dry ingredients and oil. Mix together thoroughly, then pour in the apple juice and stir again.

While the oven is heating to 325°F / 170°C (gas mark 3), line a 7½-in / 19-cm cake tin with greaseproof paper. Spoon the cake mixture into the tin and cover with foil. Bake for 1 hour. Cool a little, then turn out.

To make the filling, mix the tahini and carob powder with the honey, then add a little milk to form a paste.

Cut the cake across the centre from side to side, and spread the filling on each half. Sandwich together again.

Makes one 7½-in / 19-cm cake

Flapjacks

    3 oz / 75 g ghee
    2 tbsp clear honey
    6 oz / 175 g jumbo oat flakes
    2 oz / 50 g dates, chopped
    1 dried fig, chopped small

In a saucepan, melt the ghee gently and stir in the honey. Cool a little and mix in the other ingredients. Press into a 7-in / 18-cm greased baking tray and bake for 25 minutes at 350°F / 180°C (gas mark 4). Cut into fingers while still warm.

Makes 8

Couscous cake

    6 oz / 175 g wholemeal couscous
    1 pint / 570 ml white grape juice
    4 oz / 110 g cooked rice
    6 oz / 175 g wholemeal flour
    2 tbsp cornmeal
    4 oz / 110 g chopped cashew nuts
    2 tbsp ghee
    2 tbsp grated creamed coconut
    juice of 2 large oranges
    2 tsp honey

Put the couscous in a bowl. Heat the grape juice to boiling point and pour on to the couscous. Cover and allow to stand until the juice is absorbed (about 10 minutes). Melt the ghee with the honey and the coconut and add to the couscous with the other ingredients. Stir thoroughly.

Put in a greased tin and bake at 350°F / 180°C (gas mark 4) for about 1½ hours.

Serves 8

Yoghurt cake

Make sure you scrub the skin of the orange well before grating it, using a solution of water and a little wine vinegar. This will remove preservatives and other chemicals.

3 oz / 75 g sultanas
¼ pint / 150 ml goat's milk yoghurt
2 tsp honey
6 tbsp sunflower oil
1 tsp dried yeast
juice and grated rind of 1 orange
8 oz / 225 g wholemeal flour
2 tbsp wheat germ
1 tbsp soya flour
2 oz / 50 g ground almonds
2 oz / 50 g desiccated coconut
1 tsp ground cinnamon

Warm the sultanas with the yoghurt, honey and oil in a small pan, until evenly tepid. Stir in the yeast and leave in a warm place for 15 minutes. Add the orange juice and rind.

Put all the remaining ingredients in a large bowl, then add the yeast mixture, stir and knead for a few minutes. Cover with a tea towel and leave to rise in a warm place for about 1½ hours.

Oil and line a round cake tin approximately 7 in / 18 cm in diameter. Knead the mixture lightly again, turn into the tin, and cover with greaseproof paper. Leave to rise for another hour.

Bake at 375°F / 190°C (gas mark 5) for 45 minutes. Test with a skewer. If it comes out clean, it is done. Turn on to a wire rack to cool.

Makes one 7-in / 18-cm cake.

DINNER

Have a drink, such as a herb tea, fruit or vegetable juice, half an hour before eating. Then start your meal with a salad, to set the correct enzymes in motion for easy digestion. Choose one from the 'Lunch' section, or invent your own. If you are short of time, a grated or sliced carrot is always an excellent start to your meal, or a few beansprouts. Eat as early in the evening as possible to allow the body time to digest and utilize the nutrients while you are still awake. If you can eat your main meal in the middle of the day, so much the better. You will then have the energy available for the many demands made on your body, followed by a restful sleep at night.

Savouries

Unless mentioned, all the savoury dishes given here provide well-balanced usable protein. Only vegan recipes are included since these are the most difficult to find in other cookery books.

Spaghetti with tofu sauce

1 onion
1 tbsp olive oil
3 large tomatoes, skinned and chopped
4 oz / 110 g mushrooms, sliced
1 courgette, sliced
1 tsp oregano
1 tsp basil
1 clove garlic
7 oz / 200 g tofu, mashed
4 oz / 110 g wholewheat or buckwheat spaghetti

Using a large frying pan, sauté the onion in the oil until transparent. Add the remaining vegetables, sprinkle in the herbs and squeezed garlic, and cook gently for 5 minutes. Stir in the tofu and cook a few minutes longer, stirring from time to time.

Meanwhile boil about 2 pints / 1.1 l of filtered water in a large pan, then add the spaghetti and squeeze in some lemon juice. Continue to boil until soft (about 12 minutes). Drain immediately.

Serve the tofu mixture piled on the spaghetti.
Serves 3

Chinese rice

10 oz / 275 g long-grain brown rice
1¹/4 pints / 750 ml filtered water
2 level tsp cornmeal
1¹/2 tbsp filtered water
2 tbsp Tamari soy sauce
2 tbsp dry sherry
3 tbsp olive oil
1 tsp grated root ginger
2 medium onions, chopped
1 large red pepper, sliced
8 oz / 225 g mushrooms, sliced
8 oz / 225 g beansprouts
4 oz / 110 g broken cashews

Boil up the 1¹/4 pints / 750 ml water in a large pan, then pour in the rice and allow to simmer gently for about 25 minutes until soft.

Meanwhile, mix the cornmeal with the water, then stir in the Tamari and sherry and keep ready.

Heat the oil in a large frying pan or wok and sauté the onions until transparent. Stir in the ginger, then add the pepper slices and mushrooms and cook gently for a further 5 minutes. Add the beansprouts and cashewnuts together with the cornmeal mixture and turn up the heat a little. Stir-fry for a further 3 minutes.

Drain the rice and serve with the vegetables piled on top.
Serves 4

Black-eyed bean stew

8 oz / 225 g black-eyed beans, soaked overnight
1 tsp caraway seeds
1 tbsp olive oil
2 medium onions, finely chopped
1 clove garlic
1 large carrot, scrubbed and chopped
¹/2 swede, scrubbed and diced
¹/2 fennel bulb, chopped
2 tsp thyme
2 tsp marjoram
4 tbsp white wine
1 lb / 450 g tomatoes, skinned and chopped

2 oz / 50 g bulgar wheat
juice ½ lemon

Boil the beans rapidly for 10 minutes. Drain and cover with about 2 pints / 1.1 l filtered water. Sprinkle in the caraway seeds, bring to the boil and simmer until tender (about 30 minutes).

Heat the oil in a large frying pan and gently sauté the onions, squeezing in the garlic. Add the carrot, swede, fennel and herbs. Stir and cook for a few minutes to seal, then put in the beans with their liquid, the tomatoes and the wine. Sprinkle in the bulgar wheat and stir. Bring to the boil, cover and simmer gently for ½ hour, stirring occasionally. Pour in more stock if necessary, add the lemon juice and cook for another 20 minutes.

Serve hot with brown rice or barley.

Serves 6

Nut loaf

1 onion, chopped small
1 oz / 25 g ghee
4 oz / 110 g mushrooms, chopped small
1 tsp thyme
1 tsp marjoram
4 oz / 110 g hazelnuts, ground
4 oz / 110 g cashewnuts, ground
3 slices of wholemeal bread, crumbled
½ pint / 275 ml vegetable stock
2 tsp miso
1 tomato, sliced

Sauté the onion very gently in the ghee for about 3 minutes using a large frying pan, and then add the mushrooms and herbs. Fry until soft. Stir in the nuts and breadcrumbs and then transfer the mixture to a large bowl.

Heat up the vegetable stock and dissolve the miso in it. Gradually stir this liquid into the nut mixture until it is well moistened, but still quite stiff. (You may not need all the miso liquid.) Grease a large loaf tin and press the mixture into it. Arrange the slices of tomato on top and bake in the oven at 325°F / 170°C (gas mark 3) for about an hour.

Serve with 'Miso gravy' (see below), jacket potatoes and lightly steamed green vegetables.

Serves 4

Miso gravy

    1 dsp arrowroot
    ³/₄ pint / 425 ml vegetable stock
    2 tsp miso

Mix the arrowroot to a paste with a little cold filtered water. Stir in the vegetable stock and transfer to a small pan. Add the miso and warm gently over a low heat, stirring all the time, until dissolved. Do not boil, as this destroys the enzymes. When nicely thickened, pour into a gravy boat and serve.
Serves 3 to 4

Cauliflower with rosemary sauce

    ¹/₄ pint / 150 ml soya milk
    3 oz / 75 g firm tofu
    2 oz / 50 g ground almonds
    1 tbsp goat's milk yoghurt
    1 tsp rosemary
    1 cauliflower
    1 oz / 25 g slivered almonds

Put all the ingredients except the cauliflower and slivered almonds into the blender and whisk until smooth. Transfer to a small pan.

    Cut the cauliflower into quarters and steam until just done but still a little crisp. Meanwhile, gently heat the sauce. Put the cauliflower into a casserole and pour in the sauce. Top with slivered almonds. Bake in the oven for 15 minutes at 350°F / 180°C (gas mark 4).

    Serve on a bed of boiled millet.
Serves 4

Shepherd's delight

The amino-acids in the lentils need to be complemented by those in a grain or beancurd. So sprinkle some wheat germ on to your dessert, or follow with 'Tofu cream'.

    3 potatoes, scrubbed and halved

    1 small swede, peeled and chopped
    a little soya milk
    8 oz / 225 g red lentils
    1 carrot, scrubbed and diced
    3/4 pint / 425 ml vegetable stock or filtered water
    1 bay leaf
    1 onion, chopped small
    1 clove garlic, crushed
    1 tsp paprika
    1 tsp cumin
    1 tsp basil
    knob of ghee

Boil the potatoes and swede until soft. Drain and mash together with a little soya milk.

Meanwhile, put the lentils in a pan with the remaining ingredients, cover with the stock or water and simmer gently until soft. (Add a little extra water if necessary.)

Put the lentils in a greased casserole and pile the mashed potatoes and swede on top. Press down with a fork. Put little dots of ghee on the surface.

Bake in the oven at 350°F / 180°C (gas mark 4) for 20 minutes. Serve with lightly steamed greens.
Serves 4

Mung-bean curry

    8 oz / 225 g mung beans
    2 onions, chopped finely
    1 oz / 25 g ghee
    2 oz / 50 g creamed coconut
    1 tsp ground cumin
    1 tsp ground coriander
    1 tsp grated root ginger
    3 tbsp sultanas

In a large pan, cover the mung beans with filtered water and boil rapidly for 10 minutes. Renew water, boil again, then simmer gently for about 40 minutes until soft. Drain and reserve stock.

Meanwhile, sauté the onions in the ghee in a large frying pan until transparent. Stir in the spices. Chop up the creamed coconut and stir this in also, allowing it to melt. Pour in some of the bean stock, and stir until a fairly liquid but creamy sauce is obtained. Add the sultanas and beans.

Serve on a bed of brown rice with lightly steamed cauliflower.
Serves 4

Thunder and lightning

> 8 oz / 225 g chick peas, soaked overnight
> 1 lb / 450 g wholewheat macaroni
> squeeze lemon juice
> 1 tbsp olive oil
> 2 cloves garlic, crushed
> 1 tsp caraway seeds
> 1 tbsp basil

Put the chick peas in fresh water and boil rapidly for 10 minutes. Drain and replace with filtered water. Bring to the boil and then simmer for about 1 hour until soft.

Meanwhile, boil the macaroni in plenty of filtered water with a squeeze of lemon juice for about 8 minutes until nearly done.

Put the oil in a large pan and add the garlic and caraway seeds. Warm gently for 3 minutes. Add the drained chick peas and macaroni and stir in the basil. Cook for another couple of minutes to allow the flavours to blend.

Steamed courgettes complement this meal nicely.
Serves 4 to 6

Desserts

Honey, malt extract, dried fruits such as raisins and dates, and fruit juices can all be used as natural sweeteners. It is surprising how many imaginative desserts can be created without any sugar at all.

Grape and kiwi-fruit jelly

> 1 pint / 570 ml red grape juice 1 tbsp agar-agar flakes
> 4 oz / 110 g seedless grapes, halved
> 2 kiwi fruits, peeled and sliced

Bring the grape juice to the boil and sprinkle in the agar-agar. Simmer and stir until dissolved (about 5 minutes).

Arrange the grapes in the serving bowls together with the slices of kiwi fruits. Pour in the liquid jelly and allow to set in a cool place.
Makes 6

Apricot crumble

> 6 oz / 175 g Hunza apricots
> 1/2 pint / 275 ml orange juice
> 2 pears
>
> *Topping:*
>
> 2 oz / 50 g ghee
> 3 oz / 75 g wholemeal flour
> 3 oz / 75 g medium oatmeal
> 2 oz / 50 g desiccated coconut
> 3 tbsp sunflower oil
> 1 tbsp malt extract

Soak the apricots in the orange juice overnight. Drain, reserving juice, and take out the stones. Wash and slice the pears and place these with the apricots in a greased ovenproof dish. Pour in sufficient juice to cover the fruit.

For the topping, cut the ghee into small pieces and rub into the flour. Mix in the oatmeal, coconut, oil and honey and stir thoroughly.

Sprinkle the topping over the fruit and bake at 350°F / 180°C (gas mark 4) for 25 minutes. It tastes good with polenta custard.
Serves 4 to 6

Polenta custard

> 2 oz / 50 g cornmeal
> 1 pint / 570 ml soya milk
> 1 vanilla pod
> 1 dsp honey

Make a smooth paste by mixing the cornmeal with a little of the soya milk in a large bowl.

Heat the rest of the milk with the vanilla pod and stir in the honey. Bring almost to the boil, then pour over the cornmeal paste and mix well.

Return the custard to the pan and heat until thick, stirring all the time. Take out the vanilla pod and pour into a jug or bowl.
Makes 1 pint / 570 ml

Apple pudding

Before grating the rind, wash the orange and lemon in water with the addition of a little wine vinegar. This will remove preservatives.

> 1 tsp dried yeast
> 1/4 pint / 150 ml apple juice, warmed
> 1 dessert apple, chopped
> 4 oz / 110 g wholemeal flour
> 1 1/2 oz / 40 g brown rice flour
> 1 oz / 25 g soya flour
> 2 oz / 50 g medium oatmeal
> 2 oz / 50 g ground almonds
> 1 tsp cinnamon
> 1 tbsp sunflower oil
> 4 oz / 110 g raisins
> rind of 1/2 orange and 1/2 lemon

Dissolve the yeast in the warmed apple juice. Liquidize the apple with the yeast mixture.

Mix all the other ingredients in a large bowl and stir in the yeast and apple pulp. Transfer to a greased pudding basin and bake at 375°F / 190°C (gas mark 5) for 3/4 hour.
Serves 4

Rice pudding

> 6 oz / 175 g short-grain brown rice
> 1 oz / 25 g sultanas
> 1 1/2 pints / 900 ml soya milk
> 1 dsp malt extract
> 1 tsp ground nutmeg

Put the rice and sultanas in a pudding dish and rinse with boiling water. Drain.

Boil up the milk, stir in the malt extract and then pour over the rice. Sprinkle the nutmeg on to it.

Bake in a slow oven, 300°F / 150°C (gas mark 2) for 3 hours.
Serves 4

Poires belle Hélène

4 pears, halved and cored

Sauce:

1 tbsp cornmeal
1 dsp carob powder
1/2 pint / 275 ml soya milk
1 dsp malt extract

Steam the pears until soft, then place into serving bowls.

To make the sauce, put the cornmeal and carob powder into a bowl and stir in a little soya milk to make a paste. Bring the rest of the milk to the boil and pour into the paste, stirring meanwhile. Return to the pan, add the malt extract and reheat gently until the sauce thickens.

Pour a little over each of the pears.
Serves 4

Tofu cream

1/3 pint / 190 ml soya milk
3 bananas, peeled and chopped
2 oranges, peeled and divided
4 oz / 110 g firm tofu

Put the ingredients into the liquidizer and blend until creamy. The amount of milk can be adjusted according to the consistency desired.
Serves 4

Halvah

4 tbsp tahini
2 oz / 50 g ground sunflower seeds
3 tbsp honey
11/2 oz / 40 g millet flakes

Thoroughly mix together the ingredients. Divide into two and roll each into a 'log', about 1¹/₂ in / 3.5 cm in diameter. Cut as needed.
Makes 2 logs of 1¹/₂ in / 3.5 cm x 4 in / 10 cm

DRINKS

Juices

There is no better way of supplying yourself with instant minerals, vitamins and enzymes than by taking a glass of freshly made raw vegetable juice. Yes, you will need a juicer and this can be expensive, but an investment that will pay you dividends in terms of improved health. Carrots and dark-green leafy vegetables contain carotinoids that protect against cancer. They also help to fight infection and are good for the skin and digestive system. Celery assists in detoxifying and cleansing, while beetroot improves the blood.

I have found that juice from a single vegetable can be too strong to assimilate; mixing them avoids this problem and greatly improves the flavour. The following are my suggestions:

Carrot (5 parts) and celery (3 parts).
Lettuce (4 parts), alfalfa sprouts (3 parts), cucumber (5 parts) and mint (1 part).
Beetroot (5 parts), carrot (4 parts), chives (1 part).

You can also include fruit. Carrot and orange is delicious, or beetroot and red grapes. Now invent your own.

Protein drinks

The nut milks described in 'The peak immunity dairy' are wonderfully beneficial, especially if you suffer from hypoglycaemia or have difficulty in digesting food because of your illness. They are good enough to drink all on their own. Tofu is also highly recommended, being rich in protein, while the inclusion of fruit will provide extra vitamins and flavour. Here are a couple of ideas.

Fruit cup

³/₄ pint / 425 ml apple juice
1 pear
3 oz / 75 g tofu

2 tbsp ground cashewnuts
$1/2$ tsp cinnamon

Put in the blender and run until liquid.
Serves 3

Autumn treat

Any soft fruit can be substituted for the blackberries.

1 pint / 570 ml soya milk
3 oz / 75 g tofu
4 oz / 110 g blackberries
1 tsp clear honey

Blend together until smooth.
Serves 3

Postlude

As you will have gathered, I learnt a great deal during those months that I took off work. Not only was it a time of rest and reassessment, but my new régime became well established. I experimented with a wide variety of vegan recipes, meditated three times a day, visualised the healing of the 'hot spot', thought a great deal about why I had become so dangerously ill, and poured out my thoughts and feelings into a multi-volumed diary. However, the hospital appointment for my second bone scan was rapidly approaching and there were moments when I felt panic-stricken. Could there really be a death-sentence hanging over me? I knew I was doing everything possible to help myself and this gave me courage. Surely all those beansprouts must be working their magic by now.

While the nurse was injecting my arm with radioactive material, she asked me whether I had any aches or pains or any other unusual symptoms. I was able to tell her with some pride that I had never felt better. Nevertheless, when the letter from my consultant finally arrived, my hands were shaking so much that I could scarcely open the envelope. It was formal but friendly and explained quite briefly that the hot spot had receded and there was now definitely no evidence of secondary spread to the bones. The relief was immense. It was as if someone had given me back my life, and how precious it was to me now. I swore that henceforth I would treat myself with the greatest possible attention and care. No more self-neglect. Yes, my life is a treasured gift and I will do everything in my power to maintain it.

Now it is your turn to see how eagerly you are adopting your new immunity programme, by going through the following check list. Do this at three-monthly intervals and watch your rating improve. This is a self-scoring questionnaire. Ring the number that best matches your progress, with 3 as the highest.

Immunity checklist

	Self-rating
Are you regularly keeping a diary of your inner life?	1 2 3
Are you well aware of your deepest needs and do you get these met?	1 2 3
Do you often affirm your own worth?	1 2 3
Do you discuss your problems with a friend, relative or counsellor?	1 2 3
Do you enjoy your sex life with one long-term partner?	1 2 3
Are you moving out of a negative life position, such as victim or martyr?	1 2 3
Do you consult your Wise Being?	1 2 3
Have you set yourself achievable goals?	1 2 3
Do you practise asserting yourself?	1 2 3
Are you good at dealing with anger?	1 2 3
Are you letting go of old resentments?	1 2 3
How is your laughter quotient?	1 2 3
Do you allow time for creativity?	1 2 3
Do you set up dialogues between your subpersonalities to sort out inner conflicts?	1 2 3
Have you identified your main sources of stress?	1 2 3
Have you significantly reduced your stress levels?	1 2 3
Do you practise physical relaxation?	1 2 3
Do you meditate and practise healing visualisation?	1 2 3
Have you cut down on environmental pollutants at home?	1 2 3
Have you cut down on environmental pollutants at work?	1 2 3
Do you do flexibility and strength exercises for at least 10 minutes three times a week?	1 2 3
Do you do some form of aerobic exercise for at least 20 minutes three times a week?	1 2 3
Have you given up smoking or any other recreational drugs?	1 2 3
Have you cut your alcohol intake to less than two glasses of wine per day (or equivalent)?	1 2 3
Have you given up coffee and tea?	1 2 3
Have you cut out added salt and sugar?	1 2 3
Have you given up red meat and other sources of saturated fat?	1 2 3
Do you avoid deep-fried or barbecued foods?	1 2 3
Do you avoid smoked foods and foods with artificial additives?	1 2 3
Is your diet high in natural fibre?	1 2 3
Do you eat plenty of fresh fruit and vegetables, organically grown?	1 2 3
Do you eat whole cereals?	1 2 3
Have you given up refined foods and white flour products?	1 2 3
Do you eat plenty of fresh salads?	1 2 3
When you are ill or under stress, do you take vitamin and mineral supplements, especially beta-carotene, vitamin B complex, vitamin C, evening primrose oil, selenium and zinc?	1 2 3

SCORE _____

Rating

0 _____|_____ 100

Low
immunity

Peak
immunity

Addresses

Cancer and Aids support

BACUP (British Association of Cancer United Patients)
121-3 Charterhouse Street
London EC1M 6AA
Tel: 071 608 1785/6

BCMA (Breast Care and Mastectomy Association)
15–19 Britten Street
London SW3 3TZ
Tel: 071 867 8275

Cancer Help Centre
Grove House
Cornwallis Grove
Bristol BS8 4PG
Tel: 0272 743216

Cancerlink
17 Britannia Street
London WC1X 9JN
Tel: 071 833 2451

Dr Jan de Winter Clinic for Cancer Prevention Advice
6 New Road
Brighton
Tel: 0273 727213

Hospice Information Service
St Christopher's Hospice
51–59 Lawrie Park Road
London SE26 6DZ
Tel: 081 778 9252

Leukaemia Care Society
PO Box 82
Exeter
Devon EX2 5LP
Tel: 0592 218514

London Lighthouse (Aids)
111–117 Lancaster Road
London W11 1QT
Tel: 071 792 1200

The Marie Curie Memorial Foundation (nursing services)
28 Belgrave Square
London SW1X 80Q
Tel: 071 235 3325

National Society for Cancer Relief (grants and home care)
15-19 Britten Street
London SW3 3TZ
Tel: 071 351 7811

Support for those with other disorders

Action Against Allergy
43 The Downs
London SW20 8HG
Tel: 081 947 5082

Arthritis Care
18 Stephenson Way
London NW1 2HD
Tel: 071 916 1500

Asthma and Allergy Treatment
and Research Centre
12 Vernon Street
Derby DE1 1FT
Tel: 0332 362461

Asthma Society
300 Upper Street
London N1 2XX
Tel: 071 226 2260

British Diabetic Association
10 Queen Anne Street
London W1M 0BD
Tel: 071 323 1531

British Society for Clinical
Ecology (food intolerances)
Royal Liverpool Hospital
Liverpool L7 9XP
Tel: 051 709 0141

The Lupus Group
(see Arthritis Care)

The ME Association
PO Box 8
Stanford le Hope
Essex SS17 8EX
Tel: 0375 642466

The Multiple Sclerosis Society
of Great Britain and Northern
Ireland
25 Effie Road
London SW6 1EE
Tel: 071 736 6267

SPAID (Society for the Prevention of Asbestosis and Industrial Diseases)
38 Drapers Road
Enfield

Middlesex EN2 8LU
Tel: 081 366 1640

National Ankylosing Spondylitis Association
(see Arthritis Care)

Complementary therapies

British Acupuncture Association
34 Alderney Street
London SW1V 4EU
Tel: 071 834 1012

British Holistic Medical Association
179 Gloucester Place
London NW1 6DX
Tel: 071 262 5299

British Homoeopathic
Association
27a Devonshire Street
London W1N 1RJ
Tel: 071 935 2163

The Maxwell Cade Foundation
(biofeedback)
9 Chatsworth Road
London NW2 4BJ

National Federation of Spir-
itual Healers
Old Manor Farm Studio
Church Street
Sunbury-on-Thames
Middlesex TW16 6RG
Tel: 09327 83164

The Shiatsu Society
14 Oakdene Road
Redhill RH1 6BT
Tel: 0737 767896

Counselling and psychotherapy

Association for Family
Therapy
6 Heol Seddon
Danescourt
Llandaff
Cardiff CF5 2QX

Association of Humanistic
Psychology Practitioners
14 Mornington Grove
London E3 4NS
Tel: 081 983 1492

British Association for Coun-
selling
1 Regent Place
Rugby
Warwickshire CV21 2PJ
Tel: 0788 578328

CRUSE (bereavement counselling – many local branches)
126 Sheen Road
Richmond
Surrey TW9 1UR

Psychosynthesis and Education
Trust
92–94 Tooley Street
London SE1 2TH
Tel: 071 403 2100

Relate (marriage guidance)
Herbert Gray College
Little Church Street
Rugby
Warwickshire
Tel: 0788 73241

Westminster Pastoral
Foundation
23 Kensington Square
London W8 5HN
Tel: 071 937 6956

Social support

Alcholics Anonymous
PO Box 1
Stonebow House
Stonebow
York YO1 2NJ
Tel: 0904 644026

ASH (Action on Smoking and
Health)
5–11 Mortimer Street
London W1N 7RH
Tel: 071 637 9843

Depressives Anonymous
36 Chestnut Avenue
Neverley
N. Humberside HU17 9QU
Tel: 0482 860619

Gingerbread (one-parent
families)
35 Wellington Street
London WC2E 78N
Tel: 071 240 0953

National Council for the
Divorced and Separated (over
100 branches)
62 Stourview Close
Mistley
Manningtree
Essex CO11 1LZ

Carers' National Association
(caring for the elderly)
29 Chilworth Mews
London W2 3RG
Tel: 071 724 7776

The Outsiders Club (for the
emotionally isolated)
Box 4ZB
London W1A 4ZB
Tel: 071 499 0900

The Samaritans
(see phone book for local
contact)

Keeping fit

Amateur Athletic Association
(see phone book for local
branch)

The Biodynamic Clinic
(massage)
23 High Street
Ealing
London W5 2DF
Tel: 081 579 1904

British Orienteering
Federation
41 Dale Road
Matlock
Derbyshire DE4 3LT

British Veterans Athletic Federation (men over 40, women
over 35)
10 Higher Dunscar
Egerton
Bolton
Lancashire

Health Education Council
Look After Yourself!
Project Centre
Christ Church College
Canterbury
Kent

Society of Teachers of the
Alexander Technique
10 London House
266 Fulham Road
London SW10 9EL
Tel: 071 351 0828

Yoga for Health Foundation
Ickwell Bury

Nr Biggleswade
Bedfordshire
Tel: 076 727 271

Nutrition

BioCare (natural remedies)
20-24 High Street
Solihull
West Midlands BP1 3TB
Tel: 021 705 4975

BioMed International (hair
analysis by post)
55 Queens Road
East Grinstead
Sussex RH19 1BG
Tel: 0342 22854

Community Health
Foundation (macrobiotic
cooking)
188 Old Street
London EC1V 9BP
Tel: 071 251 4076

National Institute of Medical
Herbalists
9 Palace Gate
Exeter EX1 1JA
Tel: 0392 426022

Nature's Own (vitamins)
203–205 West Malvern Road
West Malvern
Worcs. WR14 4BB
Tel: 0684 892555

Neals Yard Apothecary (herbs
by post)
2 Neals Yard
London WC2

The Vegan Society Ltd
(cookery courses and lectures)
33 – 35 George Street
Oxford OX1 2AY
Tel: 0865 722166

Bibliography

Introduction

Brohn, Penny *The Bristol Programme: An Introduction to the holistic therapies practised by the Bristol Cancer Help Centre* (Century, 1987)

1 The Battle of the Cells

Ader, R. and Cohen, N., 'CNS-immune system interactions: Conditioning phenomena', *Behavioral and Brain Sciences*, 8:379-426 (1985)

Anderson, Dr James W., *Diabetes: A practical new guide to healthy living* (Martin Dunitz, 1981)

Atkinson, Atkinson, Smith and Hilgard, *Introduction to Psychology*, 9th edn. (Harcourt Brace Jovanovich, 1987)

Beck, Ernest W., *Mosby's Atlas of Functional Human Anatomy* (C.V. Mosby Co., 1982)

Brown, J.A.C., rev. Hastin-Bennett, A.M., *Pears Medical Encyclopedia* (Sphere Books, 1977)

Coleman, Dr Vernon, *Everything You Need to Know About Arthritis* (Severn House Publishers, 1985)

de Winter, Dr Jan, *The Truth About Cancer* (Blandford Press, 1986)

Dwyer, John, *The Body at War: The story of our immune system* (Unwin Hyman, 1988)

Gamlin, Linda, 'Another Man's Poison', *New Scientist* (15 July 1989)

Graham, Judy, *Multiple Sclerosis: A self-help guide to its management* (Thorsons, 1987)

Health Education Council, *Immunisation: Just a few moments' discomfort for years of protection* (1989)

Lacey, Dr Richard, *Safe Shopping, Safe Cooking, Safe Eating* (Penguin, 1989)

Lynch, Dr Barry, 'Save the children', *Radio Times* (2 September 1989)

Matthias, Sue, series ed., 'The Body Report', *Observer Magazine* (1988)

Melville, Arabella and Johnson, Colin, *Immunity Plus: How to be healthy in an age of new infections* (Penguin, 1988)

Nilsson, Lennart, *The Body Victorious* (Faber, 1987)

Roitt, Ivan, *Essential Immunology*, 4th edn. (Blackwell Scientific Publications, 1980)

Smith, Anthony, *The Body* (George Allen & Unwin, 1985)

Tudor and Tudor, *Understanding the Human Body* (Pitman, 1981)

Weiner, Michael, *Maximum Immunity* (Gateway Books, 1986)

2 How healthy is your personality?

Ader, Robert, ed., *Psychoneuroimmunology* (Academic Press, 1981)

Atkinson, Atkinson, Smith and Hilgard, *Introduction to Psychology*, 9th edn. (Harcourt Brace Jovanovich, 1987)

Cousins, Norman, *Anatomy of an Illness as Perceived by the Patient: Reflections on healing and regeneration* (Pathway/Bantam Books, 1987)

Cousins, Norman, *Head First: The biology of hope* (Dutton, 1989)

Dillon, K.M., Minchoff, B. and Baker, K.H., 'Positive emotional states and enhancement of the immune system', *International Journal of Psychiatry and Medicine*, 15:13–17 (1985–86)

Ferrucci, Piero, *What We May Be: The visions and techniques of psychosynthesis* (Turnstone Press, 1982)

Kobasa, S.C., 'Stressful life events, personality and health: An inquiry into hardiness', *Journal of Personality and Social Psychology*, 37: 1-11 (1979)

Le Shan, Lawrence, *You Can Fight For Your Life: Emotional Factors in the treatment of cancer* (Thorsons, 1984)

Martin, Paul, 'Pyschology and the immune system', *New Scientist* (9 April 1987)

Maslow, Abraham H., *Motivation and Personality*, 3rd edn. (Harper & Row, 1987)

McClelland and Kirshnit, 'The effect of motivational arousal through film on salivary immunoglobulin A', *Psychology and Health*, 2:31-52 (1988)

Plotnikoff, N.P. et al, *Enkephalins and Endorphins: Stress and the immune system* (Plenum Press, 1986)

Rogers, Carl R., *On Becoming a Person: A therapist's view of psychotherapy* (Constable 1967)

Schleifer, Keller, Camerino, Thornton and Stein, 'Suppression of lymphocyte stimulation following bereavement', *Journal of the American Medical Association*, 250: 374-377 (1983)

Siegel, Bernie S., *Love, Medicine and Miracles* (Arrow Books, 1988)

Simonton, O. Carl, Matthews-Simonton, Stephanie, and Creighton, James L., *Getting Well Again* (Bantam Books, 1980)

Solomon, G.F., 'Emotional and personality factors in the onset and course of autoimmune disease, particularly rheumatoid arthritis', *Psychoneuroimmunology*, ed. Ader, R. (Academic Press, 1981)

Weiner, Michael A., *Maximum Immunity* (Gateway Books, 1986)

3 Letting go of stress

Atkinson, Atkinson, Smith and Hilgard, *Introduction to Psychology*, 9th edn. (Harcourt Brace Jovanovich, 1987)

Blakemore, Colin, *The Mind Machine* (BBC Books, 1988)

Cohen and Willis, 'Stress, social support and the buffering hypothesis', *Psychological Bulletin*, 98: 310-357 (1985)

Coleman, Dr Vernon, *Overcoming Stress* (Sheldon Press, 1978)

Cooper, Cary L., Cooper, Rachel D., and Eaker, Lynn H., *Living With Stress* (Penguin, 1988)

Eagle, Robert, *Taking the Strain* (BBC Books, 1982)

Friedman and Rosenman, *Type A Behaviour and Your Heart* (Knopf, 1974)

Freud, Sigmund, *Two Short Accounts of Psycho-Analysis* (Pelican Books, 1962)

Gawain, Shakti, *Creative Visualization* (Bantam Books, 1982)

Gruber, Dr Barry L. and Hall, Dr Nicholas R. et al, 'Immune system and psychologic changes in metastatic cancer patients while using ritualized relaxation and guided imagery: A pilot study', *Scandinavian Journal of Behavior Therapy*, 17:25-46 (1988)

Hughes and Boothroyd, *Fight or Flight?* (Faber, 1985)

Jemmott and Locke, 'Psychosocial factors, immunologic mediation and human susceptibility to infectious diseases: How much do we know?' *Psychological Bulletin*, 95: 78-108 (1984)

Kirsta, Alix, *The Book of Stress Survival* (Allen & Unwin, 1986)

Laudenslager, Ryan, Drugan, Hyson and Maier, 'Coping and immuno-suppression: Inescapable but not escapable shock suppresses lymphocyte proliferation, *Science*, 221:568-570 (1983)

Le Shan, Lawrence, *How to Meditate* (Turnstone Press, 1983)

Locke, Kraus, Leserman, Hurst, Heisel and Williams, 'Life change stress, psychiatric symptoms, and natural killer cell activity, *Psychosomatic Medicine*, 46:441-453 (1984)

Maier and Laudenslager, 'Stress and health: Exploring the links', *Psychology Today*, 19, No. 8:44-49 (1985)

Martin, Paul, 'Psychology and the immune system', *New Scientist* (9 April 1987)

Meares, Ainslie, *Relief Without Drugs* (Souvenir Press, 1967)

Meares, Ainslie, *The Wealth Within* (Ashgrove Press, 1984)

Schleifer, Keller, McKegney and Stein, 'The influence of stress and other psychosocial factors on human immunity', (Psychosomatic Society, Dallas, 1979)

Selye, Hans, *The Stress of Life* (Van Nostrand Reinhold, 1979)

Selye, Hans, *Stress Without Distress* (Hodder & Stoughton, 1975)

Trauer, Dr Tom *Coping With Stress* (Salamander Books, 1986)

Weekes, Dr Claire, *Agoraphobia* (Angus & Robertson, 1977)

Which? *Understanding Stress* (Consumers' Association, 1988)

4 Man-made threats

Birkin, Michael and Price, Brian, *C for Chemicals: Chemical hazards and how to avoid them* (Merlin Press, 1989)

Bounds, Sarah, ed., 'The ultimate pollution protection plan', *Here's Health* (August 1989)

British Medical Association, *The BMA Guide to Living With Risk* (Penguin, 1990)

Brown, Phyllida, 'Aids and the Forgotten Defenders', *New Scientist* (13 June 1992); 'How does HIV cause Aids?', *New Scientist* (18 July 1992)

Dalton, Alan, *Dangerous Lives* (Channel 4 TV, 1989)

de Winter, Dr Jan, *The Truth About Cancer* (Blandford Press, 1986)

Elkington, John and Hailes, Julia, *The Green Consumer Guide* (Victor Gollancz, 1988)

Hamer, Mick, 'Cars at the Crossroads', *New Scientist* (11 July 1992)

Hildyard, Nicholas, *Cover Up: The facts they don't want you to know*, rev. edn. (New English Library, 1983)

Huey, Sara, ed., 'Air Pollution: Dirty diesel clampdown', *Earth Matters* (Summer 1989)

Lambert, Dr Barrie, *How Safe is Safe? Radiation controversies explained* (Unwin Paperbacks, 1990)

Lean, Geoffrey and Pearce, Fred, 'Poison on tap', *Observer Magazine* (6 August 1989)

Lean, Geoffrey, 'Sunshine state plans a green future', *Observer* (3 September 1989)

Melville, Arabella and Johnson, Colin, *Immunity Plus: How to be healthy in an age of new infections* (Penguin 1988)

Parker, Philip, ed., 'Air Pollution: Climate of catastrophe'; 'Car pollution – the facts', *Greenpeace News* (Spring 1989)

Parker, Philip, ed., 'Toxic pollution: White wash', *Greenpeace News* (Autumn 1989)

Parker, Philip, ed., 'Who's ozone friendly now?'; 'A sea of troubles', *Greenpeace News* (Summer 1989)

Porritt, Jonathon, ed., *Friends of the Earth Handbook* (Macdonald Optima, 1987)

Price, Brian, *Friends of the Earth Guide to Pollution* (Maurice Temple Smith and FOE, 1983)

Reader's Digest, *What our Grandmothers Knew: Hints, recipes and remedies of a bygone age* (1979)

Wilson, Des, ed., *The Environment Crisis* (Heinemann Educational, 1984)

5 Moving for immunity

Fiatarone, M.A., Solomon, G.F., et al, 'The effects of exercise on natural killer cell activity in young and old subjects', *Journal of Gerontology* (1989)

Namikoshi, Tokujiro, *Shiatsu: Japanese finger pressure therapy* (Japan Publications Inc., 1969)

Search, Gay and Denison, David, *Getting in Shape: The scientific way to fitness* (New English Library, 1988)

Shreeve, Dr Caroline, *Health Defence: Strengthen your immune defence system* (David & Charles, 1988)

Wells, Howard, gen. ed., *Start Living Now* (Lyric, 1979)

Which? 'Keeping fit' (Consumers' Association, February 1984)

Yamamoto, Shizuko and McCarty, Patrick, *The Shiatsu Handbook: A practical guide to acupressure*, rev. edn. (Turning Point Publications, 1989)

Yesudian, Selvarajan and Haich, Elisabeth, *Yoga and Health* (Unwin Books, 1966)

6 Feeding your defences

Adams, Ruth, *The Complete Home Guide to all the Vitamins* (Larchmont Books, 1972)

Anderson, Dr James W., *Diabetes: A practical new guide to healthy living* (Martin Dunitz, 1981)

Bartholomew, Alick, ed., *Turning Point* (Bristol Cancer Help Centre, Summer 1988)

Brown, Sarah, *Sarah Brown's Vegetarian Cookbook* (Grafton Books, 1986)

Cameron and Pauling, *Cancer and Vitamin C* (Weidenfeld, 1980)

Clark, L.C., et al, 'Plasma selenium and skin neoplasms: A case controlled study', *Nutrition and Cancer* (Jan-Mar 1984)

Coleman, Dr Vernon, *Everything You Need to Know About Arthritis* (Severn House, 1985)

Davies, Dr Stephen & Stewart, Dr Alan, *Nutritional Medicine* (Pan Books, 1987)

Davis, Adelle, *Let's Get Well* (George Allen & Unwin, 1974)

Davis, Adelle, *Let's Stay Healthy* (George Allen & Unwin, 1982)

de Winter, Dr Jan, *The Truth About Cancer* (Blandford Press, 1986)

Forbes, Dr Alec, *The Bristol Diet* (Century Arrow, 1986)

Gamlin, Linda, 'Another man's poison', *New Scientist* (15 July 1989)

Goldbeck, Nikki and David, *The Complete Wholefood Cuisine* (Thorsons, 1984)

Graham, Judy *Evening Primrose Oil* (Thorsons, 1984)

Graham, Judy, *Multiple Sclerosis: A self-help guide to its management* (Thorsons, 1987)

Griggs, Barbara, *The Food Factor: Why we are what we eat* (Viking, 1986)

Hodgkinson, Liz, 'ME, the mystery disease', *Woman's Journal* (November 1988)

Kenton, Leslie and Susannah, *Raw Energy* (Century Arrow, 1984)

Krause, Marie V. and Mahan, L. Kathleen *Food, Nutrition and Diet Therapy*, 7th edn. (W.B. Saunders & Co., 1984)

Kushi, Aveline and Jack, Alex, *Complete Guide to Macrobiotic Cooking* (Warner Books, 1985)

Kushi, Michio and Jack, Alex, *The Cancer Prevention Diet* (Thorsons, 1984)

Lappé, Frances Moore, *Diet for a Small Planet* (Ballantine, 1971)

Linehan, Liz, 'How potatoes and pasta can damage the bones', *Independent* (8 November 1988)

Mindell, Earl, *The Vitamin Bible*, 2nd edn. (Arlington Books, 1985)

Ministry of Agriculture, Fisheries and Food, *Manual of Nutrition* (Her Majesty's Stationery Office, 1985)

O'Brien, Jane, *The Magic of Tofu* (Thorsons, 1983)

Passwater, Richard A., *Selenium Update* (Keats Publishing Inc., 1987)

Quillin, Patrick, *Healing Nutrients* (Penguin, 1989)

Rippon, Sadhya, *The Bristol Recipe Book* (Century, 1987)

Rose, J., *Trace Elements in Health: A review of current issues* (Butterworths, 1983)

Salonen, J.T., et al, 'Risk of cancer in relation to serum concentrations of selenium and vitamins A and E', *British Medical Journal*, 290:417-20 (9 February, 1985)

Simkin, P.A., 'Oral zinc sulfate in rheumatoid arthritis', *Lancet*, 2: 539 (1976)

Smith, Dr Tony 'Polyunsaturated oils and the treatment of MS', *MS News* (Winter 1986)

Sonntag, Linda, *The Little Tofu Book* (Piatkus, 1987)

Weiner, Michael A., *Maximum Immunity* (Gateway Books, 1986)

Willett, W.C. et al, 'Prediagnostic serum selenium and risk of cancer', *Lancet*, II:130-4 (16 July 1983)

Workman, Hunter and Jones, *The Allergy Diet* (Dunitz, 1984)

Further reading

Bach, Edward, *Heal Thyself* (C.W. Daniel Co., 1931)

Bach, Edward, *The Twelve Healers and Other Remedies* (C.W. Daniel Co., 1933)

Clyne, Rachel *Cancer – Your Life, Your Choice* (Thorsons, 1989)

Diamond, Harvey and Marilyn, *Living Health* (Bantam Books, 1988)

Harris, Thomas A., *I'm O.K., You're O.K.* (Pan Books, 1973)

Hill, Diane, *Vegan Vitality: Captivating cuisine for a high energy lifestyle* (Thorsons, 1987)

Pleshette, Janet, *Cures That Work* (Century Arrow, 1986)

Skynner, Robin and Cleese, John, *Families and How to Survive Them* (Methuen, 1983)

Glossary

antigen A substance that causes the production of antibodies. Antigens may be formed within the body, or introduced artificially.

anti-oxidant Found in raw vegetable oils. Prevents oxygen from combining with other compounds and thus damaging cells.

bioflavonoids (vitamin P) Flavonoids provide the yellow and orange colour in citrus fruits. They assist the absorption and function of vitamin C and help build resistance to infection. Approximately 100 mg of bioflavonoids are needed for every 500 mg of vitamin C.

carcinogen A substance that induces cancer in a living organism.

carcinoma A malignant tumour arising from the epithelial cells of the skin and membranes. If it is classified as 'primary' there is no indication of further spread at the time of diagnosis.

cell-mediated immunity Immune reactions involving T-cells (see p.17).

DNA (deoxyribonucleic acid) Together with RNA (ribonucleic acid) this plays an important role in the synthesis of proteins and in the transmission of hereditary characteristics, since nucleic acids embody the genetic code.

endocrine system Consists of glands (such as the pituitary, thyroid and adrenal) that do not have ducts, but secrete hormones directly into the bloodstream. Fundamental to the control of growth and metabolism, sexual function, and intellectual and emotional development.

epithelium The tissue that lines the surfaces of the body, including inner surfaces such as the mouth and bladder.

free radical A molecular fragment that can cause damage to the genetic material of cells, which may result in cancer.

humoral immunity Refers primarily to the antibodies produced by the B-cells (see p. 17) that circulate in the blood and other body fluids (once called 'humours').

hypothalamus A vital part of the forebrain. It regulates temperature, body weight and appetite, blood pressure and fluid balance, and sexual behaviour.

immunoglobulin There are five types of these antibodies: IgG, IgA, IgM, IgD and IgE. The most common is IgG, which coats microorganisms, hastening their destruction by other immune cells. IgA acts as a first line of defence, especially against viruses; it guards entrances and concentrates in body fluids. IgM circulates in the bloodstream, where it destroys bacteria. IgD is present on the surface of B-cells. IgE is involved in allergic reaction.

lumpectomy Removal of a tumour and some surrounding tissue by surgery.

lymphocyte See White Cells chart on p. 17.

macrophage See White Cells chart on p. 17.

mast cells See White Cells chart on p. 17.

mastectomy Removal of the breast by surgery. This can either be simple or radical. The latter is more extensive and involves the additional removal of the muscle beneath, and lymph glands of the armpit.

metastasis Spread of cancer from the original tumour to other distant sites, generally referred to as secondary growths. The usual route is via the lymphatic system into the glands. Less commonly, the malignant cells enter the bloodstream and set up growths in the bones, lungs and liver.

milliSievert See sievert.

mutation An alteration occurs in the hereditary material, resulting in a change in the characteristics of the organism.

neuron A specialised cell forming in the basic unit of the nervous system. The human brain is composed of 12 billion or more.

neurotransmitter A chemical that carries a nerve impulse from one neuron to the next.

nigari A seawater extract from Japan, available in granules from some health-food shops. Used as a curdling agent and coagulant in the making of tofu (q.v.).

oncology The part of medical science that deals with and treats tumours.

oncologist A person who specialises in the treatment of cancerous growths.

phagocyte See White Cells chart on p. 17.

pituitary gland A gland about the size of a pea situated just above the back of the nose at the base of the brain. Secretes hormones that regulate important body functions.

psychosomatic diseases Physical illnesses in which major causative factors are mental and emotional. These act through the autonomic nervous and endocrine systems, upsetting hormone levels and other bodily functions.

rad Ionising radiation loses energy in the matter it travels through. The rad measures the radiation in terms of energy deposited, or dose absorbed, and is used, for example, when treating people medically with X-rays. In the SI system it has been replaced with the gray (Gy), which is equivalent to 1 joule of energy being deposited in 1 kg of matter. 1 Gy is equal to 100 rads.

radiotherapy Medical treatment, usually for cancers, involving large doses of X-rays (or other ionising radiation), carefully calculated to cover the affected area only.

RDA (recommended daily dietary allowances) These were first set in 1941 by the Food and Nutrition Board of the National Research Council of the Academy of Sciences in the USA. They are merely estimates of nutritional requirements of growing children and adults who are healthy. Intake at these levels will prevent nutrient depletion, but they are not meant to denote an ideal diet. Vitamin and mineral requirements vary greatly from individual to individual, particularly among those who are ill. Many nutritionists regard the RDA as inadequate.

sievert (Sv) This quantifies the potential of radiation to damage cells. The sievert measures the so-called 'dose equivalent' – the absorbed dose modified by a quality factor that depends on the type of radiation involved. Some types, in particular alpha particles, are much more damaging than others. It replaces the rem (röntgen equivalent man). 1 Sv equals 100 rem.

systemic Involving the whole bodily system; not confined to any particular part.

tempeh An Indonesian high-protein food, bought as a slab of cultured soya beans. A grey or black mould results from the *Rhizopus oligosporus* culture (similar to the moulds of blue cheeses).

tofu The Japanese for beancurd, made from soya beans and sold as a firm white slab, or with a creamier texture. Rich in protein.

vegan Vegans differ from vegetarians in that they also exclude eggs and dairy products from their diet in addition to meat. It is important to obtain sufficient protein from plant sources and to take a supplement of vitamin B_{12} which may otherwise be missing.

Index

Page references in italics refer to diagrams and charts. For recipe ingredients see under fruit, grains, vegetables etc.

acceptance: of others 67, 69; in panic attacks 97; of self 5, 69, 112, 113

acid: in stomach 11, 38; rain 141–2

additives: *see under* food

adrenal glands 80, *89*, 90, 92

adrenalin 58, *89*, 91, 94, 161; to treat anaphylaxis 37

aerobic effect *see under* exercise *and* sports

affirmations 59, 60–1, 71, 72, 260

Agent Orange 136

aggression 77, 109; getting rid of 78; *see also* anger

agoraphobia 97

Aids 5, 18, 25–7, 29, 30, 181; diet for 208–9

air: clean 116, 141; fresh, and deep breathing 160, 161; fresh, and immunity 150; effect of polluted 27; in respiration 11

alarm reaction 91, 92, *92*

alcohol 94, 173, *192*, 195, 202, 207, 260; and smoking 27; and stress 94, 96; *see also* wine

Alexander Technique 163

alertness 58; meditation and 121; stress and 93, 94

alienation 46, 57; from true self 69; *see also* loneliness

allergens 35, 36, 37

allergies 10, *17*, 30, 35–7, 127, 128, 136, 145, 146, 174, 181, 224; and food intolerance 206–7

Almond milk 243

Almond paste 239

Almond rolls 225

alpha particles 131; *see also* glossary *under* sievert

aluminium 140, 141, 197; salts 146

Alzheimer's disease 141, 146

amino-acids 170, 176–7, 179, 227, 228, 251; essential 176

anaemia 24, 35, 184; pernicious 32, 180

anaphylaxis 37, 206

anger 6, 45, 50, 53, 54, 78–9, 260; and auto-immune disease 31, 50, 51; dealing with 78–9; dispelling 77; embodiment of 163; expressing 110; freeing repressed 51; inability to express 47, 50, 109, 110; sensitivity to 50; and visualisation 123

animals: laboratory 91, 92, 171, 182; and listeriosis 39; and pesticides 177–8; *see also* pets

ankylosing spondylitis 208

antibiotics 23–4; and candidiasis 29, 30

antibodies 5, 8, 14, 15–16, *17*, 18, 19, 20, 22, 23, 25, 132, 138, 142, 176; in auto-immune disease 31; copper and 183; in diabetes 32; in food allergy 206; and HIV 26; imagery and 122; in lupus 34; from mast cells 36; receptor molecules of 16; in rheumatoid arthritis 34; selenium and 185; against sperm 26, 32; in ulcerative colitis 35; vitamin A and 178; vitamin B complex and 179, 181; vitamin C and 181; vitamin E and 182, 185

antigens 8, 15–16, 20, 21; antigenic drift 20; of HIV 26; prepared 22; *see also* glossary

anti-oxidant 181, 182, 185, 192; *see also* glossary

antisepsis, natural *10*, 11

anxiety 4, 6, 7, 34, 51, 54, 85, 94, 98, 108, 109, 111; reduction of 52, 69, 77, 115; symptoms of 96–8

appetite: loss of 95; zinc and 166

Apple pudding 255

approval 46, 47, 113; parental 108

Apricot crumble 254

Arab salad 229

arteries 150; damage to 167, 169; diabetes and 32; hardening of (atheroma) 179

arthritis 50, 207; diet and 173; exercise and 159; and folic acid deficiency 180; pantothenic acid

and 181; selenium and 189; *see also* rheumatoid arthritis
art therapy 83–4
asbestos 144, 145; asbestosis 129, 130; cancer and 27, 129, 130
aspirin 80, 180, 181
assertiveness 50, 53, 56, 68, 75, 76, 77–8, 103, 105, 108, 116, 260
asthma 36, 37, 96, 142
athlete's foot 10
atomic bomb 132
attention 75, 115, 116; gaining 70, 71, 113
authority, figure of 7, 74, 110, 113
auto-immune diseases 21, 25, 31–5, 140, 192; and psychological factors 49; and visualisation 122
Autumn treat 258

babies 22, 23, 63, 161; allergies in 36; loss of from listeria 40; and salmonella 38, 39
bacteria 10, 13, 24, 164, 182; beneficial 9, 193; definition of 9; destroyed 17, 18; in food poisoning 37, 38, 39, 40, 41; and food refinement 167; as pathogens 9, 11, 12, 13, 14, 15, 17, 22; Proteus 34; reproduction and growth of 9, 13; Staphylococcal 23; Streptococcal 23
baking soda 146
Banana and pear cake 244
B-cells 14, 16, 17, 18, 19, 25, 30, 31, 178, 179, 132, 138, 142, 184; receptors on 58; *see also* B-memory cells
beans 171, 172, 173, 174, 176, 180, 196; aduki 228; black-eyed 249; Bobby 228; Boston baked 220; butter 234; 236; and flatulence 198; haricot 221; mung 228, 232, 252; sprouting 184, 227, 228, 232, 248, 249; red kidney 229; *see also* soya beans *and* tofu
behaviour: change in 93; defects in 138; new 56, 104; patterns 55, 70, 72, 98, 108; rules for 110
belonging 56, 58
benz-a-pyrene 142
bereavement 48, 62; as stressor 99, 100, 102; *see also* mourning *and* loss
beta-carotene 189, 260; *see also* vitamin A
bile 11, 18, 19, 88–9
biofeedback 124–6; with stethoscope 163
biological magnification 178
biotin *see* vitamin H
birth defects 133, 134, 136, 143, 147

Black-eyed bean stew 249
bladder 10, 88–9; *see also* cancer, of bladder
bleach 144; bleaching 137
blindness 137; in diabetics 32, 167
blood: in biofeedback 125, 126, 126; and brain 150; calcium in 178; cancer of 28; copper and 183; circulation 13, 140; clots 19, 49; in fight or flight response 90; and immune response 24; in inflammation 12; in liver 18; mother's 23; oxygen and nutrients in 150, 184; poisoning (septicaemia) 39; pressure 37, 49, 81, 95, 117, 166, 172, 182, 185, 206; samples 69, 81; sugar in 32, 90, 166, 168, 169, 214; transfusions 26, 27; vegetable juices and 257; *see also* cells, red and white, *and* vessels, blood
bloodstream: antibodies in 16; bacteria in 15; candidiasis and 30; drugs in 26; hormones in 4, 89, 91, 126, 162; lymphocytes in 14, 179; malignant cells in 2; memory cells in 21; oxygen and 150; poison in 38, 160; salmonella in 39; substances in 19
B-memory cells 16, 17, 21
body: anger and 78; armouring 164; awareness of 6; balance in 163; and biofeedback 126; bodywork 162–4; chemistry 172, 175; connection with thoughts and feelings 4, 6, 7, 43, 59, 61, 73, 76, 119, 124, 125, 151, 156, 161; detoxifying 173; disconnection from 65; disease and 21; effect of environment on 7; exercising 152–6; and food 151; healing of 5; healing energy in 161; healthy 5, 35; infection of 19, 25, 30; language of 164; listening to 67; loss of use of 171; massage and 163; nourishment of 7; and nutrients 167, 169; and oxygen 150; recording condition of 7; relaxing 6; relaxed use of 163; shape 159; strain on 3; stress and 91, 116; vitamins and 19, 183
bones 5; breast bone 16; calcium in 178, 183; copper and 183; proteins and 176; in rheumatoid arthritis 34; visualisation and 123; zinc and 166; *see also* cancer, of bones, *also* marrow, of bone *and* scan, bone
boredom 75; stressor 90, 99, 100, 102, 105

botulism 38
brain: damage 22, 26, 142; in
 fight or flight response 90; and
 heavy-metal pollution 140, 141;
 and immunity 24–5, 58, 151;
 inflammation of 22; and oxygen
 150; relaxation and 117; right
 86; waves, tumours 58, 129; waves,
 alpha and beta 119, 125
bread 223–7; wholemeal 168, 169,
 174, 183, 194, 219, 220, 236,
 238, 239, 240, 250; white 173,
 174, 193
breakfast 177, 214–21, 236
breast 62; benign disease of 192;
 see also cancer, of breast
breathing 90, 96, 117, 150; deep
 158, 159–60; impact of music
 on 85; meditating on the breath
 120; restriction of 3; *see also*
 yoga breathing
breathlessness 95
bronchi *10*, 11, 37, *88–9*;
 candidiasis and 30; *see also*
 cancer, bronchial
bronchitis 22, 128, 141, 142, 143
Bruton's Syndrome 25
butter 167, 169, *174*, 183, 243
Butterbean pâté 236

cadmium 138, 140, 142, 189, 201
caffeine 169, 202
cakes 166, 173, *174*; sugar-free
 174, 244–7
calcium 170, 178, 183, 185,
 197, 203, 215, 219; calcium
 pantothenate *see* vitamin B₅
calories 171
cancer 2, 3, 4, 5, 27–9, 48, 51,
 63, 69, 76, 105, 132, 134, 136,
 147, 257; alcohol and 173; of
 bladder 128, 142; of breast 27,
 29, 47, 48, 183, 194; bronchial
 129; cells *17*, 28, 133; of cervix
 27, 28, 48, 143, 180; of the
 colon 167, 193; dead cancer
 cells 18; diet and 165, 166, 171,
 172, 173, 175, 208; fat and 167;
 Gerson and 175; of groin 128;
 of intestine 212; of larynx 28;
 of lip 28; of liver 143, 183; of
 lung 129, 133, 142, 143, 145;
 meditation and 121; natural
 killer cells and 151; and nitrates
 140; of oesophagus 185; among
 overweight 158, 204; and
 oxygen 150; of pancreas 27,
 143; and pesticides 135; of
 placenta (choriocarciroma) 28;
 and repressed creativity 84; and
 selenium 189; of skin 128, 132;
 of stomach 27, 139, 171; and
 stress 103; testicular 28, 129;

and unresolved feelings 62,
 109; visualisation and 122, 123;
 vitamin A and 166, 179; vitamin
 C and 181
Cancer Help Centre, Bristol 4, 43,
 62, 63, 83, 121, 124, 149, 159
 173, 175
Candida albicans 10, 24, 26, 29–30,
 190, 209; treatment for 30
capillaries: of bloodstream 150; of
 lymphatic system 13
carbohydrates 19, 168, 176, 206,
 214; of antigens 8; diabetes
 and 175; refining of 166, 167,
 171, 173
carbon dioxide, from cells 150
carbon monoxide 142, 181
carcinogens 28, 136, 137, 139, 142,
 146, 181, 182, 198; cocarcinogen
 132; folic acid deficiency and
 180; in food wrapping 200; *see
 also* glossary
carcinoma 28; primary 2; *see also*
 glossary
care 63; in need of 5, 73;
 professional 4, 75; self 5, 73;
 touch and 163
Carob cake 245
carotinoids 179, 257; *see also*
 beta-carotene
Carrot and cashew soup 234
Carrot pâté 237
cartilage 34, 176
catalytic converters 141, 142
cataracts 132, 133
Cashew and sesame milk 242
Cauliflower with rosemary
 sauce 251
cells 19, 28; abnormal 28; antibody
 producing *see* B-cells; auto-
 immune disease and 31, 32,
 34; beta-cells 32; of body 13,
 17, 21; brain 26, 150; cancer-
 fighting 69; dead *see* debris;
 dendritic 26; diet and 175;
 division of 28, 180; feeding *see*
 phagocyte; infected *17*; injury to
 12, 185; invasion of by pathogens
 9, 16, 27, 30; malignant 1, 2,
 140, 184, *see also* cancer *and*
 tumour; nerve 24; and oxygen
 150; production of 178; radiation
 and 27; red 150, 180, 184;
 responding to sound 85; swelling
 of 166; white *see under* white
 cells; *see also* mast cells *and*
 plasma cells
cereals *see* grains
CFCs (chlorofluorocarbons) 132
change: adjustment to 107;
 oneself 3, 4, 55, 56, 68, 70,
 94, 108; physiological, through
 meditation 119

cheese 180, 194, 239; fungus in 9; goat's milk 194; listeria in 40; *see also* Soya cheese

chemicals: in the air 127, 132; and allergies 37; in breast milk 37; in food 137, 178, 204, 227, 247; harmful 8, 18, 136, 139, 143, 144, 145, 146, 147, 148; pollution by 135–7; produced by white cells 14, 16, *17*; in water supplies 138

chemotherapy 28, 182

Chernobyl 130

Chestnut terrine 237

chicken 170, 176, 180, *186*, 194; battery 174; cook-chill, and listeria 40; and salmonella 38, 39; thawing of 41

chickenpox 15, 30

Chicory salad 232

childhood: feelings and beliefs from 108–9; isolation in 45; patterns dating from 70

children 21, 22; and asthma 37; behavioural disorders in 36; and emotional conflict 163; handicapped 105; leukaemia in 28; stunted in growth 59

Chinese rice 249

chlorine 30, 132; chlorinated chemicals 138

choice 71, 74, 112, *see also* will, free

cholera 9, 23, 172

cholesterol 19, 49, 172, *192*, 199

chromic acid 129

chromosome: aberrations 139; changes 134; number 6, 20

cigarettes *see* smoking

cilia 11, 128, 143

circulation 13; disease of 143; effect of music on 85; exercise and 149, 155, 157; massage and 159, 162

city 3, 36, 109, 181

claustrophobia 90, 96

clubfoot 134

coffee 173, 174, 202, 260

cold: common 5, 9, 95, 161; colds and 'flu 209–10; measles and 22; vitamin C and 181

cold sore *see* herpes

collapse 91, *92*, 97; from botulism 38

complement system *17*

concentration, poor 168, 177, 214

conditioning 24, 25

confidence 53, 56, 57, 69, 80

conflict: embodiment of 163; inner 63, 67, 69, 110–12, 113, 114

confusion 96, 114

conjunctivitis 36

conscientiousness 51, 54

constipation 167, 168, 185, 214

control 52; of anxiety symptoms 96; being in 92–3, of healing 7; loss of 93; of panic attacks 97; of stress 92, 99, 119, 125; through yoga 161

Control of Substances Hazardous to Health 129

cooking 169, 172, 180; against salmonella 39; utensils 197

coordination, loss of 33, 137

coping: behaviour 77; and hardy personality 52; and rheumatoid arthritis 50; and stress 91, 100

copper 183–4, 187

coronary attack 49, 94, 96; *see also* heart attack

corticosteroids 91, 181, 182

cortisone 85, *126*

cough 11

counselling 59, 62, 68, 69, 75, 105, 116, 192, 260; *see also* psychotherapy

courage 5, 71, 74, 75, 108

Couscous cake 246

Cousins, Norman 69, 80, 81, 85

cowpox 21

Cream of pea soup 234

creativity 46, 62, 76, 83–6, 110, 260; denial of 50, 58; repression of 84

crisis 4, 74, 105, 107

Crisp beansprout salad 228

criticism: implied 79; sensitive to 50, 54; unjust 77

Crunchy granola 216

Crunchy square 221

cushion-bashing 51, 78, 97, 104

cuts 12, 13, 179

cystitis 30

cysts 171

dairy products 170, 171, 172, 173, 180, 183, 194; cow's milk and cheese 174; ghee 173, 174; goat's milk 171; goat's milk yoghurt 173

Dairy, Peak Immunity 215, 216, 217, 219, 230, 239–44

DDT 136, 138

death 2, 58, 75, 80, 96, 105, 150, 259; from acidosis 32; from botulism 38; from breast cancer 29; from diabetes 167; early 20, 22, 25; of family member 44, 47, 62; from infectious diseases 22; from salmonella 39; smoking and 27; spiritual 75; from stress 91

debris 12, 14, *14*, 18, 33, 164

decision-making 52, 54, 70, 104

defence mechanisms *see* immune defences

degradation: biological 134, 135; of
  environment 137
depression 30, 35, 45, 50, 51, 52,
  54, 58, 79, 93, 96, 105, 108,
  110, 111
dermatitis 36, 95
desensitisation: for asthma 37; for
  phobias 97
despair 46, 69, 112
desperation, feeling of 4, 47
desserts 174, 176, 194, 195,
  242, 253–7
detergents 144, 146
detoxification 19, 204–5, 207, 210;
  system 36, 128, 143, 257, *and see*
  liver *and* kidneys
diabetes 31, 167, 175, 179, 183,
  185, 210; diet and 173; juvenile-
  onset 20; and listeria 40; among
  the overweight 32, 158, 171;
  stress and 91
diarrhoea 35, 181; from salmonella
  39; from stress 95
dieldrin 135, 136
diet: for Aids 208–9; for allergies
  128, 206; American 171; for
  arthritis and rheumatism 207;
  assessment of *see* questionnaires;
  Bristol 43, 175; for cancer
  208–9; and candidiasis 30, 209;
  change of 158; for diabetics
  210; for colds and 'flu 209–10;
  of Hunza 171; macrobiotic 172;
  mineral deficiencies in 166; for
  multiple sclerosis 33, 210–11;
  the Peak Immunity 173–5, 177,
  178, 180, 185; (changing to)
  193–5, 215; the Peak Immunity
  and special conditions 206–12;
  poor 5; refined 193; refined
  Indian 171; for rheumatoid
  arthritis 211–12; for ulcerative
  colitis 35; vegan 165, 176, 180,
  259; vegetarian 171, 172, 194;
  of Vilcabamba 171; Western
  165, 167, 170, 175, 176, 182,
  184, 185
digestion 19, 88–9, 170, 173;
  disorders of 201; poor 212
digestive system 18, 176, 257;
  cancer of 27; in lupus 35;
  penetration by bacteria 9
dinner 248–57
dioxins 137, 143
diptheria 20, 21, 23
dips 236–9, 243
diseases 76, 178; anger and 31, 78;
  childhood 22, 23; circulatory
  143; common in the West 29,
  31; degenerative 50, 55, 158,
  167, 171, 173, 175, 182, 190,
  204; fungal 29; heart 143;
  immune disorders 18; infections

15, 21; inflammatory *17*; lymph
  nodes and 14; pathogens and 9,
  15, 16, 19; repressed feelings
  and 91; resentment and 73, 77;
  serious 5; stress-related 91, 94,
  99, 116, *126* tendency towards
  20, 63; viral 22; vulnerable
  to 4; work-related 127–31; *see
  also* auto-immune diseases *and*
  immune-deficiency diseases
diverticulosis 167
DNA (deoxyribonucleic acid),
  glossary; and folic acid 180; in
  lupus 35
drinking and eating 56, 169,
  173, 201–3
drinks 257–8; colouring in 36;
  soft 184
drugs 18, 20, 25; addiction
  to 26; anti-inflammatory
  34, 35; and auto-immune
  disease 31; for hayfever 36;
  immuno-suppressive 20, 24,
  25; sulfa 24; *see also* antibiotics;
  chemotherapy; *and* steroids
dust 35, 37, 128, 145, 160
dysmenorrhoea 63, 67, 192

eating: healthy 170; out 194; too
  much 95; *see also* drinking
  and eating
eczema 36, 95
eggs 165, 173, 176, 180, 181, 182,
  183, 184, *186–8*, 199; antibiotics
  in 30; battery 174; salmonella
  and 38, 39, 41
electrical smog 134
electrical skin resistance: in
  biofeedback 124–5; in music 85
electromagnetic spectrum 133, 134
emotions: and auto-immune
  diseases 31; and biodynamic
  therapy 163; and biofeedback
  124–5; damaging negative 52,
  80; and disease 25; examining 5;
  persistent 114; positive 80; *see
  also* feelings
endocrine system 80, *89*; brain,
  immunity and 151; creativity
  and 86; *see also* glossary
endorphins 81, 151, 157
energy 110, 194; availability of 62,
  112, 115, 118; balancing through
  yoga 161; and biofeedback 126;
  and biodynamic massage 163;
  drain on 47; expending 149; and
  fat storage 158; from food 150,
  176; healing 160; implosion of
  47; and shiatsu 162; through
  visualisation 123
enkephalins 81
environment: adapted to 36; effect
  on immune system 20, 25;

polluted 127–48; shared 10; *see also* city *and* host

enzymes *13*, *17*, 18, 33, 143, 144, 146, 170, 176, 180, 194, 201, 206, 215, 248, 257; in allergic reaction 36; in phagocytosis 12

epidemic: food poisoning 37; viral 20; whooping cough 22

epithelium 9; *see also* glossary

essential fatty acids (EFAs), 36, 190–3, *192*, 223

esteem 56, 57, 59; loss of 80, 99

evening primrose oil 192, 260

events: in control of 93; negative life 93; *see also* stressors

exercise 54, 149–61; aerobic 149, 155–7; for diabetics 32; connected with feelings 7; for flexibility and strength 149, 151–5; hatha yoga 161; for health 150, 260; lack of 5; meditative 7; for multiple sclerosis 33; and natural killer cells 151; outdoor 171; to relieve tension 97, 116; for rheumatoid arthritics 34; shiatsu 162; for the unwell and disabled 158–9; warming up for 149, 157–8; for weight loss 158

exhaust fumes 140, 141–2

exhaustion 91, 92, *92*, 97

external defences *see* immune defences

eyes *10*, 11, 36, *88–9*; diet and 175; problems 132; relaxing 118; stinging 141; strain 127

faintness 94, 177, 214

family 43, 66, 74, 109

farming, intensive 37, 139

fat 18, 19, 167, 169, 170, 171, 172, 173, 175, 177, 183, *192*, 260; burning of 32; loss of 158; metabolism of 33, 211

fatigue 168; in multiple sclerosis 33; potassium deficiency and 185; when exercising 156, 214

fear 53, 54, 65, 73, 85, 90, 97; sharing 105; and visualisation 123

feelings: art therapy and 83–4; childhood 108; in connection with body and mind 4, 6, 7, 76, 85; effect on body 6, 43, 59, 62; expression of 6, 31, 46, 67, 75, 108, 116; in touch with 6; out of touch with 67; recording 7; repression of 6, 7, 48, 50, 67, 91, 108–10; about self 108; sharing 56, 58; *see also* emotions

fertilisers, artificial 139, 166, 184

fertility: decreased 133, 138; vitamin E and 182

fever 22; glandular 30; Rocky

Mountain spotted 23; yellow 23

fibre 167, 169, 170, 173, 193, 260

fight or flight response 87, 90–1, 94, 125

finger 12; cut 13; tingling during relaxation 126; thermometer 125

fish 165, 170, 172, 173, 174, 176, 180, *186–8*, 192, 194; contaminated 138, 177–8; haddock 185; halibut 179; -liver oils 179, 183; sardines 183; tinned and botulism 38

fitness: lack of 149; physical 6, 155

Flapjacks 246

flatulence 198

flora, of intestine 24, 30

flour: brown rice 255; buckwheat 225; cornmeal 218, 225, 246, 249, 254, 256; rye 224; white 166, 169, 182, 260; wholemeal 166, 182, 223, 225, 226, 240, 244, 245, 246, 247, 254, 255; *see also* soya flour

fluid, body 26; *see also* tissue fluid

foetus 23; liver of 16

folic acid 35, 179, 180, 187

food 170, 193, 195; additives 166, 169, 173, *188*, 204, 206, 215, 260; as allergen 10, 206; amino-acids in 176; to avoid *174*; canned 169, 173; chain 177-8; contaminated 39, *see also* fish, contaminated; convenience 37, 40, 170; for energy 150; fresh 40; fried 167, 168, 169, 172, 198, 260; frozen 39, 169; handling of cooked and raw 41; to include *174*; junk 173, 184; keeping hot 41, 42; nutritious 19, 34; preparation and cooking methods 198; preservatives 166, 184, *188*, processing 165, 166, 172, 173, 181, *186–8*; raw 174; refinement 165, 166, 167, 169, *186–8*, 260; reserves in biofeedback *126*; rich 171; smoked or burnt 173, 181, 198, 260; storage of 41; sufficient 56; supply 151; vitamins and minerals in 178, *186–8*; wholefoods 165, 166, 170, 173, *see also* chemicals, in food

food intolerance 36, 206–7

food poisoning 37–42, 77; avoiding 41–2; treatment for 40; *see also* questionnaires

foreign bodies 10, 14; *see also* pathogens

forgiveness 79–80

formaldehyde 127, 143, 145

free radicals 146, 192; *see also* glossary

freezing 41, 42, 182, *187*; *see also* food, frozen
Freud, Sigmund 109, 110
friendship 58, 70, 77; *see also* relationships
fruit 176, *186–8*, 193, 194, 196, 207, 215; apples *188*, 216, 230, 255; apple juice 245, 255, 257; apricots 171, 179, 184, *186*, *187*, *188*, 216, 245, 254; avocado pears 180, 182, 184, *186*, *187*, 232, 238; bananas 169, 180, 185, *186*, 197, 242, 244, 256; citrus 182; dates 180, 183, *186*, *187*, *188*, 222, 245, 246, 253; blackberries 258, dried 165, 169; figs 183, 185, *187*, *188*, 246; fresh 170, 173, 260; grapefruit 185, *187*, *188*, 232; grapes 253; grape juice 246, 253; kiwi fruit *187*, 253; locally grown 172; lemons 185, *187*, *188*; lemon juice *see individual recipes*; mango 165; melon 179, 182, *186*, *187*, *188*, 235; in muesli 216; oranges *187*, *188*, 193, 234, 242, 247, 255; orange juice 246, 247, 254; organic 166, 174; pear *188*, 244, 254, 256, 257; pineapple 165; pineapple juice 231; raisins 165, 182, 184, 185, *186*, *187*, *188*, 215, 217, 218, 253, 255; raw 173, 175, 178; rhubarb 183, *187*; satsumas 230, 247; stewed 217; sultanas 217, 218, 244, 245, 252, 255; strawberries 182, 184, *187*, *188*
Fruit cup 257
frustration 80, 81, 91, 104, 111; stressors 90, 100, 102, 106–8
fulfilment 58, 73, 76, 114
fumes: from dry cleaning 146; noxious 138, 145; from photocopiers 127; toxic 8, 145; traffic 3; *see also* exhaust fumes
fungi 9, 10, 24; spores from 35; *see also Candida albicans*
fungicide 145, 198

gammalinolenic acid (GLA) 36, 191, 192, *192*
gamma rays 133
General Adaptation Syndrome 91–2, *92*
genes 20; and auto-immune disease 31; genetic damage 133, 134, 138, 147; genetic defect 25, 137; healthy 55; genetic material of HIV 26; and multiple sclerosis 33; genetic mutation 130; genetic predisposition to cancer 27
Gerson, Dr Max 174, 175

ghee 214; to make 243–4; *and see individual recipes*
glands 228; pineal 86; salivary 22; sebaceous 11; sweat 124; swollen 30, 128; *see also* adrenal glands; endocrine system: liver; lymph nodes; pituitary; thymus; thyroid
glandular fever 30
gluten 199, 224
goals 53, 71, 75–6, 83, 260
grains 166, 172, 173, 176, *186–8*, 196, 199; barley 171, *186*, 215; bulgar 249; brown rice 170, 176, 180, 183, *186*, 198, 199, 231, 246, 250, 255; corn 185; maize 171; millet 198, 199, 215, 216, 217, 218, 220, 228, 245; oats *188*, 215, 216, 217, 218, 220, 221, 225, 243, 244, 246, 254, 255; refined 167, 174; rye *186*, 215, 224, 228; sprouting 183, 227, 228, 228; wheat 180, *187* 224, 228, 229; wheat bran 181, *186*, 190, 193, 215, 223; wheat germ 180, 181, 182, 184, *186*, *188*, 215, 216, 217, 222, 223, 237; white rice 171; whole 169, 170, 172, 173, 174, 175, 180, 181, 182, 184, 185, *186*, *187*, *188*, 260
Grape and kiwi fruit jelly 253
grief 53; expressing 105; *see also* bereavement; mourning; sadness
group 53, 59; support group 69, 105, 123; therapy 51, 63, 69, 75
Guacamole 238
guilt 54, 62, 65, 79, 109, 114

haemoglobin 139, 150, 184
hair: as allergen 10; follicle 11; of nose 8, *10*, 11; proteins and 176; of trachea *10*
halocarbon vapour 146
Halvah 256
happiness 6, 73, 74, 76, 84
Hashimoto's thyroiditis 32
hatred 79, 80; of self 114
hay fever 36, 37
headache 95, 127, 141, 162, 168, 214
healing 5, 12, 20, 117; with biofeedback 124, *126*; through breathing 160; creativity and 86; enzymes and 33; forgiveness and 79; inner 45, 62, 67; through massage 162, 163; meditation and 119–21; through relaxation 116; and self-love 59; sexuality and 65; visualisation and 121, 122, 123–4; yoga and 161
health: Alexander Technique and 163; assertiveness and

77; biofeedback and 125;
deterioration of 105; eating and
195; effect of creativity on 84;
effect of emotions on 79; holistic
5, 7, 43; inner harmony and
51, 58, 59, 74; iron and 184;
laughter and 81; maintenance of
34; mind influencing *see* mind;
of muscles and tissues 150;
natural 173; problems 171; and
ratio of T-cells 18; and reduction
of stress 75; sedentary lifestyle
and 150; selenium and 166, 185
Health and Safety Commission 129
heart 22, 150, 164; affected
by laughter 81; affected by
rheumatoid arthritis 34; attacks
91, 97, 141, 150; in biofeedback
125, 126, *126*; calcium and
183; effect on lymphatic system
13; exercise and 149, 155, 156;
disease 3, 32, 49, 99, 166, 167,
171, 174, 183, 189; in fight
or flight response 87, *88*, 90;
palpitating 96, 160; racing
95, 96, 117; slowing of 160;
weakness of 166, 185
heat, damaging nutrients 181, *186*,
187, *188*
heavy metals 136, 142; immuno-
suppressive effects of 189;
pollution by 141
help 4; asking for 54, 70, 71, 73,
75, 104, 115; inability to receive
73; self 259
helplessness 3, 54, 57, 69, 75,
76, 77, 110, 114, 115; and
cancer 48, 69
hepatitis 38, 132; B 25
herbs 174, 196; basil 221, 237, 248,
252, 253; bay 237, 252; chives
231, 257; marjoram 249, 250;
mint 185, 229, 232, 257; mixed
dried 220, 225; oregano 221,
230, 248; parsley 229, 232, 234,
236, 238; rosemary 251; sage
238; tarragon 219, 231, 232,
234; thyme 235, 249, 250; *see
also* tea, herb
Herb sausages 220
herbicide 136, 137, 147
herpes 26, 27, 30–1
histamine 12, *17*, 36, 206
HIV (human immunodeficiency
virus) 25, 26, 173
hobbies 54, 58, 105
Hodgkin's disease 28, 180, 209
holistic *see* health *and* lifestyle
home, stressors at 100, 105, 107
honey 174, 182, 185, *186*, *188*,
216, 217, 223, 225, 244, 245,
246, 253, 254, 256, 258
hope 76, 80

hopelessness 54, 70, 75, 114; and
cancer 48, 69, 93
hormones 18, *89*, 132, 176;
creativity and 86; imbalances in
20; immuno-suppressive 4, 115,
125, 181; links with immune
system 81; stress and 91; *see also*
endorphins
host 16, 19, 24; human as 8, 9, 10
hot spot 2, 195, 259
humour 53; *see also* laughter
Hummus 238
hygiene 23, 39
hypoglycaemia 175, 210, 257
hypothalamus 59, *89*

illness: among bereaved 99;
emotional conflict and 163;
laughter and resistance to 81;
massage for 162; psychological
advantages of 75; repression and
67; viral 184; *see also* disease
immune 21; cells, receptors 151;
memory *see under* memory *and*
B-memory cells; suppression 24;
tolerance 21
immune defences 19, 135; building
healthy 7; definition 8; external
defence mechanisms 8, *10*,
10–11, 160; flushing 11; folic
acid and 180; general defence
processes 12–15; healthy 26,
59; internal defences 11–18;
lymphatic system and 164;
magnesium, zinc and 166;
oxygen and 150; prostaglandins
and *192*; protein and 176;
selenium and 185; shiatsu and
162; yoga and 161; *see also*
immune system
immune-deficiency diseases 25–31,
25, 26, 29, 147
immune-efficiency 33, 52, 53, 55;
see also questionnaires
immune system 178; on alert
5; and allergies 35; and auto-
immune disease 31, 33, 34, 51;
of babies 36; and bacteria 18;
and breathing 160; and cancer
27, 28; effect of counselling
on 69; definition 8; effect
of feelings on 6, 48, 91; of
elderly 52; and exercise 149;
expectations and 24; healthy
19, 28, 135, 140, 227; and
herpes 31; and HIV 25, 26,
and hormones 81, 86, 91, 151,
157; impaired 20, 28, 30, 37,
52, 91, 114, 132, 137, 140,
147; iron and 184; magnesium
and 185; and nervous system
25; and overweight 204; the
Peak Immunity Diet and 173;

principles of 6, 8; of seals 138; specific response 8, 14, 15–18 *17*, 21, 206; stimulation of 131; suppression of by radiation 132; and relaxation 115, 116; and transplants 20; and viruses 9, 18, 20; and visualisation 121, 122; and vitamin A 178; and vitamin B$_6$ 179

immunisation, active and passive, 23; *see under* vaccination

immunity 13, 16, 22, 170; and auto-immune disease 31, 34; and brain 24, 58; cell-mediated 16, glossary; -depleting factors 165–7; destruction of 18; diet and 172, 175; and emotional support 69; -enhancing nutrients 176-93; and HIV 26, 27; humoral 140, glossary; and laughter 82; liver and 19; lowered 20, 24, 25, 30, 40, 91, 142, 182, 183, 193; natural 23; potassium and 185; recipes for 214–58; self-assertion and 77; stress and 92, 115;

immunoglobulins 23, 36, 142, 178; IgA 68, 82; IgG 28

independence 71; and lupus 35, 51

indigestion 30, 95

infections 19, 23, 176, 178, 181, 183, 257; Aids and 26; from cut 12; free from 11; glands and 14; due to immune deficiency 25; life-threatening 24; recurring 20; respiratory 174; serious 9; susceptibility to 20; of urinary tract 34; vulnerable to 150

inflammation 12, 80, 81; in multiple sclerosis 33; in rheumatoid arthritis 34; in ulcerative colitis 35

influenza 9, 20, 23, 95; *see also* colds and 'flu

ingredients, for Peak Immunity Diet 199

injection 21, *23*; of antibodies 25

injury 12, 20, 151

inoculation *see* vaccination

insects 10; allergic to 37; bites and stings 37; and food poisoning 41

insecticides 136, 137, 144, 166

insomnia 95

insulin 32, 166, 175

interferon *17*, 28

internal defences *see* immune defences

intestines 18, 23, 178, 193; bacteria in 9; candidiasis and 30; fibre and 167; listeria and 39; membrane of 36; salmonella and 38; *see also* flora, of intestine

intimacy 53, 57, 58, 67, 68; avoiding 73

invaders *see* pathogens

iron 35, 184, *188*, 193, 208, 215, 219; deficiency 166

irritability 94; *see also* anger

irritant 145, 146

iscador 202

isolation 45; *see also* loneliness

Italian salad 229

Japanese spread 239

joints: exercises for 151–5; in lupus 35; in rheumatoid arthritis 21, 34, 184

joy: 72, 80, 86; lack of 73

judgments, making no 6, 67, 68, 84

juices 257; carrot 179; fruit and vegetable 174; *see under* fruit and vegetables

Kaposi's sarcoma 26

kidneys 18, 19, 228; abnormalities in 185; and diabetes 32; environmental toxins and 31; reduced function 166; stimulation of 204; waste-disposal processes of 8

kitchen: hygiene in 41; temperature of 41, 42

knowledge, of self 5, 115

laughter 53, 80–3, 260; benefits vital organs 81; good-humour 52; and resistance to illness 81; *see also* questionnaires

lead 140, 142, 144, 147, 189, 201, 211

Leek broth 234

legs 22; jelly 96

legumes 171, 174, 176, 184, *192*; *see also* beans, lentils, peas

lentils 170, 228, 236, 252

LeShan, Dr Lawrence 29, 45, 47, 48, 57, 86

lethargy 30, 105, 172

leucocytes *17*; leucocytosis 201

leukaemia 28, 47, 129, 130, 132, 133, 134, 147, 180, 209; lymphoblastic 28

libido, loss of 95

life 2, 3, 4, 19; choice for 71; effortless 163; enjoying 50, 59; force 172; intolerable 59; meaningful 76; quality of 29, 93, 108, 114, 175; rewarding 74, 259

lifestyle: examining 5; HIV and 27; holistic 5; immunity-enhancing 4, 29, 30, 35; improved 69; lowered immunity and 26; modern 30; sedentary 32, 150, 158, 171; stressors 99–100, 104–8

limbic system 59
lindane 147
linoleic acid 191, *192*
linolenic acid 192, *192*
listeria 37, 38, 39–40, 194;
    symptoms of 40
liver *88–9*, 184, 202, 204;
    environmental toxins and 31;
    in fight of light response 90; of
    foetus 16; and food additives
    169; lobules 18; role of 18–19;
    and vitamin A 179; waste-
    disposal system of 8; yoga and
    162; *see also* cancer, of liver
loneliness 46, 57, 70, 74; and
    infections 58; *see also* isolation
longevity 171
loss 35, 45, 46, 50, 51, 80, 105; of
    self 62; *see also* death
love 56, 59, 66, 72, 74, 75;
    conditional 68; food and 193;
    as healer 68, 80; loved one,
    loss of 45; making 109; movies
    about 68; rejecting 73; of self
    5, 59, 60, 113; for true self 46;
    unconditional 67, 68
lumpectomy 2, glossary
lunch 227–33
lungs 11, 150; candidiasis and
    30; damage to 22, 182; deep
    breathing and 160; exercise and
    149, 155, 156; reduced capacity
    141; in rheumatoid arthritis 34;
    see also cancer, of lung
lupus 175; *see under* systemic lupus
    erythematosus
lymph 2, 13, 14, *14*, 15, 16, 52,
    159; nodes 1, 13, 14, *14*, 16, 24,
    35, 91, 133, 162, 164; vessels 13
lymphatic system 12, 13–15; cancer
    of 28, 133; exercise and 149;
    skin brushing and 164
lymphocytes 13, 14, *14*, 16, *17*,
    18, 20, 21, 24, 48, 134, 164;
    bereavement and 99; health
    of 190; imagery and 122;
    production of 142; receptor 16,
    24; *see also* B-cells *and* T-cells
lymphoma 28, 131; non-Hodgkin's
    147

macrophage 14, *14*, 15, *17*, 28,
    33, 181, 182, 185; damaged by
    listeria 40
magnesium 166, 184, *188*, *192*, 193
malaria 10
malignancy 25, 27; fighting off
    93, 179
malignant melanoma 69, 132
malt extract 174, 218, 222, 226,
    244, 253, 254, 255, 256
mammogram 1, 2
margarine 174

marrow, of bone 16, *17*, 24, 180
martyr, life position of 54, 73,
    260; and rheumatoid arthritis
    patients 50
massage 115, 158, 161–3;
    biodynamic 163; shiatsu 162
mast cells *17*, 36, 142, 143;
    receptor sites 36
mastectomy 1, glossary
ME (myalgic encephalomyelitis)
    174
meaning 66, 74; to life 46;
    loss of 47
measles 9, 15, 22, *23*; German
    see rubella
meat 167, 169, 170, 172, 173, 174,
    175, 176, 177, 180, 184, 194,
    212, 260; antibiotics in 30
meditation 34, 43, 74, 96, 115,
    117, 119–21, 161, 259, 260; and
    biofeedback 125
Melon and almond soup 235
membrane 36; of antibody 16;
    of brain 22; of cell 185; of
    scavenger cell 12, 15; and
    vitamin A 178
memory: loss of 141, 142, 147;
    of mast cells 36; of specific
    immune response 15, 21; *see also*
    B-memory cells
meningitis 22
menu planning 205
mercury 140, 141, 189, 211;
    poisoning 138
metabolism 19, 150, 176; of
    amino-acids 179; and auto-
    immune disease 31; fat and
    167; in multiple sclerosis 33;
    the Peak Immunity Diet and
    173; relaxation and 117; of
    vitamins 166
metastases 2, 29, glossary
methaemoglobinaemia 140
microbes 19, 184, 185; *see also*
    pathogens
micro-organisms 14, 15, *17*, 19; *see
    also* pathogens
microwaves: and electrical smog
    134; industry 130; ovens 41,
    42; and radiation 133, 134;
    safety of 135
mid-morning snack 221–3
milk: breast 23, 36, 37; cow's 36,
    180 194; unpasteurised and
    listeria 40; *see also* soya milk *and*
    Dairy, Peak Immunity
mind 7; alert 6; influencing health
    25, 43, 61, 85, 124, 151; over
    matter 126; sluggish 6; in
    unison with body 161; *see also*
    thoughts
minerals 167, 169, 172, 173, 178,
    183–90, 193, 198, 199, 203,

208, 214, 215, 227, 257, 260;
imbalance 185; immunity-
enhancing *187*, *188*; loss of 32
miso 199, 235, 239, 250, 251;
soup 199
Miso gravy 251
Miso soup 235
Mixed grain herb bread 225
molasses, black 174, 180, 183,
184, *186*, *188*, 208, 221, 222,
224, 245
monocytes 12, 13 *17*
morality, rigid 51, 54
moth-proofing 127, 144, 147
motivation, for personal change 4,
195
mourning 45, 62; forgiveness and
79, 80; *see also* bereavement;
grief; sadness
mouth: and candidiasis 30; dry 94;
as entry for pathogens 9; in fight
or flight response 87; relaxing
118; saliva in *10*, *88–9*
mucous membranes 203, 228; and
asthma 37; and candidiasis 30;
and vitamin B₆ 179
mucus *10*, 11, 37
Muesli 215; as source of calcium
183
multiple sclerosis 32–3, 105,
189, 192, 210–11; diet and
175; and personality 51; and
physiotherapy 158; and yoga 161
mumps 9, 22
Mung-bean curry 252
muscles: activity of 13; and asthma
37; botulism and 38; bulk
158; calcium and 183, 185; in
cleansing breathing 161; cancer
of 28; and diabetes 32; energy
for 150; exercises for 151-5;
in fight or flight response 90,
125; lymphatic system and
164; magnesium and 166,
185; massage and 162; oxygen
requirements 155; paralysis of
22; proteins and 176; relaxing
116, 117–19, 126, *126*; vitamin
E and 182; warming up 157–8;
wastage of 34, 159; weakness in
166, 185
music 3, 76, 84, 85, 86, 113,
156, 163
mutation 20, 27, 31, 136, glossary
mutagenic chemicals 139

National Cancer Institute,
USA 172
natto 199
natural killer cells (NK) *17*, 26,
28; and emotional hardiness 52;
after exercise 151, 157; imagery

and 122; and stress 92
nausea 95
neck 14, 16, 22; aching or stiff 95
needs 5, 48, 54, 56–9, 75, 76, 79,
80, 112, 115, 260; expressing
77, 104; Maslow's hierarchy
of 56, 58
nerves 24; calcium and 183;
endings 117, 118; fibres 33;
signals 33; vitamin E and 182
nervousness 50, 96, 97, 108;
nervous attack 98
nervous system 22, 24, 140;
autonomic *88–9*, 90, 161;
copper and 183; endocrine and
89; and lupus 35; and multiple
sclerosis 32; over-aroused 97,
98; parasympathetic 89, 117;
sympathetic *88*, 90, 94, 96, 97,
98, 115, 116, 118
neuron *89*, glossary
neurotransmitter 24, 58, glossary
nigari 241, glossary
nitrates 139, 201; and vitamin A;
nitrate time bomb 139–40
nitric acid 140
N-nitrosamines 139
noise 3, 105, 110
nor-adrenalin 58, *89*
nose: breathing through 160; as
entry for pathogens 9; hairs in 8,
10, 160; membrane of 36, 160;
in respiration 11; running 36
nourishment 58, 170, 173, 193;
emotional 68, 75; *see also*
drinking and eating; food;
nutrients
nuclear plants 143, 145; and
leukaemia 130; and radiation 27
nuclear reactions 133
nutrients 18, 19, 150, 169,
170, 178; deficiency in
165; destruction of 172;
immunity-enhancing 176;
immunity-enhancing, and
their best sources *186–8*;
leaching of 166
nuts 165, 169, 172, 173, 174,
176, 181, 184, 185, *188*,
196; almonds 165, 180, 182,
183, *186*, *187*, *188*, 216, 219,
220, 221, 222, 225, 226, 235,
239, 243, 244, 247, 251, 255;
cashew *186*, 217, 221, 222, 234,
236, 242, 246, 249, 250, 258;
chestnuts 237; coconut 216, 217,
219, 222, 242, 245, 247, 254;
coconut, creamed 236, 246, 252;
hazelnuts *187*, 216, 220, 221,
250; nut milk 216, 217, 257;
peanuts *187*; pecans 182, *187*;
pine nuts 217; roast 169; storage
of 200; walnuts 180, *186*, *187*,

217, 221, 222, 234, 236, 242, 246, 249
Nut loaf 250
nutrition, poor 20, 25
Nutty wheat germ 217

obsessions 95
oestrogen, and breast cancer 27, 64, 183
oils 169, 174, *192*; of skin 11; storage of 200; vegetable 182; olive and sunflower, *see under individual recipes*
okara 216, 239, 240–1
oleic acid 209
olives 229 230
organs: biofeedback and *126*; cancer of linings of 28; damage to from cancer 26; foreign 20; proteins and 176; target 62; vital 19, 28, 35, 81
organisms: harmless 8; in vaccination 21, 23; *see also* pathogens; bacteria
Oriental lentil pâté 236
oxygen 140, 145, 150, 184, 185; exercise and 149, 155; oxygenation 81, 158, 159, 160; usage *126*
ozone layer 132

pains: abdominal 35, 95; body 6; chest 3, 4, 95, 96, 116, 156, 161; emotional 5, 62, 113, 114; laughter and 81; low back 96, 163; menstrual 95, 192
pancreas *89*; and diabetes 31, 32; yoga and 161; *see also* cancer, of pancreas
panic 3, 87, 111, 114, 259; attacks 96
pantothenic acid *see* vitamin B₅
paralysis 9, 63, 150
parasites 10, *17*; attacks from 132
parents 48, 57, 110; approval from 68, 109
pasta 196, 229, 248, 253
pâtés and savoury spreads 183, 236–9
pathogens 8, 9, 10, 11, 12, 13, 14, 15, 16, *17*, 18, 19, 20, 21, 23, 24, 142, 149, 178, 181, 184, 185
patient 43; cancer 48, 77, 81, 86, 122; cancer, outliving prognosis 76; of HIV/Aids 26, 81; immune system of 20; on immuno-suppressive drugs 25
peas 169, 181, 184; chick 228, 232, 248, 249
peace 59, 74; through meditation 121, 122, 125; through yoga 160
pencillin 9, 24; *Penicillium notatum* 23

perfectionism 50, 51, 54, 105, 116
performance stressors 99, 101, 103, 106–7
permethrin 147
persona 112, 114
personality 5, 69; and auto-immune diseases 49–52; balance in 67, 76; benign 48; cancer-prone 43–9; conflict 49; core 111; enriching 114; and exercise 156; hardy 52; multiplicity of 110, 114; shadow of 67; subpersonalities 110, 111, 112, 113, 114, 115, 119, 120, 260; Type A 49; well-behaved, nice 47
perspiration 87, *88*–9, 90, 95, 125, 149
pertussis *see* whooping cough
pesticides 18, 135, 136, 137; in breast milk 37; on food 198; in food chain 177–8; in moth-proofing 127
pets, and food poisoning 41, 42
phagocytes 16, *17*, 18, 138, 142, 185; phagocytosis 12, 140
phobias 95, 97
phosphorus 184, 193, 215, 219
physical stressors 90, 100–1, 102–3, 106–8; eliminating 105
the Pill: and breast cancer 27; and candidiasis 29; and smoking 27; vitamin C and 181; vitamin B₆ and 180
Pitta bread 226
pituitary 59, 86, *89*
placebo 24, 25
plasma: blood 12; cells 16, *17*, 18; proteins 19
play 84
plutonium 131
pneumonia 22, 26
Poires belle Hélène 256
poison: of botulism 38; from caffeine 169; cell 122, 151, 159; in food 8; from food additives 169; poisonous chemicals 127, 135; poisonous heavy metals 140; selective, in drugs 24
Polenta 218
Polenta custard 254
poliomyelitis 22, 23
pollen, as allergen 10, 35
pollutant 19, 142, 260
pollution 147, 148; air 182; and asthma 37; chemical 128, 135–7; by heavy metals 140; of home 143, 144, 145, 146, 147; at work 127, 145
positive thinking 33, 61, 122; and auto-immune disease 31
potassium 166, 185, 188, 197, 208, 212

potential 57, 68, 93
power lines, high-voltage 133, 134, 135, 143
power stations 140; *see under* nuclear plants
preservatives *see food*, preservatives
press-ups 97, 154
problems 98, 103; emotional 5, 69, 260
prognosis 2, 63, 122; for cancers 28; creativity influencing 86; visualisation influencing 122
programme, for healthy living 6
projection 69, 74
prostaglandins 190, 192; E₁ *192*, 190–1, 202
protein 19, 167, 168, 169, 171, 175, 176, 177, 179, 194, 199, 206, 210, 214, 215, 219, 228, 236, 240, 241, 253; of antigens 8; blood 12, 19; of complement system *17*; drinks 257; foreign 26; of interferons *17*; usable, daily allowance of *177*; *see also* plasma proteins
protozoa 10, 24
psychoneuroimmunology 49
psychotherapist 25, 31, 37, 43, 69, 110, 151
psychotherapy 58, 59, 62, 67, 68, 69, 75; behavioural 97; biodynamic 163
pulse: for aerobic exercise 155; in biofeedback 125; for yoga breathing 160
pulses *see* beans; lentils; peas
Pumpernickel 224
pus 12, *17*
pyrethrum 147
pyridoxine *see* vitamin B₆

questionnaires: on diet 167–70; on food poisoning 40–2; on immune efficiency 53–5; immunity checklist 260; on laughter 82–3; on stress, physical 95, 96; on stress at work and home 99–103, on environment 143–8
Quick millet porridge 218
Quick sesame bread 223

radar 134, 135, 136, 145
radiation 131–3, 145; atomic 199; and auto-immune disease 31; and cancer 27, 133; electromagnetic 135; extremely low frequency (ELF) 133; infra-red 133; ionising 130, 132; low frequency 133, 134; non-ionising 133; 'safe' limits of 132; sickness 132; ultra-high frequency 134; ultra-violet 11, 132, 133

radioactive 2; dust 131; injection 259
radiotherapy 1, 2, 29, 43, 63, 133, 182, 199; of ovaries 63, 66
radon gas 145
rage 79; suppressed 80, 91, 109; *see also* anger
rash: from aspirin 80; of lupus 34; from radiotherapy 43
RDA (recommended daily dietary allowances) *186–8*, glossary; of folic acid 180; of vitamin B₂ 180; of vitamin B₆ 179; of vitamin C 182; of zinc 180
receptors *see under* B-cells *and* T-cells; lymphocyte; immune cells; mast cells
Red and green salad 232
redundancy 52
refrigerator, temperature of 41
relationships 58; Aids and 26; avoidance of close 50; important 46; intimate 68, *see also* intimacy; long-lasting 52, 53, 57
relaxation 60, 74, 95, 96, 97, 98, 105, 112, 115, 116, 260; through Alexander Technique 163; in biofeedback 124–6, *126*; deep muscular 117–8, 120, 122; for desensitisation 98; and herpes 30; and imagery 121, 122; and massage 162; quick 119, 122; for rheumatoid arthritis 34; and Type A personality 49
remission 29, 35, 58, 86, 175
resentment 47, 50, 73, 77, 79, 80, 104, 260; repressed 109; and visualisation 123; *see also* hatred
respiratory system: diseases of 141; passages of 22; penetration by bacteria 9, 11
rheumatism 207
rheumatoid arthritis 21, 34, 85, 184, 211–12; dependence and 50; and personality 49–50
riboflavin *see* vitamin B₂
Rice and spinach salad 231
Rice pudding 255
RNA (ribonucleic acid), *see* glossary *under* DNA; folic acid and 180
roasts, savoury 240
royal jelly 181, *186*
rubella 9, 22, *23*

sadness 6, 61; and forgiveness 79; *see also* bereavement; grief; mourning
salads 169, 170, 175, 227, 248, 260, 260; alfalfa 208, 227, 228, 257; celery 230, 238, 257; chicory 232; cress 235; cucumber 232, 257; fennel

227, 230, 249; lettuce 227, 229, 257; pepper, green 182, 230; pepper, red 236, 249; radish 228, 232; salad dressings 227, 229, 230, 231, 232; tomatoes 182, 219, 220, 221, 227, 229, 230, 232, 237, 238, 248, 249, 250; watercress 180, 232; *see also* vegetables

salt *see* sodium chloride

saliva 11, 68, 82

salmonella 37, 38

sarcoma 28

savouries 248–53

scan: bone 2, 259; liver 2; ultrasound 1, 93

scavenger 12, 13, *13*, 15, 16; *see also* macrophage; phagocyte

Scottish porridge 217

seaweeds 172, 192, 196, 199; agar-agar 253; arame 199; hijiki 199; kelp 185, 215; nori 199

security 46, 56, 57, 58; loss of 80

seeds 174, 176; *186–8;* caraway 224, 233, 249, 253; fenugreek 228; pumpkin 165, 216, 222, 229; sesame 183, 184, 215, 216, 221, 227, 242; sprouting 183, 227, 228, 232; sunflower 180, 183, 184, 215, 216, 217, 221, 222, 223, 227, 232, 256

seitan 199

selenium 166, 182, 185, 188, 189, 208, 210, 212, 260

self: ideal 61; knowledge of 108, 111, 115; and non-self 20–1, 31, 123, true to 57, 58, 75, 86, 108

self-actualisation 56, 57

self-expression 63, 86, 114

self-sacrificing *see* martyr, life position of

self-worth 57, 59, 68, 260

Sellafield 130, 133

septicaemia 39

sewage 139

sex 26, 109

sexuality 64, 65, 66, 69, 105, 109, 260; sexual functioning and zinc 166

Shepherd's delight 251

shingles 30

sick building syndrome 127, 145

Simonton, Carl and Stephanie 121

skin 21, 183, 257; as barrier *10*, 11; and biofeedback 124; *126*, *126*; broken or cut 9, 11, 12; brushing 158, 164; cancer of 28, 128, 132; and candidiasis 30; and diet 175; disorders of 91, 132, 139; irritation 136; oil of 11; and vitamin A 179

sleep 34, 35, 116, 170

smallpox 9, 21, 22

smog 141

smoke 145; from bonfires 143; and exhaust fumes 141-3

smoking 105, 142, 143, 181, 260; and cancer 27; and stess 94, 96

sneeze 11

sodium chloride (common salt) 146, 166, 170, 173, 174, 175, 185, 198, 260; sea salt 172

soil 22, 166, 184; botulism in 38; depleted 165; erosion 166, *188*

Solomon Dr G.F. 49, 50, 51, 52, 151

solvents 146, 147

soups 172, 233–5

soya: beans 167, 176, 180, 182, 183, 184, 196, 228, 240, 241; bean products 199; cheese 230, 243; flour 180, 220, 239, 243, 245, 247, 255; milk 199, 239–40 *and see individual recipes;* sauce, Tamari 249; *see also* tempeh, tofu

Spaghetti with tofu sauce 248

spices 171, 174, 196; *and see individual recipes*

spleen 14–15, 24, 161, 178, 179

spontaneity 57, 84

sporting activities 81, 86, 149; giving aerobic effect 156; and aggression 78; cycling 61, 149; footwear for 158; jogging 97, 149, 157; and lupus 51; squash 78

spreads 196

Staphylococcal *see* bacteria

steroids 25; and risk of listeria 40

Sticky bread 244

stillbirths 137

stomach 14, 21, 23, 32; acid in *10*, 11; cancer of 27, 139, 171; churning 95; delicate 174; disorders 139; in fight or flight response 87; relaxing muscles 119; ulcers 91

Streptococcal *see bacteria*

stress 5, 20, 25, 75, 77, 80, 85, *88–9*, 91, 92, 93, 96, 108, 109, 116, 132, 181, 182, 185, 260; and asthma 37; and biofeedback 124–6; and cancer 104; causes of 98–9; chronic 95, 114; and deep breathing 160; emergency action 115–6; and herpes 30, 31; lowering of 108, 112, 114, 115; and lupus 35, 51; and magnesium 166; and massage 162; and multiple sclerosis 34; and perception 91; response to 100, 119; scale 103; and ulcerative colitis 35

stressors 91, *92* 93, 116; coping with 93; internal 108–16; at work and home 100–03; *see also* bereavement; boredom; frustration; performance; physical; threat

stroke 150

subconscious *see* unconscious mind

suffering 2; psychological 73; relief of through laughter 81

sugar 166, 168, 169, 170, 171, 172, 173, 174, 175, 195, 260; and diabetes 32; fructose 169; *see also* sweeteners

sulphur dioxide 140, 141

sun: and cancer 132; radiation from 27, 131

supplements 209; *see also* minerals *and* vitamins

survival: ensuring 109; impulse for 58

sweeteners 196

symptoms: fear of 97; of panic attacks 97; of stress 94–7, 98, 99, 116

syphilis 23

systemic lupus erythematosus 34–5; personality and 51

tahini 183, 197, 236, 239, 245, 256

talents 58, 61, 74, 86

T-cells 16, *17*, 20, 25, 26, 28, 31, 33, 92, 138, 140, 142, 178, 179, 184, 211; receptors on 58; *see also* T-helper, T-killer *and* T-suppressor cells

tea 170, 171, 173, 174, 260; bancha 174, 203; fruit 165, 169, 174; herb 165, 169, 174, 202–3, 248; nettle 205

tears 7; as defence mechanism *10*, 11

teatime treats 244–7

television 135; transmitters 134

tempeh 165, 174, 198, 219, 220

Tempeh toast 219

temperature: in biofeedback 125; cold, and listeria 40; high, from listeria 40; from salmonella 39

tendons 21, 34, 176

teratogenicity 136; teratogenic chemicals 139; *see also* birth defects

tetanus 9, *22*, *23*

T-helper cells *17*, 18, 26

therapies, complementary 29; and multiple sclerosis 33; *see also* psychotherapy; group therapy

thiamine *see* vitamin B$_1$

thoughts: confused 95, 97, 115; connected with body and feelings 4, 6, 76, 119, 124, 151; in meditation 119; positive *see* positive thinking; recording 7; self-talk 6, 111, 120; sharing 58

threat stressors 90, 100, 101, 106–7

throat: sore 14, 21, 127; swollen, and asthma 37

thrombosis 182

thrush *see Candida albicans*

Thunder and lightning 253

thymus 16, *17*, 24, 91, 161, 178, 179

thyroid 21

tissues: and auto-immune disease 32; of body 11, 19, 21, 164; copper and 183; connective, in rheumatoid arthritis 34; disease of connective 80; feeding of 150; fibrous 14, *14*; fluid 13, 165; folic acid and 180; injury to 12; lymphatic *17*; oxygen and 149, 150; proteins and 176; sodium and 169; spaces 12

T-killer cells 16, 181; *see also* natural killer cells

T-lymphocytes *see* T-cells

tobacco 27, 143

tofu 165, 173, 174, 176, 198, 194, 199, 219, 230, 232, 237, 240, 241–2, 248, 251, 256, 257

Tofu cream 242, 256

touch 161, 162; healing through 163

toxic waste 130, 138

toxins 18; cleansing breathing and 161; cytotoxin 28; of diphtheria 22; environmental 31, 129–43; of listeria (listeriolysin) 40; and lymphatic system 165; produced by pathogens 9, 16, 21; and skin brushing 165; in smoke 145; of tetanus 22; produced by T-killer cells 16, *17*; in tobacco smoke 143; and vitamin A 179; *see also* poisons

trace elements 183, 185, 199, 215

traffic 3, 141, 142, 143

Trail mix 222

trans fatty acids 191, *192*

trapped 3, 49, 54, 114

treatment 2, 7; for cancer 28, 29, *see also* radiotherapy

T-suppressor cells *17*, 18, 51, 52

tuberculosis (TB) 9, 20, *23*, 26

tumours 1, 28, 51, 181, 183, 184, 185; brain 58, 130; cells of *17*; diet and 174, 175, 178; secondary 4; surveillance 92; visualisation and 121; vitamin E and 182; *see also* cancer; malignancy

2,4-D 136

2,4,5-T 136

ulcers 91; stomach 91
ulcerative colitis 35; diet and 175;
    personality and 51; repressed
    rage and 109; stress and 107
unconscious mind 67, 74, 112, 121,
    122; movement and 156
unemployed 99
unleaded petrol 142
uranium 131
urine 10, 11, 18, 32; urea 19;
UV (ultra-violet) light 180, 183; see
    also radiation, ultra-violet

vaccination 21–3, 23; against
    HIV 26
values 5, 104
vascular disease 142
vegan 180, 195, 199, 208, 214; see
    also diet, vegan
vegetables: beetroot 184, 227, 231,
    233, 257; broccoli 180, 182, 183,
    184, 227, 232; Brussels sprouts
    180, 182, 227; cabbage, red 227;
    cabbage, white 227; calabrese
    232; carrots 165, 169, 227,
    231, 234, 235, 237, 238, 248,
    249, 252, 257; cauliflower 180,
    184, 227, 232, 251; courgette
    219, 248; fennel 227, 230, 249;
    fresh 170, 172, 173, 175, 260;
    frozen and tinned 174, 180;
    green 171, 180, 182, 184, 185;
    and hormones 198; immunity-
    enhancing 186–8; Jerusalem
    artichokes 184, 227; juice 35,
    257; kohlrabi 182, 227; leek 234;
    legumes see beans; mushrooms
    180, 181, 198, 219, 220, 231,
    237, 248, 249, 250; onions 219,
    221, 229, 233, 234, 235, 237,
    238, 248, 249, 250, 252, organic
    166, 174; potatoes 185, 233,
    234, 251; raw 172, 173, 175,
    178, 182, 184, and see salads;
    spinach 179, 180, 182, 184,
    231; stock 233; swede 249, 252;
    sweet potatoes 179; turnips 180,
    182, 183, 184, 227, 231; see also
    beans; peas
vegetarian see diet, vegetarian
vein 151; hepatic portal 18, 19
vessels: blood 12, 21, 32, 150;
    lymphatic 13, 14
victim: life position of 50, 52, 54,
    70, 71, 72, 73, 76, 156, 260; of
    system 7
vinegar 174; cider 208, 221, 229,
    231, 233, 234; malt 227; wine
    230, 231
viruses 4, 5, 11, 16, 17, 26, 179,
    184; and auto-immune disease
    31; and cancer 27, 28; definition
    of 9; destroyed 18; and diabetes
    32; Epstein-Barr 30; herpes
    30, 31; and interferon 28; and
    vitamin C 181; and vitamin E
    182; see also HIV
vision: blurred in multiple sclerosis
    33; vitamin A and 166, 179; zinc
    and 166
visualisation 74, 117, 121–4,
    259, 260
vitamins 19, 167, 169, 172, 173,
    178–83, 186–7, 198, 214, 215,
    227, 257; immunity-enhancing
    186–7; supplements 260, see also
    RDA; vitamin A (retinol) 19,
    166, 169, 178–9, 181, 186, 189,
    228; vitamin B complex 166,
    179–81, 199, 208, 223, 244,
    260; vitamin B_1 (thiamine) 215,
    219; vitamin B_2 (riboflavin) 179,
    180, 186, 200, 212, 215, 219;
    vitamin B_3 (niacin) 192, 215,
    219; vitamin B_5 (pantothenic
    acid) 179, 180, 186, 187, 208,
    209; vitamin B_6 (pyridoxine)
    178, 179, 180, 186, 189, 192,
    200, 212, 228; vitamin B_{12} 180;
    vitamin C (ascorbic acid) 28, 31,
    35, 80, 169, 179, 181–2, 185,
    187, 189, 192, 200, 207, 210,
    212, 260; vitamin D 19, 178,
    183; vitamin E 19, 31, 179, 181,
    182-3, 185, 187, 189, 192, 192,
    212; vitamin F (fatty acids) 190,
    see essential fatty acids; vitamin H
    (biotin) 192, 209; vitamin M see
    folic acid
vulnerability 71

Waldorf salad 205, 230
walking 105, 116, 149, 156, 158,
    171; see also sporting activities
washing: as defence mechanism 10,
    11; of food 178, 227
water 22, 139, 174, 184; filter 141,
    197, 201; spring 172
weedkillers 144
weight 158 203-4
white cells 12, 14, 16, 17, 24, 25,
    28, 52, 122, 178, 180, 183; and
    HIV 25, 26; and imagery 122;
    protective 20; receptors 151;
    see also B-cells; lymphocytes;
    macrophage; monocytes; natural
    killer cells; T-cells
whooping cough 22, 23
will 71
windpipe (trachea) 10, 11
Windscale 130; see Sellafield
wine 195, 249
wisdom 65, 74, 75
Wise Being 74, 260
womanhood 62, 63, 64, 65,
    66, 67, 69

women: and auto-immune disease
    31, 50; and candidiasis 29;
    and diabetes 32; and lupus
    35; pregnant and listeria 40;
    pregnant and magnesium 185;
    pregnant and salmonella 39; and
    rheumatoid arthritis 34
work: change of 105, 108; physical
    169; -place hazards 127–31;
    problems at 104, 105; time off
    259; workaholics 98
worrying *see* anxiety
worthlessness 47, 60, 79
wounds 22, 161; pantothenic acid
    and 181; vitamin A and 166; *see
    also* injury

X-rays 27, 133

yeast 223, 224, 225, 226, 244, 247,
    255; brewer's 180, 181, *186*,
    188; fungus in 9; infections 174;
    see also candidiasis
yoga: breathing 96, 160–1; hatha
    161; Yogis 172
yoghurt 31, 206, 208, 209, 216;
    goat's milk 217, 232, 233, 236,
    238 247, 251, 194
Yoghurt cake 247

zinc 140, 142, 166, 178, 180, 184,
    185, *188*, 189, 190, *192*, 193,
    209, 210, 212, 260

A Selected List of Cedar Books

While every effort is made to keep prices low, it is sometimes necessary to increase prices at short notice. Mandarin Paperbacks reserves the right to show new retail prices on covers which may differ from those previously advertised in the text or elsewhere.

The prices shown below were correct at the time of going to press.

☐	7493 0791 9	**New Arthritis and Common Sense:**	
		A Complete Guide to Effective Relief	Dale Alexander £4.99
☐	7493 0046 9	**Sex and Your Health**	James Bevan £4.99
☐	7493 0938 5	**The Courage to Heal**	Ellen Bass and Laura Davis £7.99
☐	7493 0098 1	**Divorced Parenting**	Dr Sol Goldstein £4.50
☐	7493 1033 2	**Carbohydrate Addict's Diet**	Dr Rachael Heller and Dr Richard Heller £4.99
☐	7493 0246 1	**Overcoming Overeating**	Jane Hirschmann & Carol Munter £3.99
☐	7493 0322 0	**Women, Sex and Addiction**	Charlotte Davis Kasl £4.99
☐	7493 1079 0	**Help For the Bed-Wetting Child**	Dr Roger Morgan £4.99
☐	7493 0933 4	**The Amazing Results of Positive Thinking**	Norman Vincent Peale £4.99
☐	7493 0821 4	**The Power of Positive Living**	Norman Vincent Peale £4.99
☐	7493 0715 3	**The Power of Positive Thinking**	Norman Vincent Peale £4.99
☐	7493 1023 5	**The Power of the Plus Factor**	Norman Vincent Peale £4.99
☐	7493 1041 3	**How to Survive in Spite of Your Parents**	Dr Margaret Reinhold £5.99
☐	7493 1018 9	**When Am I Going to be Happy**	Dr Penelope Russianoff £5.99
☐	7493 0733 1	**When You and Your Mother Can't be Friends**	Victoria Secunda £5.99
☐	7493 0724 2	**Living with ME: A Self Help Guide**	Dr Charles Shepherd £4.99

All these books are available at your bookshop or newsagent, or can be ordered direct from the publisher. Just tick the titles you want and fill in the form below.

Mandarin Paperbacks, Cash Sales Department, PO Box 11, Falmouth, Cornwall TR10 9EN.

Please send cheque or postal order, no currency, for purchase price quoted and allow the following for postage and packing:

UK including BFPO £1.00 for the first book, 50p for the second and 30p for each additional book ordered to a maximum charge of £3.00.

Overseas including Eire £2 for the first book, £1.00 for the second and 50p for each additional book thereafter.

NAME (Block letters) ....

ADDRESS...

....

☐ I enclose my remittance for ....

☐ I wish to pay by Access/Visa Card Number ☐☐☐☐☐☐☐☐☐☐☐☐☐☐☐☐

Expiry Date ☐☐☐☐